The Practice of Clinical Supervision

Nadine Pelling   John Barletta   Philip Armstrong

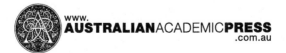

www.
AUSTRALIANACADEMIC**PRESS**
.com.au

First published in 2009 from a completed manuscript presented to
Australian Academic Press
32 Jeays Street
Bowen Hills Qld 4006
Australia
www.australianacademicpress.com.au

Reprinted in 2010.

National Library of Australia cataloguing-in-publication entry:

Title:	The practice of clinical supervision / editor, Nadine Pelling, John Barletta, Philip Armstrong.
ISBN:	9781921513312 (pbk.)
Notes:	Bibliography.
Subjects:	Clinical psychologists--Supervision of.
	Psychotherapists--Supervision of.
	Counsellors--Supervision of.
	Personnel management.
Other Authors/	Pelling, Nadine.
Contributors:	Barletta, John
	Armstrong, Philip.
Dewey Number:	362.204250683

Foreword

Christmas looms as I begin to write this foreword. My Christmas thoughts, these years, tend to centre around new beginnings, surprises, unexpected happenings and, of course, epiphanies that characterise new manifestations or insights. I am committed, at least in mind, to lifelong learning and lifelong learning as we know, includes all these themes and more. Christmas says something to me about not remaining still, not taking it all for granted and being open to the disorienting events of life that kick-start my learning once more. The festive season forces me to observe again, to look anew and be ever alert to what is growing and developing outside of my immediate awareness.

Supervision that is reflective practice is also part of these meanderings. If 'shepherds watch their flocks by night' then those of us in the helping profession remain watchful and vigilant to ensure we don't fall psychologically or emotionally asleep in the comfort stories of our work and practice (Ryan, 2004). It is so easy to do so. I am reminded that the opposite of reflection is mindlessness — how we reproduce the same routines over and over again without thinking about or asking questions of them. 'Ask me again what I am living for?' is a good life question to keep us on our toes and connect us continually to new learning. 'Ask me again why I am doing it this way?' is a good supervisory question to ensure we are open to new learning. We forget (I certainly do) and with forgetfulness comes mindlessness and apathy.

I liked this book because it woke me up (again). I had fallen asleep or at least had become drowsy. I had failed to notice some of the exciting, new, surprising developments in the field of supervision. I knew about them in theory — this book brought them home to me in practice. Schatzman (1991) coined a phrase in the area of research that is very applicable to this book, 'What *all* is involved here?' he would ask. This book widens the supervision window and gives us access to more of the 'all' of supervision. Let me explain that a bit more.

This is not meant to be a comprehensive text on clinical supervision or a step-by-step manual for either helping professional trainees or supervisor trainees. In that sense it's not 'all' here. The book is more a state-of-the-art proclamation of where supervision is today and what are some of the crucial themes we need to consider as supervisors. This will make it invaluable to the experienced supervisor who knows supervision and needs to update on what has been happening recently. However, due to its wide remit and its cross-professional application (counsellors, psychotherapists, psychologists, social workers, life and business coaches who are interested in supervision can all benefit from the contents), it will also be attractive to trainee practitioners who are beginning supervision, and to trainee supervisors who are taking their first steps as supervisors. To cater for this wide audience, the various chapters blend contemporary research with modern models and up-to-date frameworks and practical tools applied to various contexts. And that is its great strength — the breadth it provides on supervision.

I was particularly pleased to see a chapter on the effectiveness of supervision in regard to client outcome. This has been the 'blind spot' of clinical supervision research — is supervision in the least way effective in client progress? A new study on brief therapy shows it is (Chapter 7). That is good news for doubters who continually ask: Why have supervision if we have no evidence that it positively affects client progress? Other modern areas that caught my attention were: Culture-informed counselling supervision (Chapter 17), what supports supervisee learning (Chapter 8), supervisor gatekeeping anxiety and technology in supervision (Chapter 19) and another area not often discussed in supervision, administrative supervision (Chapter 2). Those are just a few of the nuggets and gems in the book that 'woke me up' and challenged me to think again, and again.

There is much more, of course. An Aladdin's cave of goodies awaits the reader. Ethical issues in supervision, supervision from various psychotherapy modalities, the organisational dimensions of supervision, research in supervision, and applied supervision to a number of contexts (e.g., drug and alcohol services, school counselling). While these are by no means new areas for supervisors, these chapters update us on the research, literature, models and frameworks available in more recent times.

The trainee features a lot in many chapters (e.g., addressing supervisee fears in Chapter 9) and purposeful assessment in Chapter 14. While much is written on supervisee development it was encouraging to see a chapter on supervisor development (Chapter 12). That is what I mean by using Schatzman's phrase 'What *all* is involved here?' This is a 'big' book that is comprehensive in walking well-trodden supervisory paths and pioneering new ones.

While the book is written primarily by Australian authors there is a substantial contribution from overseas, particularly the United States and Canada. This gives the book an international flavour.

By introducing this foreword with a Christmas note, I had not intended to imply any messianic intentions to the book, and would not want you to think of it as a be-all or end-all of supervisory literature. But as the Christmas theme directs us to think of new beginnings, changing times and hope for what it is to come, I think it is fair to say that this book does that too. It captures the past and what we have inherited from those who have led the way in supervision theory and research; it presents the present state of play of where clinical supervision is and its sets an agenda for the foreseeable supervision future.

Michael Carroll, PhD

Visiting Industrial Professor
University of Bristol, UK
December 2008

References

Ryan, S. (2004). *Vital practice: Stories from the healing arts: The homeopathic and supervisory way.* Portland, UK: Sea Change.

Schatzman, L. (1991). Dimensional analysis. In D.R. Maines (Ed). *Social organization and social process: Essays in honour of Anselm Strauss* (pp. 303–314). New York: Adline de Gruyter.

Contents

Acknowledgments

Nadine Pelling

For Professors Robert Betz (deceased), Edward Trembley (deceased), and C. Dennis Simpson as well as Dr Joseph Oldz. You have been truly amazing role models for me, and no doubt countless others, both professionally and personally. Thank you for your support throughout the years. I also thank my daughter, Jasmine Pelling-Schweis, for reminding me of the importance of play.

John Barletta

To my supervisors and mentors, particularly Professors Maurizio Andolfi and Tom Davis, from whom I learn to push boundaries. To colleagues who enable me to gather what it means to be a therapist. To countless supervisees who teach me about other worlds. To my patients who educate me about life as I endeavour to help them. To my wife, Sandra, who unintentionally shapes me.

Philip Armstrong

Without the dedication, patience and hard work of my co-editors, Dr Nadine Pelling and Dr John Barletta, this text would not have been possible. It would be remiss of me to not recognise their significant contributions — not only to this publication, but in guiding and helping me to remain focused throughout the process. I would also like to acknowledge my wife and daughter who continue to ensure I remained grounded and in touch with life outside therapy.

The authors, editors and publisher would like to gratefully credit or acknowledge the following:

That the contents of this book were informed by the 2006 Counselling Supervision class at the University of South Australia taught by Nadine Pelling. During this class Dr Pelling led the participants in an activity to create a comprehensive table of contents for a counselling supervision book using existing clinical and counselling scholarship. The result of this exercise informed the current book contents.

The introduction chapter written by Dr John Barletta is based upon:

Barletta, J. (2007). Clinical supervision. In N. Pelling, R. Bowers, & P. Armstrong (Eds.), *The practice of counselling* (pp. 118–135). Melbourne, Australia: Thomson.

Some of the information contained in the chapter on supervisor development written by Dr Nadine Pelling and Dr Elisa Agostinelli originates from the following previously published items and originally Dr Pelling's doctoral dissertation from Western Michigan University (2000):

Pelling, N. (2008). The relationship of supervisory experience, counseling experience, and training in supervision to supervisory identity development. *International Journal for the Advancement of Counselling, 30*(4), 235–248.

Schofield, M., & Pelling, N. (2002). Supervision of counsellors. In M. McMahon & W. Patton (Eds.), *Supervision in the helping professions: A practical approach* (pp. 211–222). Sydney, Australia: Prentice Hall.

The chapter on counsellor competence written by Dr Nadine Pelling was originally published as follows and is reprinted here with permission:

Pelling, N. (2006). Counsellor competence: A survey of Australian counsellor self-perceived competence. *Counselling Australia, 6*(1), 3–14.

Pelling, N. (2007). Counsellor competence (Chapter 2). In N. Pelling, R. Bowers, & P. Armstrong (Eds.), *The practice of counselling* (pp. 36–45). Melbourne, Australia: Thomson.

About the Authors

Nadine Pelling, PhD, earned her BA (Hons) Psychology from the University of Western Ontario in Canada and her MA and PhD in Counseling Psychology from Western Michigan University. Trained and experienced as a psychologist and counsellor, she has called Australia home since 2000. Nadine has produced over 75 publications and has made over 40 conference presentations. Nadine is a member of the Australian Psychological Society (College of Clinical Psychologists), a registered psychologist and enjoys being active in the scientist-practitioner tradition, which means engaging in applied as well as research/scholarly work. Nadine is a Fellow with the Australian Counselling Association and is also currently their research director. Nadine was also awarded the Australian Psychological Society's prestigious Early Career Teaching Award in Psychology in 2006. Nadine is a Senior Lecturer in Clinical Psychology at the University of South Australia, Adelaide.

John Barletta, PhD, a Clinical Psychologist in private practice, enjoys providing therapy, medico-legal reports, clinical supervision, psychometric assessments, consultation and workshops. He has supervised psychologists, counsellors, social workers, nurses, educators, clergy and administrators for many years. John earned his doctorate from Ohio University, and masters from The University of Queensland. He is an Accredited Supervisor with the Psychologists Registration Board of Queensland, a Registered Supervisor with the Australian Counselling Association, was on the editorial board of *Counselor Education and Supervision*, and is on the International Scientific Committee of the Accademia di Psicoterapia della Famiglia, Rome. A member of the Australian Psychological Society (College of Clinical Psychologists), National Board for Certified Counselors (National Certified Counselor), Queensland Association for Family Therapy (Clinical) and Queensland College of Teachers (Registered Teacher), John was awarded for Leadership in International Collaboration by the American Counseling Association's division, Association for Counselor Education and Supervision. He made significant contributions to associations including the initial development of the Psychotherapy and Counselling Federation of Australia, and was twice President of the Queensland Guidance and Counselling Association. Until recently he was a tenured senior academic in the School of Psychology, Australian Catholic University, where he was on staff for over a decade, was Clinical Practicum Supervisor, established fieldwork for counselling trainees and was Course Coordinator of the Master of Counselling. Further information available at http://www.john barletta.com

Philip Armstrong, a PhD candidate, has a graduate degree in counselling from University of New England (New South Wales), a Diploma of Applied Science (Counselling), and is a registered clinical supervisor with Australian Counselling Association (ACA). Philip has been a therapist since 1995 when he worked with veterans with whom he had an affinity due to shared experience as a member of the Australian Army. Much of his work since has centred on men's issues and relationships. He has maintained a practice but has moved into the CEO position with ACA, and is Secretary-General of the Asia–Pacific Rim Confederation of Counsellors. He is editor and founder of the peer reviewed *Counselling Australia*, and co-founder and managing editor of *Counselling Psychotherapy and Health*, an international web-based peer reviewed journal. Philip has several publications, the latest being co-editor of *The Practice of Counselling*. Philip's contribution to the counselling profession within Australia and internationally has been acknowledged through a Fellowship awarded by ACA, and membership as an Associate Fellow of the Australian College of Health Service Executives. He has been honoured with a biographical record in the 2009 *Marquis Who's Who in the World*. Philip's clinical practice, Clinical Counselling Centre, won a prestigious business award for Professional Services partly due to establishing a postnatal depression support group. He is recipient of the Defence Force Service Medal and Defence Medal. Philip lives in Brisbane with his wife and daughter, and also has a son and daughter from a previous marriage. Further information available at http://www.philiparmstrong.com.au

Elisa Agostinelli, PhD, is currently coordinating a bereavement centre for children in Brisbane. Elisa had studied and trained as a clinical psychologist in Rome, Italy. She has a bachelor and master's degree in psychology and a master's degree in family therapy. She obtained her PhD from the University of Toledo, Ohio, in Counselling and Mental Health. Her counselling experience had been with families, couples, children and adults, running individual and group sessions. Elisa also worked with clients with schizophrenia and children in a neurological and psychiatric hospital in Italy. She has trained counsellors at University of Toledo; University of New England, New South Wales; Australian Catholic University, Queensland; and at the Domestic Violence Prevention Service, Gold Coast, Queensland. She has supervised students in the master's course in counselling and master's in school psychology practicum at the University of Toledo. She has presented family therapy theory and practice on a number of occasions at the University of Queensland. Her research interests are personal and professional development of counsellors and psychologists, supervision, and multicultural counselling.

Mary L. Anderson, PhD, is Assistant Professor and Program Coordinator of the School Counseling program at Western Michigan University. She is a licensed professional counsellor, nationally certified counsellor, and earned a doctorate in counselling from Oakland University, Michigan. While at Oakland, she served on the faculty as an assistant professor, director of the Adult Career Counseling Center, and co-director of the School Counselor Academy. Before her appointment at WMU, Mary fulfilled a 3-year faculty appointment at Radford University, Virginia. She has published several book chapters, and co-authored the third edition of *Counseling Adults in Transition*. Mary is an active member of counselling associations, including the American Counseling Association and the American School Counseling Association. Her research interests include counsellor supervision, school counselling and advocacy, work/life transitions, and spirituality in counselling.

Kate Anthony, MSc, runs OnlineCounsellors.co.uk, a training company for mental health practitioners who wish to work with clients online, and is joint-CEO of the Online Therapy Institute (http://www.onlinetherapyinstitute.com). She is the author of several articles and chapters on the use of e-mail, bulletin boards, IRC, videoconferencing, stand-alone software and more radical innovative use of technology within therapeutic practice, such as virtual reality. She co-authored the 1st, 2nd and 3rd editions of the *BACP Guidelines for Online Counselling, Psychotherapy and Supervision*. She presents at an international level at conferences and is co-editor of *Technology in Counselling and Psychotherapy: A Practitioners Guide* (2003) and *The Impact of Technology in Mental Health* (2009). She is co-author of *Online Therapy* (2009) and *Clinical Supervision in Mental Health: Best Practice for Online Applications* (in press). She is Past-President and Fellow of the International Society for Mental Health Online, and Fellow of the British Association for Counselling and Psychotherapy.

Nancy Arthur, PhD, is Professor in the Counselling Psychology Program in the Division of Applied Psychology and Canada Research Chair in Professional Education at the University of Calgary, Alberta, Canada. Her teaching and research interests involve the preparation of professionals for working in global contexts and for social justice, with specific focus on multicultural counselling and career development. Nancy has developed and instructed graduate level course curriculum on career development and multicultural counselling for face-to-face and distributed learning formats. Nancy's counselling experience with diverse groups of adult learners lead to the authorship of *Counseling International Students: Clients From Around the World.* Her co-edited/co-authored book with Sandra Collins, *Culture-Infused Counseling: Celebrating the Canadian Mosaic,* received the 2006 Book Award from the Canadian Counseling Association. Her most recent book, co-edited with Paul Pedersen, is *Case Incidents in Counselling for International Transitions.*

Matthew Bambling, PhD, a clinical psychologist, is an experienced researcher who lectures in the School of Psychology at Australian Catholic University, and he is the associate editor for the journal *Psychotherapy in Australia.* In 2002 he won the prestigious Kenneth Howard Memorial award for best project awarded by the Society for Psychotherapy Research for what is acknowledged as the first randomised treatment trial that tested the effect of supervision of therapists on client outcome. At the University of Queensland in 2003 he won the Dean's commendation for outstanding research, and in 2006 *Psychotherapy in Australia*'s Writers Award for his article on the link between emotional and physical health. Matthew's research interests include psychotherapy outcomes, treatment effectiveness, depression, health and mental health problems.

Herbert Biggs, PhD, is Associate Professor and Director of Service, Innovation and Engagement in the School of Psychology and Counselling at the Queensland University of Technology. He is a Psychologist and Australian Certified Rehabilitation Counsellor. He earned his doctorate from Massey University in New Zealand, and subsequently has taken academic positions at Southern Cross University (New South Wales) and Griffith University (Queensland). Herbert was foundation member of the Australian Society of Rehabilitation Counsellors, and is a member of the Rehabilitation Counsellors Association of Australasia and the Australian Psychological Society. He serves on the editorial boards of the *Australian Journal of Rehabilitation Counselling,* the *Journal of Rehabilitation Administration, and Work: A Journal of Prevention, Assessment and Rehabilitation.*

Gary Bischof, PhD, LMFT, is Associate Professor and Program Coordinator of the Marriage and Family Therapy Master's Program in the Department of Counselor Education and Counseling Psychology at Western Michigan University. He obtained his master's degree from Virginia Tech, and PhD from Purdue University, both in Marriage and Family Therapy. Gary is a clinical member and approved supervisor with AAMFT. His research and professional interests include medical family therapy, couple therapy and brief solution-oriented therapy. He has published his work in articles in professional journals and in book chapters on these and other topics. He has also served in leadership positions in MFT state and national professional associations.

Kisiku Sa'qawei Paq'tism Joseph Randolph (Randy) Bowers, PhD, is Assistant Professor of Education and Indigenous Studies at Cape Breton University, Canada. He was former Coordinator of Counselling Programs in the School of Health at the University of New England, Australia. He received a PhD in Counselling and Health Sociology from University of New England where he has taught since 1998. He is a Certified Practicing Counsellor, Counsellor Supervisor and Honorary Member with the Australian Counselling Association. He is Founding Editor of the international research journal *Counselling, Psychotherapy, and Health*, sponsored by the Australian Counselling Association and recently taken up by the Asia Pacific Confederation of Counselling representing eight founding nations. Dr Bowers is a Managing Editor with the *Qualitative Report*, Editorial Advisor with *Counselling Australia*, Associate Scholar with the Centre for World Indigenous Studies, Scholar Contributor with the *Fourth World Eye Weekly*, Associate Editor with the *Fourth World Journal*, and invited Scholar for Special Collections at the Mi'kmaq First Nation Resource Centre, University of Cape Breton, Canada, who house a Permanent Special Collection of his scholarship under his name. Dr Bowers' over 160 published works include over 40 research publications, book and book chapters, refereed articles, conference papers, editorials, artistic essays and poetry. His scholarship focuses on marginalisation and minority studies, with an emphasis on identity and healing.

Sandra Collins, PhD, is Associate Professor and the Director of the Graduate Centre for Applied Psychology at Athabasca University, Canada. She is a counsellor educator who has taken a leadership role in the development of graduate programming in counselling for the last 11 years. She has extensive experience in the design, development and delivery of graduate curriculum. She currently manages a large graduate program in counselling psychology (over 200 students). She has been actively involved in the regulation of psychology as a board member and president of the College of Alberta Psychologists. She is currently member of the Supervision Ad Hoc Committee. She is also president elect of the Counsellors for Social Justice Chapter of the Canadian Counselling Association. Her academic research and writing has been focused in the areas of multicultural counselling, counselling women, career counselling, and social justice. She has written numerous journal articles, book chapters, and co-edited/co-authored the book, *Culture-infused counselling: Celebrating the Canadian Mosaic* with Nancy Arthur.

Stephen Craig, PhD, is Associate Professor and Unit Director of the Counselor Education Program in the Department of Counselor Education and Counseling Psychology at Western Michigan University. Stephen was recently appointed to a 3-year term on the American Counseling Association's Professional Standards Committee and serves as a site-team member/visitor for the Council for Accreditation of Counseling and Related Educational Programs. As a member of the graduate faculty at WMU, he teaches Supervision of Counseling and Psychotherapy for doctoral students in Counselor Education and Counseling Psychology. He maintains a part-time private practice with a focus on supervision for mental health professionals who are seeking licensure as professional counsellors.

Piet Crosby, MA, is a registered psychologist, registered teacher and member of the Educational and Developmental College of the Australian Psychological Society, holds a master's degree in Psychology (Educational), and is completing a doctoral degree in clinical psychology. He worked as an educational psychologist in South Australia's Department of Education and Children's Services for over 30 years in a variety of field, managerial and policy positions, including an exchange to Denver Public Schools in the United States in 1985. He held several positions in professional and community associations. Piet is an accredited supervisor with the SA Psychology Board and is listed on the APS Register of School Psychologist Supervisors. He has supervised several trainee psychologists and trainee teachers, and managed teams of psychologists and other professionals, both co-located and working in country or other offices. He is now in private practice, with particular interests in educational psychology and assessment and intervention with pervasive developmental disorders, providing services in metropolitan Adelaide and in country areas.

Thomas Davis, PhD, is Professor of Counselor Education at Ohio University. He holds a doctorate from Ohio State University in cooperation with Miami University, and a master's from Marshall University, West Virginia. Tom, a licensed professional clinical counsellor, has been a strong advocate for the counselling profession for many years by serving in a variety of leadership positions. He has been a member of the American Counseling Association Ethics Committee, and is Chair for the Council for the Accreditation of Counseling and Related Educational Program's 2009 Standards Revision Committee. Tom has been President of both the Ohio Counseling Association and Ohio Association for Counselor Education and Supervision, has served as the Governor's appointee to the Ohio Counselor and Social Worker Board, and been President of the American Association of State Counseling Boards. His areas of interest include counsellor education and supervision, legal and ethical, chemical dependency and school counselling. He co-authored with C.J. Osborn the text *The Solution Focused School Counselor: Shaping the Profession.*

Jason Dixon, PhD, is a bilingual clinical counsellor, researcher, interpreter and counsellor educator in private practice, and provides supervision to counsellors, psychologists and social workers. He holds a doctorate from Ohio University and a Master of Counselling from Australian Catholic University. He provides clinical services in Japanese to the Japanese community, taking into consideration acculturative adjustment issues. Jason specialises in the treatment of alcohol and other drug use issues using harm reduction, relapse prevention and abstinence-based approaches. His research pursuits include psychometrics, survey design, cross-cultural psychology and counselling culturally and linguistically diverse populations.

Stephen Goss, PhD, is Lecturer in Counselling at the University of Abertay Dundee, United Kingdom. He has been involved in counselling and psychotherapy for over 20 years and has been publishing on uses of technology within that field since 1999. He co-edited *Evidence-Based Practice in Counselling and Psychotherapy* and *Technology in Counselling and Psychotherapy: A Practitioners Guide* and has written a number of book chapters, conference and journal papers, articles and research reports. His other professional interests include research methodology, pluralism in the practice and study of counselling and psychotherapy and innovative practice methods.

Sally Hunter, PhD, is Lecturer in Counselling in the School of Health, University of New England, New South Wales. Sally teaches in the graduate counselling programs and is on the executive of the Society for Counselling and Psychotherapy Education. Sally's research interests include child maltreatment, trauma, vicarious traumatisation, the therapeutic relationship and counsellor education and supervision. She has two adult children of whom she is very proud.

Caleb W. Lack, PhD, is a licensed clinical psychologist and Assistant Professor of Psychology in the Behavioral Sciences Department at Arkansas Tech University. A specialist in cognitive–behavioural therapy, he completed a predoctoral internship at the University of Florida and earned his doctorate from Oklahoma State University in 2006. He is the author of over a dozen scientific articles relating to the assessment and treatment of obsessive–compulsive disorder and Tourette's disorder, and has presented across the nation and internationally on a variety of topics, including children's reactions to natural disasters, innovative teaching methods, and evidence-based psychological practice. Clinically, he specialises in the treatment of children with anxiety disorders, including OCD and phobias, and chronic tics and Tourette's disorder.

Alf Lizzio, PhD, is Associate Professor and teaches in the School of Psychology at Griffith University, Queensland. As a counselling and consulting psychologist, he has extensive experience in both the public sector and private practice in areas related to the development of people in organisations, the effective functioning of teams and the management of change. Alf has a particular interest in processes related to the support and development of professionals and leaders.

DeeAnna Merz Nagel, LPC, DCC, is a psychotherapist, consultant and international expert regarding online counselling and the impact of technology on mental health. She specialises in text-based counselling and supervision via chat and e-mail. DeeAnna's expertise extends to assisting individuals and families in understanding the impact of technology in their lives from normalising the use of technology and social media to overcoming internet and cybersex addictions. Her presentations and publications include ethical considerations for the mental health practitioner with regard to online counselling, social networking, mixed reality and virtual world environments.

Cynthia Osborn, PhD, is Associate Professor in the Counseling and Human Development Services Program at Kent State University, Ohio, where she routinely supervises masters and doctoral students in the counselling practicum and supervision of counselling experiences. She is a licensed Professional Clinical Counselor and a licensed Chemical Dependency Counselor. Publications and research activities have been in the areas of substance abuse counselling, solution-focused counselling, motivational interviewing and counsellor supervision. Cynthia serves as co-editor of the journal, *Counselor Education and Supervision*, a refereed publication of the American Counseling Association.

Zoe Pearce, PhD, a psychologist, is Lecturer in Interpersonal Relationships in the School of Psychology and Counselling, Queensland University of Technology. She completed her doctorate at Griffith University, Queensland, in the area of communication in relationships and has conducted extensive research in the area of intimate relationships and the factors that influence the development of healthy, happy coupling. Her areas of special interest include adult attachment and bonding in relationships, communication in relationships, family relationships, and the influence of child behaviour on adult relationships. Zoe is an accredited supervisor with the Psychologists Registration Board of Queensland and conducts peer supervision and organisational supervision in a private practice. She is a member of the Australian Psychological Society and the International Association for Relationship Research.

Eric Sauer, PhD, a licensed psychologist, is Associate Professor, Co-Director of Counseling Psychology Doctoral Program, and Director of the Center for Counseling and Psychological Services-Grand Rapids in the Department of Counselor Education and Counseling Psychology at Western Michigan University. He earned his doctoral degree from Michigan State University. He completed his predoctoral internship at the University of Iowa and postdoctoral training at the University of Wisconsin-Madison. He was recently elected president of the Association for Directors of Psychology Training Clinics. He is also currently serving on the editorial boards of the *Journal of Counseling Psychology* and *The Counseling Psychologist*. At WMU, he teaches a master's level field practicum course. His professional interests include counselling psychology, counselling process and outcome, attachment theory and supervision and training.

C. Dennis Simpson, EdD, is Professor and Director of the Specialty Program in Alcohol and Drug Abuse at Western Michigan University. He is nationally Board Certified as a neuropsychopharmacologist. Dennis is also the Senior Clinician of the University Substance Abuse Clinics. He serves on the President's Council on Alcohol and is a consultant to numerous corporations and agencies on the provision and supervision of substance abuse counselling.

Brian Sullivan, PhD, is a lecturer in the Master of Counselling Program, in the School of Social Work and Human Services at the University of Queensland (UQ). He was instrumental in the development and design of that program launched in 2004. He has a Masters in School Counselling from UQ, and completed his doctorate at the University of Toledo, Ohio, in 2000. He has a strong interest in the evolution and legitimacy of counselling in Australia as a distinct profession in its own right. He is involved in a number of professional counselling organisations, at the national and international level. His work extends to community and organisational settings where he has trained police domestic violence liaison officers, probation and parole officers, social workers, psychologists and counsellors in working with involuntary clients who are perpetrators of domestic violence. He is the author of the recent text: *Counsellors and Counselling: A New Conversation* (2008). Brian has a select private practice in counselling and consultancy in Brisbane, Queensland.

Keithia Wilson, PhD, is Associate Professor in the School of Psychology at Griffith University, Queensland. She has worked for over 25 years as a consultant, educator and counsellor in organisational and community settings. Her organisational work with clients focuses in particular on improving interpersonal and team effectiveness. Her individual work with clients focuses on issues of loss and grief, and personal and spiritual development. She is active in the supervision, mentoring and training of novice and experienced practitioners, and is a consultant on the implementation of a range of supervisory systems in the community and public sectors. Keithia received the 2007 Prime Minister's Award for the Australian University Teacher of the Year.

—++++—

Introduction

The Introduction is a section comprised of two chapters that encourage the reader to reflect on the major issues associated with therapists accessing and providing professional supervision. Chapter 1 essentially establishes the domain of clinical supervision and generally sets the scope for the remainder of the textbook. It surveys the literature to provide an informative snapshot that will encourage greater reflection of processes which have often become mindlessly habitual. Chapter 2 gives confidence and knowledge to those considering the option of establishing clinical supervision as a service, within the scope of their practice, to helping professionals.

Chapter Overview

CHAPTER 1

'Introduction to Clinical Supervision' by John Barletta sets the context for supervision and clearly establishes supervision as an integral part of clinical practice for all of the helping professions. The chapter methodically works its way through introducing the goals, roles and models in supervision, so the reader quickly develops a framework for understanding the specialty, and also to anticipate what will be explored in greater depth in later chapters. Given the anxiety and misperceptions some practitioners have about supervision, this chapter clearly articulates the opportunities people have available to them as they receive and/or provide clinical supervision via respectful consultation. The supportive and challenging nature of the supervisory relationship is possibly best highlighted through Barletta's presentation of the mentor role, with the hope and optimism embedded in such a caring model.

Chapter Themes

In this chapter you will explore the following themes:

- clinical supervision
- administrative supervision
- overview of clinical supervision
- aims of clinical supervision
- need for clinical supervision
- roles of the clinical supervisor
- methods in clinical supervision
- process of clinical supervision
- techniques in clinical supervision
- beneficiaries of supervision
- maximising supervision
- current practices.

CHAPTER 2

'Administration and Marketing of Supervision' by Philip Armstrong offers the reader a pragmatic view of the considerations that need to be addressed as one establishes themselves as a provider of supervision to the professional community. His experience as a businessman shines through. Although the international market of this text means that individuals will still need to explore their local laws and regulations, it provides a useful sense of what questions to ask and which areas to explore to ensure a legal and ethical supervision practice is maintained. The sample client and supervision contracts provided are useful models to copy until one develops their preferred and individualised style and format for such documents.

Chapter Themes
In this chapter you will explore the following themes:
* supervision definitions
* supervision as a paid professional activity
* administration is not a dirty word
* sample clinical supervision contract
* sample counselling contract and confidentiality charter.

chapter one

Introduction to Clinical Supervision

John Barletta

The professional duties of those who conduct therapy are multi-dimensional, just as those who conduct therapy are from multiple disciplines. Counsellors, psychologists, social workers and, in some instances, nurses all engage in psychologically therapeutic activities. There is a view that those who do counselling simply attend to 'worried well' middle-class clients with change and success being the common outcome from the process. This is only a small part of the reality. Indeed counsellors, psychologists, social workers and those who counsel, in general, usually have a broad range of clients from differing backgrounds, with a complexity of issues, varying levels of capacity and motivation, and inconsistent or unknown outcomes. This is coupled with an increased demand for paperwork, accountability, effectiveness and efficiency.

Typically a counsellor's responsibilities include:

• individual, couple and family therapy

• group sessions

• intake appraisals and assessment

• program development and evaluation

• resource coordination

• consultation and report-writing

• professional development

• mediation

• referrals

• administration, financial and clerical responsibilities.

These tasks can include involvement with clients' family members, administrative personnel, managers, bureaucrats and professionals external to their own system. Such a demanding role necessitates counsellors to monitor their personal functioning, professional practice and to review their effectiveness. One reality, constant over time, has been that counsellors regularly practise in isolation from professional peers. Counsellors without the support and encouragement of colleagues run the risk of stagnating relative to their growth and development. Thus, the need to be involved with a relevant counselling association and ongoing supervision is essential as these can minimise the feeling of isolation and increase self-care behaviours.

Counsellors have become increasingly aware of risks such as compassion fatigue, vicarious traumatisation, burnout and legal action related to professional malpractice. These issues are increasing in the helping professions. Counsellors need to have access to a range of professional supports, including peer assistance, managerial considerations, consultation, counselling and increasingly, clinical supervision. Currently, a huge amount of writing on the topic of supervision for counsellors exists and includes the specialty journals *Counselor Education and Supervision* (American Counseling Association) and *The Clinical Supervisor* (Haworth Press).

Various types of supervision have been described in the literature and the commonality existing in descriptions centres around the name and function of two types, clinical supervision and administrative supervision. To move forward in our discussion of supervision, it is imperative that a definition of the specialty activity be established. We will then examine clinical supervision in a broad manner, outline the aims, needs and benefits of supervision and examine the applied aspects of supervision.

Clinical Supervision

Although each scholarly writing on clinical supervision offers an altered characterisation, numerous elements remain common. For the purpose of clarity, clinical supervision is considered to be a process whereby colleagues of a similar profession regularly engage in a prepared meeting for the intention of developing understanding, skills and a professional orientation, while concurrently focusing on enhancing client wellbeing. Such supervision has both a preventative and corrective function.

The clinical supervisor monitors the appropriateness of the individual counsellor's practice, while also serving as a preceptor of the profession. The dual role of ensuring the quality of services, as well as the development of the counsellor, is indeed a challenging task for the clinical supervisor. Essentially, this form of supervision enables a practitioner to have a supportive colleague help them to examine their clinical interventions and effectiveness. Due to the significance and magnitude of the role, and the reality that supervision is often recognised as a professional specialisation, clinical supervision is now usually only carried out by an accredited individual, or a senior professional, who has recognised training and expertise in supervision theory and techniques. This chapter serves as an introduction to this specialty.

Administrative Supervision

The second type of supervision for counsellors is administrative supervision. Where the focus of clinical supervision is concerned with counselling and aims to be educational, the focus of administrative supervision is involved with organisational, managerial and procedural issues. Administrative supervision includes the managing of areas such as service evaluation, financial issues, time considerations, record keeping, role and function, professional development, policy and procedures, resource allocation, information technology and organisational issues.

In a work environment, it is probably not imperative that administrative supervision be managed by another counsellor, but could be handled by a manager or member of an administrative or management team. The purpose of administrative supervision relates to organisational issues, hence an administrator might realistically be the preferred choice for this role as they would be capable of attending to the issues raised during the process.

The focus of this opening chapter is on clinical rather than administrative supervision, as the practical issues related to administrative supervision require a discussion more from a management perspective rather than a counselling viewpoint. This is quite different to that taken when considering clinical matters, and outside the scope of this text's discourse.

The diagram below (Figure 1.1) provides a snapshot of these two categories of supervision and identifies a range of methods reviewed briefly in this chapter and explored in more detail later in the text. It serves to provide the reader with a snapshot from which supervision may be examined within counselling and perhaps even non-counselling professionals alike.

Overview of Clinical Supervision

Clinical supervision stimulates and challenges the practitioner to examine their professional decisions and explore practice issues in a methodical way. As this chapter provides an overview of the roles and processes in supervision, it becomes apparent the activity is invaluable for all stakeholders, particularly in nurturing the supervisee to examine the interface between theory and professional practice.

Professionals in all cultures are customarily held to extraordinary standards by the public. The community expectation is for professionals to be

Clinical supervision
Techniques and methods:
- *self-report*
- *log review*
- *audio tape*
- *video tape*
- *live observation*
- *role-playing*
- *sitting-in*
- *co-counselling*

Administrative supervision
Organisational and management issues:
- *in-service training*
- *professional development*
- *program development*
- *attendance*
- *role statement*
- *progress notes*
- *record keeping*
- *caseload*
- *fiscal issues*
- *resource allocation*

FIGURE 1.1
Ways counsellors are supervised, managed and evaluated (Barletta, 1996).

trained to superior standards and to behave in exemplary ways. Hence, professionals need to engage in processes that ensure they continue to grow in knowledge and competence. This has seen professionals routinely attending training programs, participating in scholarly conferences, subscribing to peer-reviewed journals, affiliating with professional associations and consulting with expert colleagues. Increasingly, practitioners have found an effective way to foster their lifelong learning is by formalising a supervisory relationship with a practitioner who has more and different experiences from them and is also aptly qualified in the specialty of supervision.

Although counselling is a well-established independent profession in the United States, and accordingly produces a plethora of resources, it has only been in recent years that other countries, including Australia, have experienced the steady growth of the profession (Schofield, Grant, Holmes, & Barletta, 2006). This development has seen an explosion of counselling programs aimed at preparing competently trained practitioners. In these training programs, fieldwork is an opportunity for reappraisal of career choice, development of key competencies, learning the culture of the profession and exploration of practical interest areas. In conjunction with the institution's fieldwork handbook, both this initial and final chapter will help guide the trainee counsellor, hereafter referred to as supervisee, on the path to their development as a safe and helpful entry-level professional.

Within the context of the supervisory relationship, the supervisee in the practical environment presents cases, highlights their treatment modalities, reviews clinical interviews, presents assessments, examines psychopathology issues and explores a mixture of personal and professional challenges raised by their work. These broad topics will arise for discussion with supervisees who are in a range of settings such as community agencies, hospitals, government departments, private practice and schools.

As supervisees move through a course of counselling study, they are regularly exposed to an assortment of educative and evaluative processes and procedures aimed at ensuring they have requisite knowledge and skills to practise carefully and effectively. Although writing essays, presenting seminars and taking examinations are methods typically used by counsellor educators to assess learning outcomes, processes to enhance learning about clinical issues and to augment the professional orientation of supervisees vary enormously. When supervisees are involved in practical experiences (e.g., communication skills sessions, clinical placement, fieldwork practicum, counselling internship) techniques such as analysing learning journals, reviewing session tapes, discussing client cases and examining critical incidents are commonly and well employed. It is in these applied areas that emerging professionals are introduced to the aims and methods of clinical supervision.

In these practical endeavours, the clinical practicum supervisor, usually a senior counsellor with considerable applied experience and supervision training, is responsible for the supervisee. The supervisor ensures the supervisee is involved with an array of activities, increasing in complexity. These are processed in ways that enhance the supervisee's learning. These early supervisory experiences are an amalgam of education and evaluation and are intended to be extremely supportive as well as challenging.

With appropriate consultation and well-planned feedback, the supervisee is fostered in developmental growth and professional awareness. This progression occurs by way of various modes such as individual supervision, within a group forum session and in conversation with peers.

Aims of Clinical Supervision

Some supervisees and practitioners hold concerns about supervision relative to it being offered as a predominantly evaluative process. These anxieties rapidly dissipate when supervisees experience a quality supervisory relationship and are able to negotiate clear goals for their sessions. The mistaken belief that supervision is focused on evaluative judgments, which may impact on identity, relationships, duties, tenure, salary and promotion may be minimised by clinical supervisors being accessed from outside the agency. In this situation supervisees can benefit significantly from a greater sense of confidentiality and privacy. Generally, the purpose of evaluation is to confer opinions of value and is limited in its utility. Conversely, supervision aims to increase self-awareness and enhance professional competence. The aspiration for supervision is ongoing development of capabilities in an environment of honesty and trust in a close relationship where the focus is on professional experiences.

With regard to the specific goals of supervision, irrespective of location or specialty of the professional (e.g., addictions, community, corrections, education, health, mental health, private practice, or rehabilitation), the focus to enhance, extend and develop remains similar. The aims of supervision include:

- monitoring client safety and outcomes
- developing realistic self-evaluation
- integrating research, theory and skills
- increasing scope of practice
- exploring values, beliefs and creativity
- encouraging and ensuring legal and ethical practices
- developing a sense of collegial and professional support
- updating innovative, current perspectives and best practice
- improving perception and developing clinical wisdom
- observing agency policies and procedures
- facilitating and enlarging self-awareness
- promoting team perspective and multidisciplinary orientation
- encouraging an evidence-based approach
- identifying gifts and barriers to development
- developing critical reflection skills
- clarifying work preferences and personal priorities
- developing and managing short-, intermediate- and long-term goals
- monitoring lifelong learning
- promoting an orientation to the profession
- supporting self-care and ensuring wellbeing.

The above aims will serve as the basis for discussions between the supervisor and supervisee as they consult and negotiate to develop the practicalities (e.g., goals, context, methods, duties, procedures, scope) contained within a supervision contract (Osborn & Davis, 1996). Educational institutions may label a supervision contract a learning covenant or agreement of understanding. If a third party is involved or interested in the supervisory process — that is, employer, training provider, registration body or professional association — additional input into the development of the aims for the contract must be considered. Additional contributors frequently encourage or direct the supervisor to ensure the supervisee is developing the knowledge, skills and dispositional qualities that are representative of what is required to operate independently in the profession.

Need for Clinical Supervision

The variety of responsibilities required of counsellors makes it essential for appropriate support to be provided by the employer or educational institution; or if in private practice, is organised by the practitioner. Training, consultation, professional development, counselling and clinical supervision aims to offer support to the counsellor while also developing professional competencies. There is a chance that supervision may increase stress due to the time commitment that takes the counsellor away from an already busy schedule. Typically, this becomes merely a short-lived concern.

Receiving clinical supervision facilitates more effective service delivery for the practitioner while simultaneously ensuring some quality control for the employer or institution and the public. The counsellor may be in a situation of having to provide services in a field in which they have little experience. In such cases, the counsellor can call on the assistance of a colleague who has such experience to offer consultation through supervision until an acceptable level of ability is developed. The employer or institution takes responsibility for providing supervision for the counsellor, since it is from required activities the need for supervision arises and high standards of professional practice are expected. Some associations in Australia (e.g., Australian Counselling Association, Psychotherapy and Counselling Federation of Australia, Queensland Counsellors Association) mandate that those providing therapy services continue to engage in clinical supervision by an appropriately trained practitioner.

Roles of the Clinical Supervisor

To enable the aims of supervision to be realised for the supervisee and the full range of benefits to emerge, the supervisor employs a multitude of positions or roles, namely:

• teacher
• evaluator
• consultant
• facilitator
• counsellor
• mentor.

Clinical supervisors should be experienced practitioners who have the ability to join with a diversity of people quite quickly and with relative ease. They create a congenial and safe environment in which supervisees can explore and learn. That is not to suggest supervision is only characterised by care and support. Without challenging and appropriately provoking supervisees, learning and development will be constrained.

Good supervisors make an effort to understand how the supervisee learns, how they like to connect in professional contexts, where they are situated developmentally and what they want and need from supervision at this time in their career. This invariably means in the first session, or at initial phone contact, the supervisor spends time gaining a sense of the identity of the supervisee, their experience, what their broad goals are and where it is that they would like to journey professionally. This clarifying process is invaluable in starting the supervisory relationship in an appropriate and sustainable way.

Supervisors use a variety of roles in supervision, but typically the teacher (instructor/educator) and evaluator (monitor) roles come to the fore with supervisees who developmentally have much to learn and are dependent, for example, students and novice practitioners. These roles need to be carried out sensitively so supervisees feel supported, relaxed, empowered, extended and develop the vital habit of self-reflection. As clinical cases and critical incidents for the supervisee are being explored, the supervisor spends a lot of time allaying the supervisee's anxieties, while simultaneously being instructive and clear in their directions for subsequent client contact. At this stage, supervisees need considerable structure and unambiguous plans to implement. Supervisors cannot risk being viewed as condescending as there is a critical need to ensure supervisees connect with them so they carry out what is negotiated.

With supervisees who are practitioners with extensive training, significant experience, exceptional insight and justified confidence, supervisors are more typically a consultant and facilitator to these autonomous individuals. Such clinical supervision is very challenging to provide and engage with, but the collegial nature of these sessions is invigorating for all involved. As a consultant or facilitator the supervisor provides less structure and prescriptions, rather the confidence and competence of the supervisee is validated and integrated as they discover new insights into cases and their own development and awareness. In this scenario supervision is less hierarchical and more companionate.

Given that most clinical supervisors of counsellors are, or have been, a practising counsellor, this brings the potential of overusing or inappropriately employing the counsellor role in supervision. Supervisors must be mindful of this possible dilemma and realise supervisees are not their counselling clients and going deeply and intrusively into their personal history or issues is neither ethical nor appropriate. However, during supervision, if an awareness develops that a supervisee's personal issues are a significant part of the impasse or learning, a supervisor may address the issue in a cursory fashion and encourage the supervisee to seek counselling for themselves, before moving on with supervision. It is the supervisor's responsibility, as a quality assurer and gatekeeper to the profession, to develop the supervisee while showing them respect and privacy.

Although the counsellor role is minimised when providing supervision, having advanced training in counselling theories and skills adds enormously to interactions with supervisees. Supervisors draw on communication and helping skills, the use of which ensures supervisees feel heard and understood. It is important for novice and experienced practitioners alike that personal feelings, as well as professional concerns, are addressed. It is by acknowledging and working through a supervisee's apprehensions that they openly offer and explore the genuine issues that need to be scrutinised. Using specific praise, targeted reinforcement and constructive feedback, supervisees are encouraged in their development and movement toward established goals.

The final supervisor role is based on Greek mythology. When Odysseus, the King of Ithaca, went to fight with the alliance in the Trojan War, he left his son Telemachus with Mentor, an older wise man who acted as teacher and personal friend to provide guidance in developing values and education in the ways of the world. In an analogous style, people at various stages of their professional career can work closely with someone in a supervisory, mentoring relationship for the purposes of being coached, guided, comforted, supported and sustained. In these ways, the mentor role serves psychosocial, role-modelling and vocational functions.

Irrespective of whether the role being performed is that of teacher, evaluator, consultant, facilitator, counsellor or mentor, for the supervisory relationship to be useful specific factors are essential. The supervisor must be able to listen and encourage, occasionally nudge, appropriately share, provide opportunities for learning, and examine and modify the supervisory program regularly. There are also responsibilities for the supervisee to maximise the benefits of the supervisory process. It is imperative the supervisees set measurable goals and be willing to review and adjust them, pledge time and motivation, reflect on practice, dedicate themselves to self-assessment and explore possibilities. It is by each individual involved in supervision taking shared responsibility that greatest benefit is achieved.

Methods in Clinical Supervision

Although clinical supervision is typically offered on an individual basis, it can be arranged with peers or conducted in small groups (e.g., five supervisees). The advantages of peer and group supervision are the containment of costs, a convenient supportive context and the vicarious learning that emerges as members observe others and interact with discussions. The disadvantages include that the presence of peers may inhibit sharing, individuals have less time available for their own concerns and mediocre group dynamics will be counterproductive. Regardless of how many supervisees are present, the supervisor will promote experiential learning so supervisees have a life-changing, affirming experience.

Self-report, as unpredictable as it may be, remains the standard method used in sessions. The supervisee starts a conversation regarding cases, critical events, the impact of practice on themselves and recurring themes. Supervisors, using a case management approach, suggest or require supervisees bring to sessions case annotations, process notes, reports and client files for review. Although this indirect approach to supervision is fraught with difficulties, with regard to taking agency files and supervisees distorting information, it remains a pragmatic and realistic mode for professional exploration. As the supervisory relationship flourishes, the supervisee invariably becomes more open and honest as they realise these behaviours hold them in good stead.

As part of training supervision, the review of an audiotape, videotape or digital versatile disc (DVD) of supervisees' sessions is customary. Supervisors processing sessions using this technology can use a sensitive inquiring method where the supervisee listens/watches the recording of their clinical work with the supervisor observing. Either person stops the recording at various points to encourage reflection on what the supervisee recollects experiencing during the session. Supervisees speculate about what was occurring and explore how they were functioning. With a positive supervisory alliance established, this method of interpersonal process recall (Kagan, 1980) can use discovery learning to excellent effect.

For many years, mail, telephone, facsimile, text messages, email and the internet have been used routinely to communicate interpersonally and transmit professional information. In the context of supervision methods, these systems are used for the supervisee and supervisor to stay in contact and convey records and requests, which now requires being very mindful of confidentiality issues. If significant issues arise between sessions, telephone and email contact ensures support and guidance can be dispensed swiftly and efficiently.

Direct methods of supervision are strongly encouraged but are often difficult to arrange for a host of reasons. Live observation by the supervisor in the session, co-counselling with the supervisor and live observation (e.g., two-way mirror, walk-in, phone-in, consultation breaks) are the classic ways supervisors get an authentic impression of how the supervisee is performing and progressing. Although there are issues of cost, resources, confidentiality and time to perform direct methods, it is critical supervisees have at least some experience of these approaches.

Finally and possibly most importantly, client feedback provides the most accurate information about the impact, skills and disposition of the supervisee. Given that counselling is a process that seeks to help clients understand and grow, it follows that opinions from the recipients of the service are highly regarded. Although counsellors could be seeking feedback at every session, there has been an increasing trend to have clients complete questionnaires at the cessation of the therapy and/or at a follow-up time (e.g., 3 months). Additionally, feedback from the supervisee's trusted colleagues, collected with caution, is useful as they observe supervisees engage in various activities in the workplace.

Process of Clinical Supervision

The customary procedure for supervision is to initially develop a positive working alliance between supervisee and supervisor, being clear about what each expects and prefers in supervision, and then engage with clinical material to increase capability, awareness and self-assurance. Although many people do not like to admit experiencing difficulties, supervisors hope supervisees volunteer cases where they are most 'stuck' as this is when greatest learning will transpire. Supervisees will realise that mistakes simply highlight what they need to learn and it does not suggest they are fundamentally inadequate. To increase the likelihood of staying focused during supervision sessions to ensure supervisees' needs are met, a supervisor clarifies what the supervisee has done in the past with regard to practice and supervision, and asks where they would like help. After learning about what their practice consists of, and that they want from supervision, and if it is reasonable in terms of their development and professional requirements, working with clinical cases and applied issues commences. Issues discussed in supervision predictably include:

- client issues and goal-setting
- case conceptualisation and progress
- intervention strategies and future plans
- supervisee–client alliance and boundaries
- ethical and legal issues
- counsellor professional development
- supervisor–supervisee relationship.

In processing practical cases, the supervisor avoids moving too quickly towards solutions, but rather acts simply as a guide on the path of learning. A series of basic structured questions can be helpful for supervisees (and novice supervisors) to consider as they prepare for and conduct supervision. Initially seeking responses to the following questions will be helpful:

- What are the significant details I need to know about the case?
- Where do you feel most trapped?

- What are you thinking and feeling about these issues?
- What assistance would you like?

Towards the end of the supervision session, seeking reactions to the following queries will be valuable:

- What new understanding and ideas have been helpful?
- What patterns have emerged for yourself and your clinical practice?
- What obstacles may you encounter as you take the next steps?
- What will you do now given this additional learning?

It is beneficial and appropriate for the supervisee and supervisor to take notes during sessions to have an ongoing record of clients discussed, issues, plans, themes, struggles, learning and progress. These notes will be invaluable as the supervisory relationship continues over an extended period of time. Throughout the supervision process, the supervisee is encouraged in seeking to:

- understand the dilemma and its complexities
- find connections among the information
- formulate a working hypothesis (to avoid an explanatory fiction)
- develop a reasonable treatment plan to implement.

It is an important part of the development of a supervisor to regularly gain feedback on the impact and quality of their supervision. Excellent supervisors develop the habit of asking supervisees to at least give verbal feedback at the end of each session (e.g., How was our session for you today?) and also use specialised supervision inventories at regular intervals (e.g., annual reviews). Although supervisors may prefer to avoid considering negative feedback about their efforts, particularly early in their careers, as they develop over time they are potentially more able to integrate even harsh feedback from supervisees. After sincere reflection and with additional training and reading, experienced supervisors become committed to continuing education in this specialty so they can improve their style of relating and roles in supervision.

Techniques in Clinical Supervision

Within a nurturing supervisory environment founded on a bond of trust, the supervisor debriefs the supervisee's issues and responds in ways that are supportive and educational. The supervisor uses various techniques aimed at encouraging reflection and increasing the impact of processing clinical material. Despite some people's erroneous beliefs that supervisors provide a lot of advice, in reality advice is provided only sparingly. This is usually reserved for significant issues of almost life- or career-threatening magnitude with the supervisee clearly unaware of what action to take. More often a supervisor will use subtle influencing techniques such as explorative questioning, encouraging statements, clarification skills, empathic confrontation, self-disclosure and interpretations. These interventions convey to the supervisee the nature of the supervisor's concerns and potential areas for exploration.

When the characteristics of a case presentation are such that the supervisee has something clinical they need to learn, the supervisor may use modelling and role-play to show the supervisee what could be attempted. In addition to information and skills being reviewed via a didactic approach, the supervisor's challenges and confrontations will facilitate the supervisee's critical reflection and learning. It is this area of augmentation of critical reflection that promotes the supervisee to see themself developing as an autonomous professional.

Irrespective of the developmental stage of the supervisee and the type of issues or themes being explored in sessions, the setting of and agreeing to between-session activities (i.e., homework) is common and universally valuable. Given that supervision is only part of lifelong learning and self-improvement, homework tasks such as research, reading, reflection and writing are critical supplements. Supervisees' engagement with between-session tasks is parallel to what they routinely suggest to clients and benefits all involved.

Beneficiaries of Supervision
There are a multitude of individuals and organisations who profit from the provision of quality clinical supervision. Given that the heart of supervision focuses on ensuring the client is not being harmed and is, additionally, helped to achieve established goals in professionally appropriate ways, the recipient of counselling services is the first to benefit. Most discussions in supervisory sessions focus on interventions being used for the client and advance to how the supervisee is struggling with some aspect of the case.

As the supervisor interacts to clarify the situation and explore potential explanations and interventions to consider, another person is being supported — the supervisee. This is where the supervisee's scope of practice, expertise and insight is being deliberately and incrementally (often exponentially!) expanded. Engaging supervisees in the desire for understanding is valuable for deep learning to occur. In this sense it is the clinical material that is the teacher, not just the supervisor themself. Supervision can insulate the supervisee from work-related stress, variously referred to as burnout, rust-out, compassion fatigue, emotional exhaustion or vicarious trauma.

Furthermore, if the supervisee is a trainee at an educational institution, or if they are an employee at an agency, the organisation itself benefits with the development of a more proficient and safe practitioner. This has the potential to decrease the likelihood of the organisation being involved in accusations of not supporting or not appropriately training the people in their charge and maintains their collective reputations.

With supervision providing clear benefits to the client, practitioner, educational institution and employer, the positive impact will also be more broadly experienced by the profession, its members and the community generally. There is, however, one often forgotten individual who profits from supervision, the clinical supervisor. Although it is seldom mentioned for fear of being misconstrued, the supervisor benefits enormously from offering supervision. As they support supervisees, their understanding of clinical work, human nature and themselves improves enormously and the sense of satisfaction of being additive to so many is indeed gratifying and fulfilling. It must be reiterated, however, that it is the needs of the supervisee and client that are always the primary focus in supervisory sessions.

Maximising Supervision

There are a few requirements for supervisees to increase the likelihood of supervision being genuinely beneficial to personal and professional growth. Supervisees need to gain an awareness of where they are developmentally, be as honest as possible in sessions and understand what supervision can and cannot provide. Being prepared for sessions with material and reflections, being committed to regular supervision (e.g., one hour session per fortnight), and reading before and after sessions is highly desirable. During their formal studies, supervisees have little or no choice of supervisor. After graduation, the emerging professional could find a supervisor by asking colleagues who they respect for guidance or search databases of professional associations that maintain lists of accredited supervisors.

Having an effective supervisor who is optimistic, caring, curious, self-evaluative, self-aware, can develop and maintain trust, provides clear and useful feedback, sets and monitors realistic goals and uses power appropriately, is indeed a blessing for any supervisee. The supervisor needs to ensure the practice of supervision is not seen as part of a paternalistic guild ritual, rather a collegial initiative to develop quality clinical practice. Supervisors need to be competent in many areas, that is, professional content and the learning process, but also know the limits of their expertise and consult appropriate people when the supervisee or they are in difficulty.

Current Practices

Although increasing numbers of counsellors are participating in clinical supervision, many report they receive more supervision that is administrative rather than clinical in nature. This situation is usually not their preferred position. Counsellors indicate they find clinical supervision revitalising as they review and discuss clinical practice. If supervisory provisions fall short of desirable standards and best practice, this raises a host of legal, ethical and professional concerns in an increasingly litigious and demanding cultural context. If counsellors are to receive professional support, appropriately qualified personnel must be provided by the system or accessed externally.

Concluding Statement

Every piece of scholarly work has limits to its scope and this chapter is no different. A range of issues that have not been covered in a significant way, or at all, include diversity (e.g., age, culture, gender, religion), power, conflict, learning styles, therapeutic schools, contexts of practice, conflict, and legal and ethical issues. Some of these issues, however, are thankfully addressed in following chapters. Supervisees with a significant interest in any of these topics are also encouraged to review the plethora of theory and research initiatives in the professional literature.

For many years, supervision for counsellors was on the periphery of professional discussion. A structured and well thought-out approach to both clinical and administrative supervision is imperative to facilitate the process of increased professional credibility. Counsellors should be highly trained professionals who are confident in dealing with the range of psychological issues impacting clients. Professional competence is developed initially through formal academic or in-service training. All counsellors need to broaden their competence and, in the work setting, newly acquired skills can be nurtured and developed by a supervisor who has broad expertise. In this scenario, the supervisor performs the role of teacher, consultant and mentor.

Quality supervision seldom occurs by accident. Rather it is the result of strategic planning by counsellors, administrators and supervisors working in partnership. The aim of such collaboration is to find a practical and appropriate process of supporting the counsellor in the workplace. Without a precise approach to supervision, counselling services are destined to remain out-of-step with best practice. Counsellors need support services commensurate with their training, responsibilities and other professionals; hence, supervision must be seen as an integral component of their practice. Regardless of setting, counselling issues remain similar and the majority of counsellors desire, and benefit from, clinical supervision.

Considerations of time, personnel and cost should be the responsibility of the employer or training provider.

I have had a number of supervisors during my career, including professionals in different countries (i.e., Australia, United States of America, Italy), a variety of disciplines and assorted models (e.g., Psychiatry — systemic-relational; Social Work — contextual; Counselling — psychodynamic, humanistic, solution-focused; Psychology — psychoanalytic, social constructivism, cognitive–behavioural therapies), and modes (individual, peer, group). These diverse people and approaches have profoundly impacted me, influenced my professional awareness and clinical work. Learning from supervisors' stories was enhanced through their authenticity and the relationship.

Socrates wondered if learning was analogous to kindling a fire or filling a bucket. The following comments that supervisees have made in reference to their experiences in supervision indicates their fires have been kindled. One supervisee suggested supervision was 'a great discussion about a good conversation'. Another said it was 'a robust challenge toward integration', while one supervisee said it was 'the place for true growth', 'the only safe space to share mistakes' and 'a time when play is encouraged'.

Supervision is not an add-on service nor is it a luxury that can be neglected. Rather it is a necessity to ensure that a responsive and comprehensive counselling service is offered to the public. To ensure optimal client care, the focus for supervision must be on counsellor growth. Counsellors choose the profession because they have a desire to help others, as well as aiming to stay mentally stimulated. As a profession, if client welfare is kept foremost in deliberations, it follows that the need for supervision will be high on the professional agenda. Counsellors and professional associations should take responsibility for communicating supervision needs to the appropriate people as there should not be practitioners providing mental health services without receiving some guidance. With attention to supervision, the emerging professional can be protected from their euphoria of a grand vocational adventure dissolving into the despair of a fading dream.

Educational Questions and Activities

After reviewing this chapter and additional readings on the topic, respond to the following questions based on your experiences of, or plans for, clinical supervision. When you have developed some notes on each of the questions, share and discuss your reflections with a colleague.

• Where and with whom did you experience supervision?

• What were the stated and implicit aims?

- What was the focus of the interaction?
- What was the frequency, intensity, duration and location of the supervision?
- What format, style or model did the supervisor use?
- What and how was material discussed?
- What was the fee and who paid for the sessions?
- What were all the beneficial aspects of the experience?
- What were all the unhelpful aspects of the experience?
- What are some of the lasting effects of the encounters?
- If you have never received supervision, what do you think you need for it to be additive to your personal and professional growth?

Selected References for Further Reading

Australian Psychological Society. (2003). *Guidelines on supervision.* Melbourne, Australia: Author.

Barletta, J. (2007). Clinical supervision. In N. Pelling, R. Bowers, & P. Armstrong (Eds.), *The practice of counselling* (pp. 118–135). Melbourne, Australia: Thomson.

Barletta, J. (1995). *Legal and ethical issues for school counselors: Supervision as a safeguard.* Athens, OH: Ohio University, Department of Counselor Education. (ERIC Document ED379577)

Barletta, J. (1996). Supervision for school counsellors: When will we get what we really need? *Australian Journal of Guidance and Counselling, 6,* 1–7.

Barletta, J. (2001). An uncommon family therapist: A conversation with Maurizio Andolfi. *Contemporary Family Therapy, 23*(2), 241–258.

Barletta, J. (2006). An exceptional psychotherapy researcher: A conversation with Michael Lambert. *Psychotherapy in Australia, 12*(2), 66–70.

Barletta, J., & Vecchione, T.P. (2004). Enhancing the training of counselling professionals: A process approach. *Australian Journal of Guidance and Counselling, 14*(2), 186–194.

Bernard, J.M., & Goodyear, R.K. (2009). *Fundamentals of clinical supervision* (4th ed.). Upper Saddle River, NJ: Merrill.

Borders, L.D., & Leddick, G.R. (1987). *Handbook of counseling supervision.* Alexandria, VA: American Counseling Association.

Carroll, M. (1996). *Counselling supervision: Theory, skills and practice.* London: Cassells.

Haber, R. (1990). From handicap to handy capable: Training systemic therapists in use of self. *Family Process, 29,* 375–384.

Holloway, E.L. (1995). *Clinical supervision: A systems approach.* Thousand Oaks, CA: Sage.

Holloway, E.L., & Carroll, M. (1999). *Training counselling supervisors: Strategies, methods and techniques.* London: Sage.

Kagan, N. (1980). *Interpersonal process recall: A method of influencing human interaction*. Houston, TX: Mason.

Loganbill, C., Hardy, E., & Delworth, U. (1982). Supervision: A conceptual model. *The Counseling Psychologist, 10*, 3–42.

McMahon, M., & Patton, W. (Eds.). (2002). *Supervision in the helping professions: A practical approach*. Sydney, Australia: Prentice Hall.

Osborn C.J., & Davis T.E. (1996). The supervision contract: Making it perfectly clear. *The Clinical Supervisor, 14*, 121–134.

Queensland Guidance and Counselling Association. (2003). *Supervision practice guide*. Brisbane, Australia: Author.

Ronnestad, M.H., & Skovholt, T.M. (1993). Supervision of beginning and advanced graduate students of counseling and psychotherapy. *Journal of Counseling and Development, 71*, 396–405.

Schofield, M.J., Grant, J., Holmes, S., & Barletta, J. (2006). The Psychotherapy and Counselling Federation of Australia: How the federation model contributes to the field. *International Journal of Psychology, 41*(3), 163–169.

Spence, S., Wilson, J., Kavanagh, D., Strong, J., & Worrall, L. (2001). Clinical supervision in four mental health professions: A review of the evidence. *Behaviour Change, 18*, 135–155.

Stoltenberg, C.D., & Delworth, U. (1987). *Supervising counselors and therapists: A developmental approach*. San Francisco: Jossey-Bass.

Stoltenberg, C.D., McNeill, B., & Delworth, U. (1998). *IDM supervision: An integrated model for supervising counselors and therapists*. San Francisco: Jossey-Bass.

—++++—

chapter two

Administration and Marketing of Supervision

Philip Armstrong

There is common agreement in the provision of supervision that there are two components to, or types of, supervision, these being clinical and administrative supervision (Barletta, 2007; Bernard & Goodyear, 2004). The primary difference between the two is that clinical supervision refers to working with the supervisee in relation to client issues, therapy and self, whereas administrative supervision refers to working primarily with practice/organisational issues centred around paperwork, accounts, policy and procedures, administration, organisational and the employee's role (Haynes, Corey, & Moulton, 2003). The two overlap in many cases and are not distinct from each other. Having said that, it is important that a supervisor has a sound working knowledge of their differences and is able to separate the two and articulate to a supervisee which component is being addressed. Or, in some cases, which component is being offered as supervision as some supervisors may be unable to offer both. A supervisor whose whole experience lies within the realms of academia may struggle to competently understand the administrative needs of a supervisee whose primary work is undertaken in private practice.

When I consult with a supervisor I see a professional mental health worker who has worked intensely, gained significant experience and quali-fications, and also carries the scars of battles. Supervisors come from varying backgrounds, disciplines and deliver supervision from different perspectives, but in the main they are veterans of the mental health sector. Veterans are able to distinguish between the romantic notions of being pro-active, making a difference, helping others with the necessary reality of paperwork and threading their way delicately through protocols and politics. Most clinicians maintain the status quo, survive and practice somewhere between the two, helping others while enduring the accompanying paperwork. Supervisors are able to help make the journey for most as painless as possible as clinicians learn from their own experiences. As a supervisor, and also one who undergoes regular supervision, I look forward to the interactions of supervision and the intellectual and emotional challenges it provides. However, I have also learned that what some may see as being the 'dark side', administration within the supervisory process can be as challenging and important as clinical supervision.

There is common agreement that for supervision to be effective there needs to be a level of training in supervision theory and models, and assessed competence (Haynes, Corey, & Moulton, 2003). Incompetent supervisors may not be aware of their poor practices and therefore supervisees learn poor practices themselves, which can be passed on from one generation of professional supervisors and supervisees to another (Worthington, 1987). A lack of experience and poor training in administrative tasks and protocols would be one area where an incompetent supervisor could unintentionally sabotage the futures of many highly skilled supervisees. This is why training in administrative skills needs to be a core subject in the training of supervisors. The challenge of keeping students awake, while spending time discussing what many possibly see as a very boring subject, certainly exists. It is difficult to compete and deliver a lecture on administration when the previous lecture was on 'theories in action'.

There is one definite strategy that I find works to capture and maintain students' attention and that is to focus first on what the potential outcomes might be for a clinician or supervisor who does not keep on top of administrative tasks. One of the leading causes of bankruptcy for small businesses in Australia, according to the Australian Bureau of Statistics, is a combination of lack of business ability, lack of capital and personal reasons. All these issues should be comprehensively covered through supervision. No-one is suggesting a supervisor should become a financial adviser. However, directing a supervisee who wishes to go into private practice to seek the advice of a financial adviser in regard to capital and financial issues would fall under the duties of supervision. Bankruptcy due to poor skill levels by trades people or professionals is actually uncommon. Regardless in which sector you work, the worst case scenarios are the same; loss of your job and income if employed, loss of your business if self-employed, and potential action by the tax office, a government watch dog such as Australian Securities and Investment Commission, legal action (civil or criminal) and potential deregistration by your professional body or licensing board. Many of these actions can lead to penalties that can impact on you for years, as well as the potential loss of any assets such as your home. Supervisors and supervisees need to understand competent administration is a business, professional and ethical requirement and supports the provision of clinical work. It is also in the financial interest of the supervisor to ensure their supervisees remain financially solid.

Graduates rarely have any real notion of administrative responsibilities when first employed as counsellors. Many experienced therapists who come from noncommercial sectors also lack the appropriate administrative and marketing knowledge required to set up and maintain a private practice. The reliance on supervision at this stage of career development or change in career direction is critical, and for good reason. However, what happens if your supervisor is not well versed in administrative requirements or does not include this in their educational support? A therapist whose family is dependent on their income is generally not in a position to lose large amounts of monies due to a lack of direction from their supervisor. The developing focus of supervision definitions to include the administrative aspects of supervision illustrates the growing importance of administration. The following definitions are provided to illustrate this point.

Supervision Definitions

Bartlet's (1983) definition of counselling supervision discusses the mentoring aspect of supervision in which experienced individuals help more beginning-level practitioners. In contrast, the definition proposed by Stoltenberg and Delworth (1987) focuses on the interpersonal aspect of supervision to facilitate development and competence. McMahon& Patton's (2002) definition describes three aspects including relational, developmental and learning environment. More recently Bernard and Goodyear (2004) discuss supervision as an intervention provided by a more senior member of a profession to a more junior member or members of that same profession that is evaluative, extends over time, and enhances both professional functioning and monitors the quality of professional service provided to clients. Barletta (2007) echoes this multitasking nature of supervision and outlines no less than 20 aspects including encouraging and ensuring legal and ethical practices, and promoting an orientation to the profession — items that clearly address administrative components. Thus, from the above, we can see that definitions of counselling supervision over time have begun to incorporate administrative aspects.

Supervision as a Paid Professional Activity

Many experienced practitioners add the provision of supervision to their professional services during their career. Before actually engaging in supervision as a paid professional activity, there are a number of considerations one must address. Assuming that the individual who is contemplating adding supervision to their repertoire of professional activities is experienced and trained to be sufficiently competent, these considerations tend to be related to the business aspects of providing supervision. This section will review several considerations.

Reality

The provision of supervision services as a full-time paid professional activity is generally not viable as a replacement for clinical practice in countries such as Australia or New Zealand, primarily due to their small populations only a small market demand exists. The profession is underdeveloped in most countries within our region. Therefore a lack of demand as a full fee-paying service is a real consideration for any supervisor within the region. In many developed countries the reliance on voluntary and para-counsellors inhibits the development of supervision as a potential full-time paying profession. There are a few exceptions to this consideration; however, these are professionals who have spent much of their life building their creditability through research and publishing. In general, the demand for clinical services by the public far outweighs the demand for supervision by clinicians. Your target market, clinicians, is not only smaller but limited further by your own skill levels. It would be inappropriate for a supervisor who has worked primarily in the field of drug and alcohol to offer supervisory services to therapists who work primarily with children who suffer from autism.

Credibility

A supervisor's credibility can be the difference between success and failure financially, especially for a new supervisor starting out providing supervision. Credibility is especially important regarding supervision, as the target group to whom the supervisor is marketing themselves is comprised of colleagues and peers. Initial credibility, before a reputation is established, can be aided via listing on an appropriate supervisor register (or certification or licensure depending on the region and professional speciality to which the supervisor belongs). A register itself can be a strong marketing tool. Of course, supervision registration necessitates that the supervisor hold appropriate credentials in their area of practice.

Supply and Demand

Engaging in supervision as a paid professional activity is only likely to be successful if there is a viable supply of professionals that create a demand for such services. Supply is not necessarily the primary issue as counselling is a developing profession in many regions and, as such, growth is ongoing. Demand as a full fee-paying service is possibly the real issue. It is the burden of cost for many clinicians that is the leading issue. Particularly for those who work with clients from low socioeconomic communities or in low paid community not-for-profit organisations. Many large suppliers of counselling services (predominantly phone services) in Australia use volunteer counsellors who are unable to pay for professional clinical supervision and rely on in-house supervision. Rod Stinson, an independent labour market researcher who has analysed Australian Bureau of Statistics data in his most recent study, *What Jobs Pay 2008–2009*, found counselling to be one of the lowest paid professions in Australia. Yet registered counsellors, in the main, have an ongoing requirement to maintain annual supervision requirements. In contrast, fully registered clinical/counselling psychologists in Australia do not have an ongoing mandatory requirement to undergo ongoing supervision and are a relatively well-paid profession.

Arguably the greatest demand within psychology comes from interns and psychologists in training. Again this group is made up of low paid or, in the case of many students, unpaid workers. Demand is not on its own a good indicator of potential income, it is important to ensure any identified group are able to pay for a fee-paying service. Professional organisations, or your own market research, can help determine if supervisors are needed where you intend to provide services. Being accessible via phone, internet, as well as in person (individual and/or group) is likely to widen your potential target market and prove more popular than having limited availability. If one chooses to limit their provision of supervision to one specific modality or mode of delivery, such as face-to-face, they are likely to limit their supervisees to those living within a relatively close geographical area. In contrast, a supervisor willing to deliver services via the phone is likely to gain a greater number of supervisees from a wider geographical area. For an in-depth review of this topic the reader is referred to Chapter 18 in this textbook regarding the use of technology in the provision of supervision.

Marketing

Due to the limited demand for supervision, as discussed previously, many traditional marketing strategies are of minimal value and generally not cost-effective. Strategies such as advertising in the local paper are generally not a viable option and could also be seen as being unprofessional. Additionally, certain professions in various locations have legislative restrictions placed upon them regarding the type of marketing in which they can engage. Thus, the best way to market yourself as a clinical supervisor is to raise your profile within your professional community. Such a profile can be developed via contributing to newsletters or journals, engaging in research, contributing to scholarship such as textbook publications, presenting at conferences as well as conducting professional workshops. If you deliver supervision using modern technology your potential market is not limited by geography. However, if you cross borders you do need to be aware of any legislative, legal and reporting requirements within different regions. You will also need to check with your insurers any limitations in this regard to your cover.

Once a professional has reviewed their position, competence and the above considerations, as well as others that are relevant to their profession and location, and has decided to add supervision to their suite of professional services, there are a few significant decisions to be made. How much to charge a supervisee needs to be based on the needs of the supervisor as well as the resources of the supervisee. For example, is the supervision to benefit a volunteer counsellor or one providing services to a low socioeconomic group or to very affluent clients? You may also consider charging a one-off annual fee to an organisation that employs multiple clinicians, as opposed to individual hourly rates. Contracting supervision services to organisations that specialise in working in disaster zones and/or critical incidents can lead to a steady flow of reasonably paid work. Once a fee rate has been determined, and there may be several rates for different groups, one needs to consider how the fee will be collected, especially when services are rendered over the phone, in the field or on the internet. Fees can also reflect the type of supervision offered. Obviously fieldwork will attract a higher fee than services offered from a clinic where the client comes to you. Of course, one can decide to offer supervision services pro bono, or organise group supervision sessions via a professional organisation for the benefit of the emerging professionals.

Administration is not a Dirty Word

I suggest that administration is not a four letter word, but rather a necessary part of any supervision, and it is now prudent to outline some of the more common, important and necessary administrative facets encountered in any counselling or psychological practice.

Contracts

There are two contracts needed in a supervisory interaction. First is a Supervision Contract that outlines the requirements and responsibilities of both the supervisor and supervisee. Secondly, a Counselling Contract between supervisee and their client that needs to be reviewed by the supervisor to ensure it meets professional requirements and adequately protects the supervisee and consumer. A standard supervision contract has six main components, yet additional components can be added to personalise them. These six components can be found in the sample supervision contract included in this chapter (Figure 2.1). A Counselling Contract also contains six main components and an example of such a contract is shown below (Figure 2.2).

> HINT: Ensure any provisions you place in a contract are appropriate to your jurisdiction and do not breach the rights of your supervisee/client.

Invoicing and Receipting

Providing professional counselling or psychological services is a business, and as such one needs to be aware of the importance of invoicing and bookkeeping. Not only does accurate invoicing and receipting assist clients in gaining possible refunds for the expense incurred, but also assists the professional in preparing their mandatory business assessment statements (a tax office requirement in Australia) and end-of-year tax assessments. Although specific requirements vary by region and country, in the Australian context an invoice must include an Australian Business/ Company Number (ABN or ACN) issued by the Australian Tax Office and include the phrase 'Tax Invoice', or 'Tax Invoice/Receipt' if used in the dual role of being both an invoice and a receipt. This helps to min-imise paperwork by using the one document for two purposes. It is an invoice when given to the client and then becomes a receipt when payment is made, and saves the need to generate a separate proof of payment. Within Australia, Goods and Services Tax (GST) may be paid on certain professional services and, if applicable, must be shown on related invoices often with the phrase 'GST Included'.

If a therapist delivers services that do not attract GST then 'GST Exempt' should be noted on the invoice. Regular payment of invoices is also important as not only does this mean the electricity will not be unex-pectedly cut off but you can keep an eye on your incoming and outgoing costs. Without this information you will not be able to maintain an up-to-date balance sheet, an essential piece of paperwork if you are to keep the wolves from baying at your front door. A good balance sheet will ensure you are aware at all times of your financial position, good or bad. Readers are specifically referred to a professional accountant for relevant local details and more detailed accounting information, as these guidelines are provided for basic informational purposes only.

> HINT: To maximise cash flow and keep balance sheets relevant:
> a. dispatch and pay invoices on a weekly basis
> b. sent invoices should notate payment is on a 14-day basis
> c. if you are a procrastinator in regard to maintaining your books, engage a bookkeeper.

Sample Clinical Supervision Contract

The following contract is between Dr Mary Smith (Supervisor) and Mr John Brown (Supervisee).

1. Purpose, Goals and Objectives of Supervision:

- Monitor and promote the welfare of clients seen by Supervisee;
- Promote the development of Supervisee's professional identity and competence;
- Fulfil the requirement for Supervisee registration and accreditation; and
- Fulfil ACA membership requirement.

2. Context and Content of Supervision:

- Individual monthly supervision at Supervisor's office (via the phone on an as needs basis);
- In the case of a crisis, an appointment can be made for as soon as possible outside this time; and
- A variety of methods will be used within a multi-facet framework.

3. Method of Evaluation:

Feedback will be provided at each session. Records will be limited to session details and major issues relevant to the supervision of the case. A formal evaluation will be conducted every six months. Supervision notes (if kept) may be shared with Supervisee at Supervisor's discretion and upon request of Supervisee. An unedited video of a one-hour counselling session or attendance by the supervisor at a session may be required if the supervisor needs to view a session to continue appropriate clinical supervision. This will be discussed with the supervisee before a request is made. Written permission from the client will be required at these times.

4. Duties and Responsibilities of Supervisor/Supervisee:

a. Supervisor

Encourage ongoing professional education;

Challenge Supervisee to validate approach and technique used;

Monitor basic micro-skills and advanced skills including transference and counter-transference;

Provide alternative approaches for the Supervisee;

Intervene where client welfare is at risk;

Ensure ethical guidelines and professional standards are maintained;

Provide consultation when necessary;

Discuss administrative procedures and marketing strategies where appropriate.

FIGURE 2.1

Sample clinical supervision contract.

b. Supervisee
Uphold ethical guidelines and professional standards;
Discuss client cases with the aid of written case notes and video/audio tapes;
Validate diagnoses/assessments made and approach and techniques used;
Be open to change and alternative methods of practice;
Consult Supervisor or designated contact person in cases of emergency;
Implement Supervisor directives in subsequent sessions;
Maintain a commitment to counsellor education and the profession.

5. **Procedural Considerations:**
   a. Supervisee's written notes, diagnoses, action plans and tapes may be reviewed in sessions.
   b. Issues related to the Supervisee's professional development will be discussed.
   c. It is understood that important issues experienced in the clinical setting will be raised and addressed in supervision. Failure to raise such issues in a reasonable timeframe will be considered a breach of contract.

This contract is subject to revision at any time upon request by either Supervisor or Supervisee. The contract will be reviewed each six months on the approval of both the Supervisor and the Supervisee.

The price per one hour session is $150 (GST Inclusive), which will be invoiced monthly.

Confidentiality
All information gathered by the Supervisor during Supervision will remain confidential except when:

1. It is subpoenaed by a court of law or requested by a Government Department/Agency under the appropriate legislation, or
2. Failure to disclose the information would place you, a client and/or another person at risk, or
3. Your prior approval has been obtained to either provide a report to another professional or agency (e.g., physician, lawyer), or to discuss the clinical material with another person (e.g., parent, employer).

You will be immediately informed of the circumstances and to who at any time that notes that relate to this contract are released without your prior knowledge.

Cancellation policy
No penalties exist if you cancel a session with a minimum of 24 hours notice prior to the supervision session. If you do not keep an appointment

(continued over)

FIGURE 2.1 (continued)
Sample clinical supervision contract.

time and have not cancelled the session, you will incur the $150 consultation fee. As practising counsellors there is an expectation to commit fully to the supervision process and this includes keeping appointments. Unexpected emergencies can be discussed on an individual basis.

Contact outside of appointment times

There may be occasions when you need to consult your supervisor outside of appointment times. There is no guarantee that contact outside can always occur. If emergency contact can be done, by telephone when necessary, calls that are within a 10-minute time span will not attract any fee for service. Phone calls that go over 10 minutes will be considered as a supervision session at the regular fee plus 50% surcharge will be charged.

Agreement

We agree, to the best of our ability to uphold the guidelines specified in the supervision contract and to manage the supervisory relationship process according to the ethical principles and code of conduct of the ACA.

Supervisor:................................... Supervisee:...................................
    Mary Smith, PhD   John Brown, MCouns
    Date: 01/01/2009

(Contract adapted from Osborn C.J., & Davis T.E. (1996). The supervision contract: Making it perfectly clear. *The Clinical Supervisor, 14*, 121–134.)

FIGURE 2.1 (continued)
Sample clinical supervision contract.

Record-Keeping

There are many issues that need to be considered in regard to how you write up your case notes and keep records of clients (for additional information see Armstrong, 2006 and/or Bond & Mitchels, 2008). Regarding administration, however, there are certain considerations of which one should be aware. Additionally, different geographical regions and insurance companies may limit or require certain specific practices. For tax and auditing purposes, notes should be kept for between 5–7 years in Australia. Your professional indemnity insurance provider may also have a requirement that supervision records be kept for a certain period of time. Professional indemnity coverage may need to be maintained for a certain period after ceasing practice, which will also require your records to be kept.

In the case of clients who are minors, there may be a need to keep records for an extended period of time. Such a time lag needs to take into consideration minors who reach adulthood may seek some form of legal action against others, which could necessitate access to clinical records. A therapist's duty of care does not necessarily cease when therapy has terminated. The Australian Psychological Society Code of Ethics under Record Keeping, B.2.2 states 'Psychologists keep records for a minimum of seven years since last client contact unless legal or their organisational requirements specify otherwise' and code B.2.3 covers in further detail that 'In the case of records collected while the client was less than 18 years old, psychologists retain the records at least until the client attains the age of 25 years of age'. This is probably a good rule of thumb for supervisors whose supervisees discuss issues related to clients under 18 years of age.

A court of law requesting or demanding notes from therapists is not rare. Individuals who have participated in past couple/relationship/family therapy may also request copies of notes many years after they have ceased therapy. It is also possible that a past difficult client who has experienced a recent negative event may look to apportion blame for their predicament onto their past therapist. I am personally aware of several therapists who have had complaints made against them by past clients. These complaints may be obviously misdirected and dated, but they still have to be processed. In Australia, the majority of professional associations for counsellors and psychotherapists do not have time limits imposed for complaints against their members. Again, a supervisor may need to keep notes on supervisees for an extended period of time to cover such occasions. Professionals need to be aware of such record-keeping requirements. Another aspect of record-keeping includes the long-term archiving of client notes off-site and provisions to be made for their disposal upon the death of the professional or cessation of practice. For space savings one can have records electronically stored on electronic disks. However, one should note that the saving of notes to hard drive disks could have privacy and confidentiality implications. No hard and fast rules can be made regarding such record-keeping as such matters will depend on legal and insurance requirements, as well as the client base involved. However, I highly recommend that client notes not be destroyed, but rather archived.

> HINT: Always date entries and never use correction fluid (white-out) or delete entries as you may leave yourself open to claims of falsifying records.

Confidentiality and Its Exceptions

Confidentiality is often taken for granted by clients and new practitioners. However, there are many limits to confidentiality and these can vary according to profession (e.g., counselling, psychology, social work) as well as region. First, legislative limits to confidentiality include state or federal requirements particularly in relation to privacy laws. A good example of

Sample Counselling Contract

Counselling Services

As part of providing a counselling service to you, your counsellor Mr John Brown will need to collect and record personal information from you that is relevant to your current situation. This information will be a necessary part of the assessment and treatment that is conducted.

Access

You may access the material recorded in your file upon request in line with national privacy legislation. There may be instances where records collected for insurance purposes will be restricted.

Confidentiality

All personal information gathered by the counsellor during the provision of the counselling service will remain confidential and secure except when:

1. It is subpoenaed by a court of law or Government Department/Agency under the appropriate legislation, or
2. Failure to disclose the information would place you, and/or another person at risk, or
3. Your prior approval has been obtained to either provide a report to another professional or agency (e.g., physician, lawyer), or to discuss the clinical material with another person (e.g., parent, employer).

Consultation Fee

The cost of a one hour therapy session is $175 (GST Included), which is payable at the end of the session by cash, cheque or credit card.

Cancellation Policy

If, for some reason you need to cancel or postpone the appointment, please give me at least 24 hours notice, otherwise you will be charged the full fee.

Charter for Clients of Counsellors

The attached Charter explains your rights as a client of a counsellor.

I, (print name) ...., have read and understood this Counselling Contract. I agree to these conditions for the counselling service provided by Mr John Brown.

Signature: ....

Date: ....

Please Note: If, after reading this contract you are unsure about any aspect, please feel free to discuss this with me.

FIGURE 2.2
Sample counselling contract.

this is in Australia where legislation exists, of which many clinicians are unaware, that states the Australian Bureau of Statistics can access notes for statistical purposes. Second, the policies and procedures of the specific organisation for which one is working will have its own written requirements within their policy and procedures manuals. Clinicians need to be aware these do not subordinate legal and legislative requirements. Third, each professional body or registration/licensure board may also have requirements and members agree to abide by these requirements.

A dilemma exists when two or more of these requirements conflict. This is a very common dilemma, particularly in community not-for-profit organisations whose policies and procedures are written by volunteer management committees who may not have a solid understanding of legal and professional requirements. I have also seen government department policies that are in contradiction with legislative requirements, so it is very important supervisors are au fait with their regional requirements. It is only with skilful negotiation and interpretation that such conflicts are resolved. Such difficulties should be recorded in writing, so too the process used to resolve the difficulties. Confidentiality for supervisees is an important issue that needs to be discussed in detail and agreements documented. This is especially the case if a supervisee works in an area where there is more grey, than black and white, in regard to legislative guidelines. Supervisees need strong direction by their supervisors in this regard. A supervisor needs to document for the supervisee and make clear any cases where confidentiality may be breached, just as a counsellor would for a client (see Figure 2.3).

> HINT: Never dispose of any document that may contain information on supervisees or clients in a general waste bin, always shred documents or place in a specially provided secure confidential document receptacle. Consider making provisions for notes in your will.

Insurance

This information is as a guide only and is not intended as advice. All insurance issues should be directed to your insurer in the first instance. If a supervisor operates in a country where insurance is not a requirement, legally or by their professional body, they need to ensure they are aware of potential legal issues if they offer supervision services via the net or phone to supervisees in other regions. For supervisors who do carry insurance, it is in the supervisor's best interest to ensure that they notate they are practicing supervisors on their insurance policy to ensure their insurance coverage includes the provision of supervision as a separate service to counselling. The two primary types of insurance required in most countries for therapists are professional indemnity insurance and public

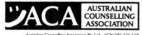

Australian Counselling Association Pty Ltd - ACN 085 535 628

PO BOX 33
Kedron Qld 4031
Suite 4, Heritage Place
634 Lutwyche Road
Lutwyche Qld 4030

telephone: 1300 784 333
facsimile: 07 3857 1777
email: aca@theaca.net.au
web: www.theaca.net.au

Confidentiality Charter for ACA Counsellors

Counselling is an unregulated industry, therefore the public can only be guaranteed appropriate practice by counsellors who abide by a Code of Conduct. All ACA registered counsellors must practice by the ACA Code of Conduct. Part of the Code of Conduct is client confidentiality. This Charter explains confidentiality and the clients rights. Your counsellor should be displaying his or her current membership certificate as a member of the Australian Counselling Association (ACA), which is the peak professional association of counsellors in Australia. Clients should be asked to sign a consent form prior to counselling.

As a client of a counsellor, you have a right to expect that:

- You will be treated with respect
- You will receive a clear explanation of the service you will receive
- Your consent for any service will be sought by the counsellor prior to the service commencing and as it progresses
- You will receive an explanation about the nature and limits of confidentiality surrounding the service
- You will receive competent and professional service
- You will receive a clear statement about fees
- You will be clear about the outcome that you and the counsellor are working toward
- You will receive an estimate of the number of sessions required to achieve the outcome
- You will receive a service free from sexual harassment
- You will be shown respect for your cultural background and language tradition

NOTE:
If you have any concerns about the conduct of your counsellor, call the Australian Counselling Association on 1300 784 333.

FIGURE 2.3
Confidentiality charter for ACA counsellors.
(Reprinted with permission from the Australian Counselling Association)

liability insurance. Some insurers may not automatically include supervision in their policies. Professional indemnity covers the professional and provides recourse for clients harmed by the actions of the professional relationship. It is important to note that professional indemnity insurance provided by an employer may not cover an employee for practice outside of the employment situation. For example, a therapist employed within an agency will be covered by the agency for work within the agency but will not be covered for work in another sector or setting outside the agency, such as a part-time practice.

Public liability insurance protects the public from harm due to property of the owner and should be held by anyone working in private practice. If a professional also lends materials, books or recordings, they should also be covered by a product liability policy, should harm result from the use of a product (i.e., a computer disk containing a virus destroys a client's computer). Finally, run-off insurance is required. Specifically, if you change your insurance company and/or policy, you need to be certain that new policies cover past actions. Similarly, professionals need to investigate their retrospective coverage once they cease practice as professionals, often based on a statute of limitations for various issues, and you do not want to leave any part of your professional practice not covered. Not only do supervisors need insurance (various types), but they also need to ensure that their supervisees are adequately insured. Often the best place to gain your professional insurance policies is via professional associations that have usually negotiated policies to cover their members' needs at a reasonable price.

HINT: If you are self-employed ensured you consider salary protection insurance and work cover.

Professional Associations

From an administrative perspective, once a therapist has joined a professional association they generally need to do two things to maintain membership. First, one must pay an annual membership fee. Second, one must generally engage in continuing professional development, sometimes including clinical supervision. These activities need to be recorded for later reporting purposes. The simplest way to keep professional development and supervision records is to obtain from your professional body, or develop one yourself, a logbook to note such activities. Such a logbook can help a professional avoid having to laboriously reconstruct their professional training and supervision if audited by their professional body. Unfortunately, it is common for busy professionals to fail to keep records of their professional development and not pay the membership fees on time.

> HINT: Always ensure you receive a certificate of attendance when you engage in any professional development activity for your records, regardless of whether it is web-based or in person.

Professional Diary

Professionals should keep a diary/calendar/agenda for work-related appointments that includes with whom they meet and a contact telephone number. Diary entries should include a short description regarding the nature of the meeting (e.g., supervision, counselling, professional development training). Diaries must be kept for record and auditing purposes and need to be archived. Past diaries can be important supporting documentation regarding tax audits or complaint procedures. Due to confidentiality and privacy issues, a professional diary used by a group of practitioners in a clinic setting must be protected from unauthorised access. For instance, clients/supervisees should not be able to see other client/supervisees names in the diary when the professional is making an appointment. Moreover, if a diary is used by multiple private practitioners in a private practice setting, using only first names in the group diary should be considered. Furthermore, if one is using an electronic diary (e.g., personal digital assistant) one should be aware that saving material to the hard drive could pose a potential threat to confidentiality if the computer is linked to the internet or if the computer is accessible to another person (there are limits to the protection offered by computer security programs).

> HINT: At the end of the year add up your client contact and supervision hours and note the totals on the last page. This will help in regard to data collection for possible future needs.

Conclusion

Although often overlooked, the administrative aspects of professional supervision are critical. While complaints and legal action are generally the result of harmful clinical practice, which can be addressed via supervision, training and experience, haphazard administration practices can also result in difficulties and need also to be addressed in supervision. Indeed, administration practices can impact on the disposition of a complaint or legal action as good practices in this area can support a clinician's actions.

Educational Questions and Activities

1. List 3 types of insurance that may be needed for a private practitioner.
   (a) public liability
   (b) professional indemnity
   (c) product liability

2. True or false?
   Providing coverage for Clinical Supervision is automatically covered in all Professional Liability insurance policies.
   False. This is not an automatic inclusion in many policies and may have to be specifically requested.

3. Name two items that by law in Australia (or in your region) must be included on an invoice for professional services.
   (a) ABN or ACN
   (b) whether the service is inclusive or exclusive of Goods and Services Tax.

4. Name two factors that must be considered before offering confidentiality in your client counselling contract?
   (a) privacy legislation
   (b) policy and procedures of the organisation for whom you work
   (c) ethical codes.

5. In relation to keeping clinical notes and records, what is a major consideration in regard to keeping notes if your client base includes minors?
   Minors may take legal action (criminal or civil) many years in the future. If any clients are in this group, the courts of law may expect you to still have copies of your notes.

Selected References for Further Reading

The Attorney-General's Department: Office of Legislative Drafting. (2004). *The Federal Privacy Act, 1988*. Retrieved June 10, 2009, from http://www.privacy. gov.au/publications/privacy88_030504.doc

Armstrong, P. (2006). *Establishing an allied health service*. Sydney, Australia: Cengage.

Barletta, J. (2007). Clinical supervision. In N. Pelling, R. Bowers & P. Armstrong (Eds.), *The practice of counselling* (pp. 118–135). Melbourne, Australia: Thomson.

Bartlet, W.E. (1983). A multidimensional framework for the analysis of supervision of counseling. *Counseling Psychologist, 11*, 9–17.

Bernard, J.M., & Goodyear, R.K. (2004). *Fundamentals of clinical supervision* (3rd ed.). Upper Saddle River, NJ: Merrill.

Bond, T., & Mitchels, B. (2008). *Confidentiality and record keeping in counselling and psychotherapy*. London: Sage

Grauel, T. (2002). Professional oversight: The neglected histories of supervision. In McMahon, M., & Patton, W. (Eds.), *Supervision in the helping professions: A practical approach* (pp. 3–15). Sydney, Australia: Prentice Hall.

Haynes, R., Corey, G., & Moulton, P. (2003). *Clinical supervision in the helping professions: A practical guide.* Pacific Grove, CA: Brookes/Cole Thomson Learning.

Lane, R.C. (1990). *Psychoanalytic approaches to supervision.* New York: Routledge.

McBride, N., & Tunnecliffe, M. (2002). *Risky practices: A supervisees guide to risk management in private practice* (2nd ed.). Palmyra, WA: Bayside Books

McMahon, M., & Patton, W. (Eds.). (2002). *Supervision in the helping professions: A practical approach.* Sydney, Australia: Prentice Hall.

Osborn, C.J., & Davis T.E. (1996). The supervision contract: Making it perfectly clear. *The Clinical Supervisor, 14*, 121–134.

Powell, D.J., & Brodsky, A. (1998). *Clinical supervision in alcohol and drug abuse counseling: Principles, models, methods.* San. Francisco, CA: Jossey-Bass.

Stoltenberg, C.D., & Delworth, U. (1987). *Supervising counselors and therapists: A developmental approach.* San Francisco: Jossey-Bass.

Worthington, E.L. (1987). Changes in supervision as counselors and supervisors gain experience: A review. *Professional Psychology: Research and Practice, 18*(3), 189–208.

———————

Professional Issues

'Professional Issues' is a section comprised of three chapters, each with a unique professional focus but with all presenting supervision related domains in our contemporary context. Chapter 3 outlines resources that can be used by supervisees and their supervisors to explore professional and regulatory aspects of counselling and psychology in various countries worldwide. Chapter 3 can thus serve as a starting point for supervisee and supervisor further explorations of our helping professions across the globe. Chapter 4 presents the ethics relating to clinically supervising the use of the popular and timely evidence-based practices. This ethical examination is in-depth and includes a case study application. Chapter 5 is a unique presentation of the current nature of scholarship in supervision and provides recommendations as to where research and scholarly activities should be directed. This chapter serves as a timely reminder that supervision is not only an applied speciality but also a research and scholarly focus.

Chapter Overview
CHAPTER 3
'Professional Organisations and Resources in Counselling and Psychology', written by Nadine Pelling is a practical chapter presented in two sections. First, a listing of professional organisations and regulatory bodies along with their contact details is presented. Second, this chapter provides references for some of the existing scholarship related to descriptions of counselling and psychology as professions in various countries worldwide. Both supervisors and therapists in training will find these resources helpful in beginning to explore counselling and psychology as professions across the globe. Such a global perspective can only aid in one's broad view of counselling and psychology and is necessary for supervising trainees in a global and mobile market place.

Chapter Themes
In this chapter you will explore the following themes:
* professional organisations
* professional resources
* a limited selection of counselling and psychology resources worldwide
* internationalisation in counselling and psychology.

CHAPTER 4
'Ethical Issues in the Clinical Supervision of Evidence-Based Practices' by Cindy Osborn and Tom Davis delivers a timely and provocative chapter that steps up to the challenge of professionals needing to empirically vali-

date the services they provide. The chapter offers a wonderfully applied case study approach that brings to life clinical imperatives and research-informed challenges in a charming way. Although they are best known to many for their seminal work on the supervision contract, (and some of that area is thankfully explored in this chapter), this particular writing explores the nexus between practitioners and researchers. While this is a lengthy chapter, the reader will find the clinical case, and the questions that are provided to explore it, an invaluable resource, so too the comprehensive references to quality research literature.

Chapter Themes
In this chapter you will explore the following themes:
- types of supervision
- training supervision
- remedial supervision
- ongoing supervision and peer consultation
- evidence-based practices
- ethical issues in the supervision of evidence-based practices
- purpose of supervision
- managing multiple relationships and interpersonal dynamics
- format of supervision
- supervisor qualifications and competence
- evaluation
- ethics in action: Developing and maintaining written supervision contracts.

CHAPTER 5

In her chapter 'Recent Supervision Scholarship', Nadine Pelling asserts that supervision is not just an applied specialty area but also one that can be the focus of research and scholarly efforts. Supporting the scientist-practitioner model of training and practice, Nadine Pelling reviews the results of two literature searches of standard counselling and psychological library databases. She indicates by whom, in which areas, and using what methods some supervision scholarship being produced. Nadine Pelling's findings lead her to suggest more research and less commentary be produced and that collaborative efforts be used across countries to explore supervision as a focus of research endeavours.

Chapter Themes

In this chapter you will explore the following themes:

- clinical supervision: An applied activity and research focus
- method
- results
- Table 5.1
- Table 5.2.

chapter three

Professional Organisations and Resources in Counselling and Psychology

Nadine Pelling

Professional Organisations

In clinical supervision we enhance and develop knowledge, self/other awareness and skill. We hope that this development continues outside of clinical supervision and that continuous lifelong learning is the result. One way to encourage continuous learning as well as the development of collegial support amongst therapists is to promote membership in various professional organisations as beneficial. It is my firm belief that all counsellors, therapists, psychologists and social workers should belong to at least one professional organisation for easy access to a developed code of ethics, collegial support and continuing professional development via the availability of workshops, conferences or the production of professional journals. I believe that such membership promotes reflective practice and continuing professional development. Professional organisations are also a very valuable resource for investigating what types of training and experience are needed in various professional areas and regions. Indeed, many professional organisations have links to regulatory boards that provide information on legislative, or voluntary, requirements when they are present. As a result, an incomplete listing of psychological, counselling and social work-related professional organisations is presented as follows for your convenience (Table 3.1). This information was as accurate as possible at the time of printing and information has come from a variety of sources, including to a large part the internet.

TABLE 3.1

A Limited Listing of Counselling and Psychology Organisations Worldwide

Region	Discipline	Service Area	Name	WWW site	Address	Contact
North America	Counselling	National United States of America	(ACA) American Counseling Association	http://www.counseling.org	5999 Stevenson Avenue, Alexandria, VA 22304, USA	Ph: (800) 473 6647 Fax: (800) 473 2329 membership@ counseling.org
North America	Counselling	National United States of America	Listing of American Counseling Boards via the ACA	http://www.counseling.org/counselors/licensureandcert/tp/staterequirements/ct2.a http://www.counseling.org/Counselors/LicensureAndCert.aspx		
North America	Counselling	National United States of America	(ACES) Association for Counselor Education and Supervision	http://www.acesonline.net		Ph: (800) 347 6647 ext 222 aces@counseling.org
North America	Counselling	National United States of America	(NBCC) National Board for Certified Counselors	http://www.nbcc.org	PO Box 77699 Greensboro NC 27417–7699 USA	Ph: (336) 547 0607 Fax: (336) 547 0017 nbcc@nbcc.org
North America	Psychology	National United States of America and Canada	Association of State and Provincial Licensing Boards	http://www.asppb.org http://www.asppb.org/about/boardcontactstatic.aspx	PO Box 251245 Montgomery, Alabama 36124–1245 USA	
North America	Psychology	National United States of America	(APA) American Psychological Association	http://www.apa.org	750 First Street, NE Washington DC 20002–4242 USA	Ph: (800) 374 2721

TABLE 3.1 (continued)
A Limited Listing of Counselling and Psychology Organisations Worldwide

Region	Discipline	Service Area	Name	WWW site	Address	Contact
North America	Psychology	National United States of America	(APA) American Psychological Association – Journals	http://www.apa.org/journals	750 First Street, NE Washington DC 20002–4242 USA	Ph: (800) 374 2721 Fax: (202) 336 5502 journals@apa.org
North America	Psychology	National United States of America	(APA) Division 17 – Society of Counseling Psychology	http://www.div17.0rg/	Division 17 Administrative Office American Psychological Association 750 First Street, NE Washington, DC 20002–4242 USA	Ph: (202) 216 7602 Fax: (202) 218 3599 kcooke@apa.org
North America	Counselling	National Canada	(CCA) Canadian Counselling Association	http://www.ccacc.ca	16 Concourse Gate, Suite 600 Ottawa, On K2E 7S8 Canada	Ph: (613) 237 1099 Fax: (613) 237 9786 info@ccacc.ca
North America	Counselling	National Canada	Canadian Counselling Certification	http://ccacc.ca/e_certification.html	16 Concourse Gate, Suite 600 Ottawa, On K2E 7S8 Canada	Ph: (613) 237 1099 Fax: (613) 237 9786 info@ccacc.ca
North America	Counselling	National Canada	(CPCA) Canadian Professional Counsellors Association	http://www.cpca-rpc.ca/	#203, 3306 – 32nd Avenue Vernon, BC V1T 2M6 Canada	Ph: (250) 558 3323 jgwright@telus.net
North America	Counselling	National Canada	(CCPCP) Canadian College of Professional Counsellors and Psychotherapists	http://www.ccpcp.ca/	PO Box 39001 RPO Lakewook Common Saskatoon SK S7V 0A9 Canada	Ph: (866) 704 4828

TABLE 3.1 (continued)
A Limited Listing of Counselling and Psychology Organisations Worldwide

Region	Discipline	Service Area	Name	WWW site	Address	Contact
North America	Psychology	National United States of America and Canada	Association of State and Provincial Licensing Boards	http://www.asppb.org http://www.asppb.org/about/boardcontactstatic.aspx	PO Box 251245 Montgomery, Alabama 36124–1245 USA	Ph: (613) 237 2144 Fax: (613) 237 1674 cpa@cpa.ca
North America	Psychology	National Canada	(CPA) Canadian Psychological Association; Societe Canadienne de Psychologie	http://www.cpa.ca/	141 Laurier Avenue West, Suite 702 Ottawa, Ontario K1P 5J3 Canada	
Europe	Counselling	National United Kingdom	(BACP) British Association for Counselling and Psychotherapy	http://www.bacp.co.uk	British Association for Counselling and Psychotherapy BACP House 15 St John's Business Park Lutterworth LE17 4HB England UK	Ph: 01455 883300 Fax: 01455 550243 enquiries@bacp.co.uk
Europe	Counselling	National United Kingdom	(UKCP) United Kingdom Council for Psychotherapy	http://www.psychotherapy.org.uk	UKCP 2nd Floor Edward House 2 Wakley Street London EC1V 7LT England UK	Ph: 020 7014 9955 Fax: 020 7014 9977 info@psychotherapy.org.uk

TABLE 3.1 (continued)
A Limited Listing of Counselling and Psychology Organisations Worldwide

Region	Discipline	Service Area	Name	WWW site	Address	Contact
Europe	Counselling	National United Kingdom	(BACP) British Association for Counselling and Psychotherapy — Supervision	http://www.bacp.co.uk	British Association for Counselling and Psychotherapy BACP House 15 St John's Business Park Lutterworth LE17 4HB England UK	Ph: 01455 883300 Fax: 01455 550243 enquiries@ bacp.co.uk
Europe	Psychology	National United Kingdom	(BPS) British Psychological Society	http://www.bps.org.uk	The British Psychological Society St Andrews House 48 Princess Road East Leicester LE1 7DR England UK	Ph: +44 (0)116 254 9568 Fax: +44 (0)116 227 1314 enquiries@ bps.org.uk
Australasia	Counselling	National Australia	(ACA) Australian Counselling Association	http://www.theaca.net.au	P.O. Box 88 Grange Qld 4051 Australia	Ph: (07) 3356 4255 Fax: (07) 3356 4709 aca@theaca.net.au
Australasia	Counselling	National Australia	(PACFA) Psychotherapy and Counselling Federation of Australia	http://www.pacfa.org.au	290 Park Street Fitzroy North VIC 3068 Australia	Ph: (03) 9486 3077 Fax: (03) 9486 3933 admin@ pacfa.org.au
Australasia	Counselling Psychology	National Australia	(AGCA) Australian Guidance and Counselling Association	http://www.agca.com.au		
Australasia	Counselling	National Australia	(SCAPE) Society of Counselling and Psychotherapy Educators	http://www.scape.org.au		edavis@ jni.nsw.edu.au

TABLE 3.1 (continued)
A Limited Listing of Counselling and Psychology Organisations Worldwide

Region	Discipline	Service Area	Name	WWW site	Address	Contact
Australasia	Psychology	National Australia	(APS) Australian Psychological Society	http://www.psychology.org.au	PO Box 38 Flinders Lane VIC 8009 Australia	Ph: (03) 8662 3300 Fax: (03) 9663 6177 contactus@psychology.org.au
Australasia	Counsellors	National New Zealand	(NZAC) New Zealand Association of Counsellors	http://www.nzac.org.nz	PO Box 165 Waikato Mail Centre Hamilton, 3240 New Zealand	Ph: (07) 834 0220 Fax: (07) 834 0221 office@nzac.org.nz
Australasia	Psychology	National New Zealand	(NZPsS) New Zealand Psychological Society	http://www.psychology.org.nz	PO Box 4092 Wellington 6143 New Zealand	Ph: 64 4 473 4884 Fax: 64 4 473 4889 office@psychology.org.nz
Australasia	Psychology	National New Zealand	(NZPB) New Zealand Psychologists Board	http://www.psychologistsboard.org.nz	PO Box 10–626 Wellington 6143 New Zealand	Ph: 64 4 471 4581 Fax: 64 4 471 4580 info@nzpb.org.nz
Australasia	Counselling	Hong Kong	Hong Kong Professional Counsellors Association	http://www.hkpca.org.hk	c/o College of International Education Hong Kong Baptist University (Shek Mun Campus) 8 On Muk Street Shatin, NT	
Australasia	Psychology	Hong Kong	Hong Kong Psychological Society	http://www.hkps.org.hk	c/o Department of Psychology, University of Hong Kong, Pok Fu Lam Road, HK	

TABLE 3.1 (continued)
A Limited Listing of Counselling and Psychology Organisations Worldwide

Region	Discipline	Service Area	Name	WWW site	Address	Contact
Australasia	Counselling	Malaysia	Malaysian Counselling Association	http://www.perkama.org/		
Australasia	Psychology	Malaysia	Malaysian Psychological Association	http://www.uum.edu.my/psima/msg%20fromthe%20presdnt.htm	D/A Malaysian Psychology Department, University of Malaysia, 43600 Bangi, Selangor	
Australasia	Counselling	Singapore	Singapore Association for Counselling	http://www.sac-counsel.org.sg/	93 Toa Payoh Central #05–01, Toa Payoh Central Community Building, Singapore 319194	
Australasia	Psychology	Singapore	Singapore Psychological Society	http://www.singapore psychologicalsociety.org	93 Toa Payoh Central #05–01, Toa Payoh Central Community Building, Singapore 319194	

Professional Resources

Students often ask me, 'What do I need to do in order to be a professional therapist?', to which my first answer is generally a compound question, 'Where and in what area do you intend on working (i.e., Canada or Australia and psychology or counselling)?' as regulations differ across the globe and professions. I then refer those seeking international counselling or psychology information to the relevant country's professional organisations as previously presented. Luckily, I also keep a file of article copies regarding counselling and psychology in different countries. These have proven to be helpful starting points for those interested in exploring a specific helping profession in a specific country. It is beyond the scope of the present chapter to outline the nature of psychology and counselling across the globe and thus I have chosen to simply present some of the references in my file I have collated in the following sections for your review. This is not an exhaustive bibliography but simply a starting point for those interested in gaining more information.

A LIMITED SELECTION OF COUNSELLING AND PSYCHOLOGY RESOURCES WORLDWIDE

United States

Council for Accreditation of Counseling and Related Educational Programs. (n.d.). Available at http://www.cacrep.org

Munley, P.H., Duncan, L.E., McDonnell, K.A., & Sauer, E.M. (2004). Counseling psychology in the United States of America. *Counselling Psychology Quarterly, 17*(3), 247–271.

Pope, K.S. (n.d.). *Psychology Laws & Licensing Boards in Canada & the United States.* URL: http://kspope.com/licensing/index.php

Weinrach, S.G., & Thomas, K.R. (1993). The National Board for Certified Counselors: The good, the bad, and the ugly. *Journal of Counseling and Development, 72*(1), 105–109.

Canada

Canadian Counselling Association. (2005). *Certification of Canadian counsellors.* URL: http://www.ccacc.ca/cocc.htm

Canadian Counselling Association. (2005). *CCC main page.* URL:http://www.ccacc.ca/ccacc.htm

Janel, G. (2002). Facilitating mobility for psychologists through a competency-based approach for regulation and accreditation: The Canadian experiment. *European Psychologist, 17*(3), 203–212.

Lalande, V.M. (2004). Counselling Psychology: A Canadian perspective. *Counselling Psychology Quarterly, 17*(3), 273–286.

United Kingdom

Aldridge, S. (2006, February). Update on regulation. *Therapy Today,* 34–35.

Balfour, F.G.H. (2000). The statutory registration of psychotherapists. *British Journal of Guidance & Counselling*, *16*(3), 311–320.

British Psychological Society. (2006). BPS acts on new adoption supports regulations. *The Psychologist*, *19*(5), 298–301.

British Association for Counselling and Psychotherapy. (n.d.). *Accreditation*. URL: http://www.bacp.co.uk/accreditation/index.html

British Psychological Society. (n.d.). *Home Page*. URL: http://www.bps.org.uk

British Psychological Society. (n.d.). *Statutory Regulation — FAQs*. URL: http://www.bps.org.uk/the-society/statutory-regulation/faq.cfm

British Psychological Society. (2005). Statutory regulation: Some questions answered. *The Psychologist*, *18*(4), 238–239.

British Association for Counselling and Psychotherapy. (2005, December). Regulation: The mapping project. *Therapy Today*, 37–39.

Brown, S. (2005, December). Editorial. *Therapy Today*, 2.

Denburg, M.L. (1969). Registration of applied psychologists. *Bulletin of the British Psychological Society*, *22*(74), 19–20.

Dryden, W., Mearns, D., & Thorne, B. (2000). Counselling in the United Kingdom: Past, present and future. *British Journal of Guidance & Counselling*, *28*(4), 467–483.

Fontana, D. (1982). The registration of psychologists: An unhelpful distinction between teachers and practitioners. *Bulletin of the British Psychological Society*, *35*, 377–378.

Inskipp, F., & Johns, H. (2003). A visionary in British counselling. *International Journal for the Advancement of Counselling*, *25*(2–3), 115–118.

Joseph, S. (2005). Interview with Professor David Lane entitled 'Registering Interest'. *The Psychologist*, *18*(4), 228–229.

Jacobs, M. (2000). Counselling in the United Kingdom: Past, present and future. *British Journal of Guidance & Counselling*, *28*(4), 451–466.

Latak, K. (2006, May). Studying Psychology in Europe. *The Psychologist*, 297.

Lunt, I., & Lindsay, G. (1993). Professional psychologists in the United Kingdom: Current issues, trends and developments. *European Review of Applied Psychology*, *43*(2), 91–98.

Musgrave, A. (2006, May). The onward march of regulation. *Therapy Today*, 10–12.

Steering Committee on Registration, British Psychological Society. (1984, January). Recommendations for the registration of psychologists. *Bulletin of the British Psychological Society*, *37*, 1–7.

Steering Committee on Registration, British Psychological Society. (1983, April). Registration and academic psychologists: A consultative paper. *Bulletin of the British Psychological Society*, *36*, 120–125.

Tholstrup, M. (1999, May). Professional registration: A contentious debate. *Counselling Psychology Review*, *14*(2), 15–20.

Walsh, Y., Frankland, A., & Cross, M. (2004). Qualifying and working as a counselling psychologist in the United Kingdom. *Counselling Psychology Quarterly*, *17*(3), 317–328.

Woolfe, R. (1999). Training routes for counsellors, counselling psychologists and psychotherapists. In R. Bor & M. Watts (Eds.), *Trainee handbook: A guide for counselling and psychotherapy trainees* (pp. 6–18). London: Sage Publications.

Australia

Brown, J., & Corne, L. (2004). Counselling psychology in Australia. *Counselling Psychology Quarterly, 17*(3), 287–299.

Helmes, E., & Wilmoth, D. (2002, March). Training in clinical psychology in Australia: A North American Perspective. *Australian Psychologist, 37*(1), 52–55.

Journal Special Issue: Counselling in Australia. (2006). Guest edited by Nadine Pelling. *International Journal of Psychology, 41*(3), 153–215.

Littlefield, L., Giese, J., & Katsikitis, M. (2007, April). Professional psychology training under review. *InPsych, 29*(2), 6.

Pelling, N. (2006). Getting a global perspective: Counselling Australia. *Counseling Today, 48*(7), 35.

Pelling, N., & Sullivan, B. (2006). The credentialing of counselling in Australia. *International Journal of Psychology, 41*(3), 194–203.

Pelling, N., & Whetham, P. (2006). The professional preparation of Australian counsellors. *International Journal of Psychology, 41*(3), 189–193.

New Zealand

Shouksmith, G. (2005, January). Psychology in New Zealand. *The Psychologist, 18*(1), 14–16.

Stanley, P., & Manthei, R. (2004). Counselling psychology in New Zealand: The quest for identity and recognition. *Counselling Psychology Quarterly, 17*(3), 301–315.

Hong Kong

Hong Kong Social Workers Association. (n.d.) *Home page.* URL: http://www.hkswa.org.hk

International Counselling and Psychology Resources

Marsella, A.J., & Pedersen, P. (2004). Internationalizing the counseling psychology curriculum: Toward new values, competencies, and directions. *Counselling Psychology Quarterly, 17*(4), 413–423.

Okorodudu, R.I. (2006, June). Global citizenship: Implications for guidance and counselling innovations in developing nations. *International Journal for the Advancement of Counselling, 28*(2), 107–120.

Pelling, N. (2004). Counselling psychology: Diversity and commonalities across the Western World. *Counselling Psychology Quarterly, 17*(3), 239–245.

Other Countries

Iliescu, D., Ispas, A., & Ilie, A. (2007, January). Psychology in Romania. *The Psychologist, 20*(1), 34–35.

Forster, P. (2005, May). Psychology in Vanuatu. *The Psychologist, 18*(5), 288–289.

Gómez, B. (2007). Psychotherapy in Argentina: A clinical case from an integrative perspective. *Journal of Clinical Psychology, 63*(8), 713–723.

Jain, A.K. (2005, April). Psychology in India. *The Psychologist, 18*(4), 206–208.

Biruski, D.C., Jerkovic, I., & Zotovic, M. (2007, April). Psychology in Bosnia and Herzegovina, Croatia and Serbia. *The Psychologist, 20*(4), 220–222.

Sato, T., & Fumino, Y. (2005, March). Psychology in Japan. *The Psychologist, 18*(3), 156–157.

Internationalisation in Counselling and Psychology

I encourage both supervisors and supervisees to explore how different countries regulate their chosen profession and/or how their country regulates professions related to their own. Having an international and/or multidisciplinary perspective can aid in developing self/other awareness and you never know when the information may by requested by a colleague or supervisee.

Educational Questions and Activities

1. As an individual or a group list all of the possible benefits and drawbacks of being a member of a professional organisation.

2. Ask a trusted colleague or supervisor what they think the benefits and drawbacks of being a member of a professional organisation entail.

3. Look up one professional organisation in your area in your home country and one in a country in which you are interested. What do the respective organisations say about your professional area in those countries?

4. How much does it cost for a student or a beginning professional to join the professional organisation most relevant to your work?

Selected References for Further Reading

Pelling, N. (2006). Professional counselling organisations. In N. Pelling, R. Bowers, & P. Armstrong (Eds.), *The practice of counselling* (pp. 442–453). Melbourne: Thomson Publishers.

Pelling, N.J. (1998). Record keeping to ease the internship, practicum, and job application process. *Counseling Today, 40*(11), 36.

English, S., & Marino, T. (1998). Update: Professional counselors and managed care. *Counseling Today, 1*, 18.

Association of Psychology Postdoctoral and Internship Centers. (2009). Internship Application (AAPI). Retrieved June 5, 2009, from http://www.appic.org/match/5_3_match_application.html

Connelly, A.R. (2006, April). Resume or vita? What's the difference? *Counseling Today*, 11.

chapter four

Ethical Issues in the Clinical Supervision of Evidence-Based Practices

Cynthia J. Osborn and Thomas E. Davis

For as long as some form of psychotherapy has been taught, the supervision of the implementation of that psychotherapy has been practised. The earliest model of supervision, originating from the teaching and learning of psychoanalysis, resembled a master–apprentice interaction between supervisor (master therapist) and supervisee (novice therapist or apprentice; see Binder & Strupp, 1997). As the practice of counselling and other forms of psychotherapy has expanded and evolved, so has supervision. This is particularly true with the emergence of innovative therapeutic practices, including evidence-based practices (EBPs). No longer can clinical supervision be considered a well-defined practice, one typically confined to a student's formal academic training (e.g., during practicum), or representing the guidance or shepherding of a therapist in the early phase of his or her career. As Milne (2007) contended, Bernard and Goodyear's (2009) longstanding definition of clinical supervision may no longer capture the varied types of counselling and the concomitant functions of supervision, nor satisfy the need for empirical support that 'the evidence-based movement' has created.

Although clinical supervision is now considered a discipline separate from psychotherapy or counselling, the two retain a symbiotic relationship: one cannot exist without the other. This entanglement — as with any type of professional relationship, particularly, in the intimate function of counselling — has always brought with it ethical and legal issues. However, as the type, function and setting of therapy has changed, so has the supervision of that therapy and, in the process, new ethical considerations have arisen.

This chapter focuses on ethical issues in clinical supervision (rather than administrative supervision), particularly in the era of EBPs. Although certain ethical issues remain 'standard' in clinical supervision (e.g., evaluation, power, multiple relationships) regardless of the type, function and setting that is supervised, therapy and supervision practiced in an EBP milieu raise further ethical considerations.

The following case involves Leah, Laurie and Dr Bennett — all of whom are connected in the training and implementation of one EBP, multisystemic therapy (MST). After reading through the case, review the questions that follow that are intended to stimulate ethical considerations that are discussed throughout the chapter.

Case Study

Leah earned a Master of Counselling degree 3 years ago and has worked in a juvenile correctional facility since graduation. Tired with what she considered to be a more punitive and less remedial treatment philosophy, she pursued employment elsewhere. She was recently hired as a therapist at a community-based mental health facility, 'Horizons', that serves adolescents and families. Funding sources have required the facility to render treatment services that have empirical evidence to support their efficacy and effectiveness, so-called evidence-based practices (EBPs). One of these, multisystemic therapy (MST; Henggeler & Borduin, 1990), has been adopted by the facility, requiring all frontline clinicians to obtain intensive training and ongoing supervision. The facility has contracted with a small, private training and research group, 'Ignite', comprised of clinicians and university faculty with expertise in MST and other EBPs (e.g., cognitive–behavioural therapy, motivational interviewing).

MST is a comprehensive treatment approach for adolescents and their families, conducted by a team of professionals, that includes home-based therapy. This treatment approach is pragmatic and goal-oriented and was initially designed for serious juvenile offenders. Today, MST is appropriate for adolescents who struggle with both mental health and substance use concerns and, in the process, have become involved in the legal system. Service providers receive ongoing group supervision for 6 months after completing an initial and intensive 5-day MST training.

As a recruit, Leah has been assigned an internal supervisor, Laurie, a social worker with 15 years of experience, who oversees clinicians working with youth who have co-occurring mental health and substance use disorders. Laurie is new to MST whereas Leah had learned about MST as a graduate student. Both Leah and Laurie just completed the 5-day MST training conducted by Dr Bennett, one of Ignite's trainers and a lecturer at the university where Leah earned her degree. He taught several counselling courses in which Leah was a student.

Due to the severe, chronic, and complex nature of problems that families appropriate for MST present to treatment, a multidisciplinary treatment team approach is indicated and is the norm for direct care in MST. Each team is typically comprised of two to four practitioners, and Laurie and Leah are on the same MST team. Although each is responsible for four to six client cases (i.e., four to six adolescents and their families), MST practitioners meet regularly as a team to coordinate services to all families. Team members provide coverage when the primary therapist for a family is on vacation or otherwise not on-call and all team members have met all the families served by their colleagues.

MST supervision is intended to mirror that of MST direct care and thus supervision is provided to a team. Group supervision — rather than individual supervision — is therefore the standard format of MST supervision. The group format for MST supervision allows therapists to learn from one another, to work collaboratively and as a cohesive unit (as therapists are teaching families to do) and to practice a new skill set with colleagues. To remain consistent with MST training guidelines, both Laurie and Leah will participate in ongoing MST group supervision for at least 6 months and Dr Bennett will be serving as their MST team supervisor. The purpose of supervision is to ensure therapist fidelity with or adherence to MST practice principles.

The introduction of an EBP to a mental health facility like Horizons can 'shake up the system' and therefore it can have the effect of clinicians re-evaluating their priorities and practices. 'Treatment as usual' may no longer be an option. 'Standard supervision practice' also may no longer exist, or be unrecognisable. As a result, clinicians may feel out of their comfort zone or even lost, uncertain as to how to address the new configurations and possible dilemmas that an EBP — a new and perhaps unfamiliar 'standard of practice' — has ushered in.

In the preceding case, the administration at Horizons has adopted MST as the new standard of practice. How does this affect the practice of supervision? What ethical and possibly legal issues does it raise? Specifically:

- Should Leah and Laurie participate in and be members of the same MST supervision group?

- Should Dr Bennett serve as Leah's individual MST supervisor?

- Who should (or can be) ultimately be responsible for welfare of Leah's clients — Laurie or Dr Bennett?

- How can and should Leah's clinical skills be assessed? Would someone (Laurie or Dr Bennett?) need to accompany her to clients' homes to observe her interactions with clients and their families?

- Who is responsible for Leah's clinical evaluation?

- What happens if Leah's MST skills do not meet minimum requirements at the end of the 6-month training/supervision period?

Types of Supervision

The case of Leah, Laura and Dr Bennett illustrates some of the complexities of clinical supervision, particularly in the current era of EBPs. What is the purpose of supervision of an EBP such as multisystemic therapy (MST)? How is supervision conducted? Who gets to decide? Who is ultimately responsible for the professional development of supervised therapists and for the welfare of their clients? There is clearly not one way to conduct supervision and supervision fulfils various functions. We briefly discuss four types of supervision, each of which may raise unique ethical considerations given the purpose or intent of supervision.

Training Supervision

Supervision is regarded primarily as the required teaching and clinical oversight or monitoring of persons (e.g., trainees) preparing to enter a helping profession during their formal/academic training. When students are enrolled in a practicum or an internship and are delivering counselling services to clients, they are required to be supervised by a faculty member and a practitioner in the field. This is the predominant understanding of supervision and is exemplified in Bernard and Goodyear's (2009) definition of clinical supervision as:

> … an intervention provided by a more senior member of a profession to a more junior member or members of that same profession. This relationship is evaluative, extends over time, and has the simultaneous purposes of (1) enhancing the professional functioning of a more junior person(s), (2) monitoring the quality of professional services offered to the client(s) she, he, or, they see(s), and (3) serving as a gatekeeper of those who are to enter the particular profession. (p. 7)

In this definition of supervision, the power differential between supervisor and supervisee is made explicit and a master–apprentice model is implied. Although this type of supervision 'extends over time', its purpose is to ensure client welfare and, at the same time, determine whether a counsellor-in-training is prepared to practice and be recognised by a credentialing body as a professional counsellor. In this sense, supervision is time-limited and corresponds to a period of apprenticeship or probation. The supervisee must be able to demonstrate that he or she is ready to function as a professional independent of close monitoring or supervision and the supervisor must be able to assess the supervisee's preparedness, fulfilling the role of 'gatekeeper', the one who may hold the key to the trainee's induction into the profession.

Given the purpose of training supervision, evaluation is understandably an integral function of supervision and the source of much anxiety for supervisees and supervisors alike. Gould and Bradley (2001) offered some explanation for what Nelson, Barnes, Evans and Triggiano (2008) described as 'supervisor gate-keeping anxiety', including discomfort with what some supervisors may construe as the authoritarian and dictatorial role of evaluator. Supervisors may also be uncertain as to how to evaluate and may therefore shirk this important responsibility. This is suggested in Ladany, Ellis and Friedlander's (1999) survey of 151 psychologists-in-training. The most frequent ethical violation of their supervisors reported by these supervisees (by 33.1% of respondents) was that of 'performance evaluation and monitoring of supervisee activities'. Specific supervisor evaluation practices supervisees deemed unethical included 'gives me little feedback' and 'never listened to my audio tapes'. One supervisee in Ladany et al.'s study reported, 'At the end of the semester I was very surprised to find that she was unsatisfied with my work ... I had never been evaluated or critiqued'.

Remedial Supervision

Not only is evaluation integral to training supervision, it is an essential function of remedial supervision. By remedial supervision we refer to supervision that a credentialing body or professional association may require to restore to 'good standing' an independently licensed therapist who has been found to be in violation of an ethical code or standard. Cobia and Pipes (2002) described mandated supervision as a mechanism 'to rehabilitate impaired professionals' (p. 143). As with training supervision, remedial supervision may also be time-limited and encompass a probationary period. Unlike training supervision, however, remedial supervision is intended to be restorative, whereas training supervision is designed to be foundational and generative (i.e., launching a new clinician into professional practice).

Although it appears that remedial supervision is not an uncommon practice (see Rapisarda & Britton, 2007), it is rather surprising that very little has been discussed in the literature about its purpose and how it should be conducted. In terms of research, Rapisarda and Britton attempted to interview supervisors in one state who provided what they referred to as sanctioned supervision, but were not successful. They conducted a focus group instead with clinical supervisors about sanctioned supervision. Participating supervisors ($N = 8$) who had *not* provided remedial or sanctioned supervision to a colleague envisioned several concerns about this type of supervision including supervisor liability (e.g., what happens if the supervisee continues to practice unethically?), evaluation practices and payment for supervision. The need for more training in conducting this type of supervision was also shared among supervisors. In their discussions of sanctioned supervision, several participants indicated this particular intervention resembled 'clinical monitoring' rather than supervision.

Ongoing Supervision and Peer Consultation

Compared to training supervision and remedial supervision, ongoing supervision and peer consultation are typically voluntary and initiated by an independently licensed therapist for the purpose of continuous professional enhancement. The British Association for Counselling and Psychotherapy (BACP, 2007), however, requires that all accredited therapists (i.e., counsellors, psychotherapists, trainers and supervisors) receive 'regular and on-going formal supervision/consultative support for their work' (p. 5). Sometimes referred to as peer supervision and conducted in a group setting (see Bernard & Goodyear, 2009; Borders, 1991), ongoing supervision may be characterised as a form of clinical consultation for experienced clinicians to offer one another support and guidance. This is particularly true for clinicians in private practice as an antidote to professional isolation. It is also true for clinicians in a group practice or a community-based agency who desire additional support and assistance with ethical dilemmas. In Australia all practising counsellors registered with the peak professional body, Australian Counselling Association (ACA) and the umbrella association, Psychotherapy and Counselling Federation of Australia (PACFA) are required to undergo ongoing clinical supervision to maintain their membership (ACA, 2009; PACFA, 2009).

From interviews with 30 social workers in Australia who were willing to discuss an ethical dilemma they had experienced, McAuliffe and Sudbery (2005) found that 21 were provided with supervision (primarily administrative) by their employing organisation (often referred to as the 'immediate line manager' and not necessarily social workers). Four of the 21 elected to obtain additional, external, private and ongoing supervision to focus more on professional development and emotional support. Of the nine social workers without access to internal supervision, all had accessed external supervision from social workers, an indication that clinicians may pursue continuous supervision from members of their own profession.

Peer consultation has been proposed recently as a means of fostering supervisor development, specifically enhancing critical thinking skills when working with challenging client cases. Granello, Kindsvatter, Granello, Underfer-Babalis and Hartwig Moorhead (2008) described their supervisory peer consultation group that met on a periodic basis to generate multiple perspectives on specific supervisory experiences of group members. One member served as the ethics consultant and offered guidance in ethical decision-making. The purpose was to generate multiple perspectives about specific clinical (including supervisory) issues. In so doing, Granello et al. reported that they each learned to think more complexly about supervision and realised the importance of investing in their own development as supervisors, 'with more than lip service to the idea that development must be lifelong' (p. 42).

Targeted and Skill-Specific Supervision

A fourth type of supervision is practiced for reasons similar to ongoing supervision and peer consultation (i.e., professional support and development) but is associated with specific skill sets and therapeutic approaches, namely evidence-based practices (EBPs). The adoption of any EBP and other forms of innovative practices requires initial, periodic and often ongoing supervision to ensure fidelity to the treatment protocol. Heaven, Clegg, and Maguire (2006) referred to supervision of an EBP as the 'bridge between the classroom and workplace following ... training' (p. 314). With respect to cognitive–behavioural therapy (CBT), Pretorius (2006) described supervision as 'quality control ... during initial training and throughout therapists' careers' (p. 413).

Dialectical behaviour therapy (DBT; Linehan, 1993) has become an EBP in the treatment of borderline personality disorder (see Linehan et al., 2006). Of the five functions of a standard DBT 'package' is that of therapist skill enhancement and motivation. Regular (i.e., weekly) therapist training/consultation team sessions are held specifically to reduce burnout, provide therapy for therapists, improve therapist empathy for clients and offer skills training to therapists regarding specific client difficulties (Lynch, Trost, Salsman, & Linehan, 2007). Supervision in DBT is therefore not only for the purpose of ensuring that therapists deliver DBT-consistent services to clients and that clients are receiving quality care. It is also intended to 'treat' the therapists at the same time that clients are being treated by DBT therapists. The focus of these DBT team meetings and ongoing supervision is on therapist fitness and wellbeing and less on client difficulties (Lynch et al., 2007), illustrating the importance Linehan (1993) has placed on therapeutic humility. Fruzzetti, Waltz, and Linehan (1997) asserted that supervision in DBT is designed to anticipate, minimise or even prevent burnout by enhancing 'therapist training, effectiveness, and competence, and also satisfaction and enjoyment with [their] work' (p. 85). Supervision is also continuous when practicing DBT. This means that as long as a clinician is practicing DBT, he or she is receiving and participating in regular supervision.

As mentioned earlier in this chapter, supervision of multisystemic therapy (MST) is intended to 'facilitate therapists' acquisition and implementation of the conceptual and behavioral skills required to achieve adherence to the MST treatment model' (Henggeler & Schoenwald, 1998, p. 1). As with CBT, therefore, MST supervision serves as a 'quality assurance' measure, designed to ensure treatment fidelity; in other words, the purpose of MST supervision is to ensure that services clinicians have been trained to deliver to clients are actually being implemented. This function of supervision is also true for the supervision of nonclinical staff trained in a standard practice adopted by a treatment or correctional facility. For example, the supervision of probation officers is a required element in New Zealand's Department of Corrections (see Norrie, Eggleston, & Ringer, 2003) to ensure implementation of the department's 'best practices' (interpreted as providing the best services to offenders, Departmental Services and the community).

Supervision of EBP often has a specific purpose: to provide further and extended training in EBP so as to facilitate the application of a specific skill set to clinicians. In this way, supervision targets a specific counselling approach or style and is intended to help clinicians transfer or apply new counselling behaviours to their work with clients. If the clinician fails to meet minimum criteria for treatment adherence or fidelity, additional and perhaps intensive supervision may be required. Although some EBPs may require supervision only until the supervisee has achieved a certain level of proficiency (i.e., time-limited supervision), other EBPs (e.g., DBT) consider supervision an essential component of the therapeutic approach and is therefore ongoing. It seems that EBP supervision contains features of the first three types of supervision discussed in this chapter: training supervision, remedial supervision and ongoing supervision.

Evidence-Based Practices

The American Psychological Association (APA) has defined evidence-based practice (EBP) as 'the integration of the best available research with clinical expertise in the context of patient characteristics, culture, and preferences' (APA Presidential Task Force on Evidence-Based Practice, 2006, p. 273). The purpose of EBPs has been to 'raise the bar' by providing clients with services that have research support, services that have 'passed the test' and can be trusted to yield beneficial therapeutic outcomes. Despite its laudatory purpose to prioritise only those therapies that have been proven to be effective, the EBP 'movement' has been criticised for several reasons. These include (a) what appears to be an exclusive focus on treatment interventions rather than client or therapist factors, (b) a seeming lack of consensus as to what constitutes 'evidence' (i.e., results of randomised clinical/control trials only?) and (c) the mandatory manner in which EBPs are marketed (see Cormier, Nurius, & Osborn, 2009, pp. 278–279).

Negative views of EBPs are therefore understandable, particularly when clinicians are required by their superiors (who may also represent sources of funding) to adopt a new skill set and to be monitored over a period of time to ensure fidelity or treatment compliance. Bohart (2005) has accused advocates of EBPs as dictatorial because they restrict alternative practices. Indeed, he referred to the 'hegemonic tendencies' of EBPs (p. 51) and has implied that this strong-arm approach is unethical. Depending on how

EBPs are introduced to clinicians and how training and supervision are presented, clinicians may feel 'manualised'. It may be that Laurie, an experienced clinician introduced at the beginning of this chapter, may feel this way about her 'assignment' of having to learn and practice MST under Dr Bennett's supervision. This may be particularly true because she is expected to participate in MST training along with Leah, Laurie's new supervisee who is also new to the profession.

Although highly controversial, the focus on EBPs appears to have opened up lines of communication between practitioners and researchers, has prioritised care that is 'in the best interest of the client', and has ushered in a more integrative perspective about client care. In addition, EBP has challenged clinicians to be more accountable in their practice. That is, simply following 'intuition' when making practice decisions is no longer acceptable. Indeed, Reamer (2006) defined as 'non-traditional and unorthodox' those interventions that are 'not based on sound theory and research-based evidence' (p. 192) and argued that social workers who practice these interventions make themselves vulnerable to ethics complaints, lawsuits and criminal charges. Falender and Shafranske's (2007) delineation of competency-based supervision is consistent with what we suspect is the increasing expectation for supervisor accountability.

Gambrill and Gibbs (2002) found that of a sample of social workers (n = 83) and social work students (undergraduate and master's degree; n = 124), the majority reported relying on intuition in making practice decisions (e.g., treatment planning with clients) rather than evidence- or science-based information, even after receiving training on integrating research into practice. Furthermore, the majority of this same sample acknowledged wanting their physician to make decisions about their medical care based on research findings rather than their (the physicians') intuition. Gambrill and Gibbs interpreted their findings to mean that

> Social workers want their physicians to rely on scientific criteria when they make recommendations for treatment, but rely on weak evidentiary grounds such as tradition when working with clients ... [or, in other words] what's good for the goose is not viewed as good for the gander. (p. 39)

This suggests that clinicians in the behavioural sciences (e.g., counselling, psychology) may have conflicting views of EBPs, believing that EBP may apply to the work of other professionals but not to their own work.

The emphasis on EBPs has at least two implications for the practice of clinical supervision. First, many if not the majority of EBPs seem to require some form of supervision to facilitate or ensure clinician proficiency in the EBP. This implies that supervisors are competent themselves in the EBP. It is unclear whether the supervisor of an EBP is required to receive training specifically in clinical supervision, and whether such training is separate from the EBP itself (i.e., training supervisors to provide training supervision). In multisystemic therapy (MST), it appears that supervisor training is specific to MST and that such training is provided by 'MST consultants' (see Henggeler, Schoenwald, Liao, Letourneau, & Edwards, 2002).

A second implication of EBP in the practice of supervision pertains to what may be the fracturing of supervision due to the possible splintering of clinical practice itself. To explain this we refer to the case of Leah, Laurie and Dr Bennett presented at the beginning of this chapter. If Leah will be supervised by both Laurie and Dr Bennett, how will the supervision she has received from both of them differ? If one will focus on her MST skills, what will the other supervision focus on — her overall professional skills, including clinical documentation, openness to supervision, collaboration and cooperation with colleagues? We wonder if Leah will be confused, not knowing who her 'actual' or 'ultimate' supervisor is and what she is expected to do. In addition, Laurie is an experienced clinician and is new to MST. By focusing specifically (and perhaps exclusively) on MST interventions, what effect this might have on her foundational skills, such as empathy. A concern might be that Laurie will be so focused on adhering to a specific skill set and protocol that certain pre-existing counsellor qualities (e.g., patience, positive regard) may suffer. This splintering may not be noticed or be of concern to Dr Bennett if his primary focus is on ensuring that Laurie demonstrates proficiency in MST skills. Laurie's ongoing and holistic professional development — including working through ethical dilemmas that may not be specific to MST — and personal growth may therefore get overlooked.

Yet a third implication of EBP supervision is that just as EBPs have demonstrated effectiveness or even efficacy in research trials, so too may the supervision of EBPs need to demonstrate effectiveness beyond supervisee satisfaction or even supervisee competence. Although client improvement has long been proposed as the intended and defining outcome of clinical supervision, linking client improvement to supervision has proven difficult, if not impossible. Supervisors of EBPs, however, increasingly need to supply evidence that their work with clinicians yields beneficial results for clients. This is apparent in Henggeler et al.'s (2002) investigation of MST supervision in which families (i.e., clients) measured therapist effectiveness, therapists who were supervised by MST supervisors according to the MST supervision manual.

The entrée of EBP into the lexicon of counselling and psychotherapy practice will have additional implications for the practice of clinical supervision. Not only will supervisors need to be conversant in, and perhaps proficient with, evidence-based *therapeutic* practices, they will need to demonstrate competence in supervision and practice according to certain evidence-based *supervisory* practices, practices that have not yet been established. Falender and Shafranske's (2007) discussion of competency-based supervision, however, may represent one effort toward determining such supervisory practices. One of their 12 recommendations for implementing competency-based supervision is that supervisors commit to supervision according to certain values, one of which is EBP (see p. 238). Furthermore, Milne (2007) offered a definition of supervision that he contends fulfils four criteria of empiricism (i.e., precise, specific, operational and supported by research or corroboration): 'The formal provision by senior/qualified health practitioners of an intensive relationship-based education and training that is case-focused and which supports, directs and guides the work of colleagues (supervisees)' (p. 438). These discussions in the literature, coupled with increased emphasis on EBP in counselling and psychotherapy, will continue to influence how supervision is practiced, and ethical issues are an integral part of this evolution.

Ethical Issues in the Supervision of Evidence-Based Practices

Our discussion thus far of supervision of evidence-based practices (EBPs) has only hinted at specific ethical issues. In this section we briefly discuss five ethical issues related to the supervision of EBP: (a) purpose of supervision, (b) managing multiple relationships and interpersonal dynamics, (c) format of supervision, (d) supervisor qualifications and competence and (e) evaluation. These do not exhaust the list of potential ethical issues but do serve to concentrate the discussion.

Purpose of Supervision

Treatment fidelity is an essential aspect of any EBP. In ongoing research investigations, ensuring treatment fidelity (or construct validity) allows researchers to state with a certain degree of confidence that what was tested was indeed the actual treatment. Studies conducted on the supervision of certain EBPs have demonstrated that supervision does increase a clinician's proficiency with the specific skill set associated with an EBP. For example, Smith et al. (2007) reported that following a 2-day training in the EBP of motivational interviewing (MI; Hettema, Steele, & Miller, 2005; Miller & Rollnick, 2002), clinicians who received individual supervision of five counselling sessions they conducted demonstrated an increase in MI-adherent behaviours (e.g., empathic reflections). Supervision in this study was conducted using a live and interactive teleconference format: MI supervisors wore a modified headset to allow them to hear the live counselling session and speak directly into an earpiece worn by the supervisee. During a mid-session break and at the conclusion of each counselling session, the supervisee and supervisor spoke directly to one another. Each clinician received a total of 7.5 hours of individual supervision and skill level was assessed at 20 weeks post-training and then 3 months later.

As already stated, it appears that a primary purpose of supervision of certain EBPs is to ensure clinician adherence to a specific EBP skill set. This focus could be viewed as *coercive* and also *exclusive*. By coercive we mean the practice of supervision that restricts supervisee and also supervisor innovation and creativity. Following a supervision manual may have this effect. Indeed, it seems somewhat ironic that EBPs could be accused of discouraging or even outright obstructing innovation when most, if not all, EBPs began as innovative practices themselves, approaches that challenged or at least offered alternatives to the accepted standards of care at the time.

The focus of supervision of EBPs also appears to be exclusively on supervisee skill performance, which resembles the practice of 'clinical monitoring' that participants in Rapisarda and Britton's (2007) study associated with sanctioned or remedial supervision. In their review of the supervision literature, Morgan and Sprenkle (2007) identified several dimensions of, or common factors in supervision, one being emphasis. They determined that the emphasis of supervision (primarily training supervision) appears to be on clinical competence (i.e., knowledge of and demonstrated skill in applying specific interventions, strategies) or professional competence (e.g., emotional management, personal growth, understanding and practice of ethical standards) or a combination of the two. They describe these emphases on a continuum, with clinical competence on one end and professional competence on the other. The purpose of supervision of EBPs is more than likely closer to the clinical competence endpoint than the professional competence endpoint. A concern with this exclusive focus is, as mentioned earlier, the potential oversight of a supervisee's professional development, such as his or her ability to work respectfully and constructively with other professionals. Any type of supervision should not only be concerned with how well the supervisee is able to apply techniques that are consistent with an EBP; supervision should also attend to and encourage supervisee personal growth.

Such a happy medium' may be the purpose of at least one EBP — dialectical behaviour therapy (DBT). As mentioned, supervision or consultation in DBT is not only intended to ensure that clients are receiving quality care but that counsellors are also being cared for (see Lynch et al., 2007). Weekly DBT consultation meetings often include practising self-care strategies (e.g., deep breathing, mindfulness exercises) and communication strategies (e.g., striving to be 'radically genuine' with other members of the team), the same strategies taught to and practised with clients in DBT. It could be said, therefore, that the purpose of DBT supervision is to achieve and maintain a balance of both clinical competence and professional competence. This balance itself seems to be consistent with dialectical philosophy and practice wherein a synthesis of acceptance and change is achieved. An ethical issue arises, however, when DBT supervision is more like therapy than consultation.

Managing Multiple Relationships and Interpersonal Dynamics

Managing multiple relationships is an ethical issue in any type of supervision and refers to the interactions between supervisor and supervisee, as well as relationships both parties have with others in the execution of counselling and supervision (e.g., clients, clinical director, other supervisees who are members of the same consultation team or supervision group). These professional relationships can be compromised and ethical concerns raised when personal interests become primary. An extreme example of this is when supervisors and supervisees engage in a sexual relationship with each other. Due to the inherently hierarchical nature of most types of supervision (specifically training, sanctioned, and targeted/skill-specific supervision), the ethical issue may be how the supervisor uses or exerts his or her power in interactions with the supervisee and reciprocally, how the supervisee responds to or operates within this power dynamic. Moreover, these interactions are influenced by the predominant or preferred power base from which the supervisor operates.

Power can be thought of as the potential and actual influence that a supervisor has on a supervisee. Robyak, Goodyear and Prange (1987) applied three types of power to supervision that Strong and Matross (1973) had originally applied to the therapeutic relationship. *Legitimate power* refers to the supervisor's sanctioned or designated position and the supervisee's perceived trustworthiness of the person in this role. Dr Bennett, the assigned multisystemic therapy (MST) supervisor mentioned earlier, may be thought to have legitimate power by virtue of his contract with Horizons, the facility that hired him for his expertise. *Referent power* derives from the supervisor's interpersonal style and the supervisee's attraction to, resonance with, or agreement with the supervisor's values, opinions, experiences or practices. Dr Bennett's referent power will depend on his personal qualities and how he facilitates his interactions with Laura and Leah, particularly in group supervision. The third type of power, *expert power*, would be based on Dr Bennett's advanced or specialised knowledge and skills in MST. Although Dr Bennett may be knowledgeable in MST, his success as an MST supervisor may be evaluated by Laura and Leah according to how well he is able to assist them in learning and applying MST to their clients; that is, his supervisory knowledge and skills.

Gottlieb, Robinson and Younggren (2007) reinforced the notion that multiple relationships are to be expected in supervision and should not be avoided unequivocally. This is true for Dr Bennett, Laura, and Leah. Dr Bennett is one of Leah's former professors and is now her assigned MST supervisor. Because Leah is a new clinician at Horizons, Laura has been assigned as her internal supervisor and has 12 years' more experience in mental health than Leah. Laura and Leah, however, attended the 5-day MST training together and are now members of the same MST treatment team and supervision group at Horizons. In this sense, they may be considered equals. Laura is new to MST and therefore is not able to supervise Leah's MST application. For these three to be able to work together effectively, and for client care not to be compromised, Dr Bennett and Laura may need to agree and collaborate on a distribution of power or, more precisely, how each will use power as a supervisor. It may be that Dr Bennett's power will be restricted to or prioritised as his MST expertise, whereas Laura's power will derive from her clinical mental health experience and her familiarity with Horizons and their clients. It appears that Dr Bennett's power will be time-limited (at least 6 months), whereas Laura's power as Leah's supervisor will extend beyond that time.

Format of Supervision
Henggeler et al. (2002) suggested that 'The effective transport of evidence-based models might require a major shift in current mental health supervisory and quality-assurance practices' (p. 165). This shift may include ongoing rather than time-limited supervision (consistent with DBT supervision), conducting group supervision as standard practice rather than individual supervision (consistent with MST and DBT supervision), and incorporating other means of interactions to typical face-to-face supervisory communication (e.g., live teleconference supervision; Smith et al., 2007).

The importance of ongoing supervision in learning a new skill set associated with an EBP has been suggested in studies of motivational interviewing (MI). Miller, Yahne, Moyers, Martinez and Pirritano (2004) found an increase in MI skill proficiency among clinicians who participated in up to six 30-minute individual telephone 'coaching sessions' following a 2-day MI training. Schoener, Madeja, Henderson, Ondersma and Janisse (2006) reported similar findings in their study of therapists who received approximately eight biweekly small group supervision sessions following a 2-day MI training. The results from these and other MI supervision studies (e.g., Smith et al., 2007) indicate that posttraining supervision in an EBP is a critical component for skill retention. Indeed, in Miller et al.'s study, clinicians who attended the 2-day workshop but did not receive supervision actually demonstrated *diminished* MI skill levels at 4, 8, and 12 months after the 2-day training, essentially erasing skills learned at the workshop.

The need for ongoing supervision of an EBP beyond initial training may be explained by Heaven et al.'s (2006) study of clinical nurse specialists in the United Kingdom. Although the nurses received training in communication skills and not an EBP, the results are consistent with those of MI supervision research. Specifically, nurses who received 12 hours of supervision over 4 weeks after a 3-day training improved their use of specific communication skills (i.e., open questions, negotiation, psychological exploration and response to cues) from baseline (preworkshop) to 1 month after supervision had concluded. When compared to nurses who did not receive supervision, however, there was no evidence of transfer of skills. Heaven et al. explained that some of the nurses were 'deeply embedded in a philosophy of care that was diametrically opposed to the model being taught' (pp. 322–323) and supervisors lacked time to challenge in a supportive fashion these 'entrenched defences' (p. 323). They speculated that 'a longer period of supervision would have [provided] an opportunity to challenge more entrenched longstanding beliefs' (p. 323).

Although ongoing supervision, and specifically group supervision, may be essential to attain proficiency in an EBP, ethical issues arise in coordinating services. For example, if MST supervision would continue beyond the first 6 months, would Dr Bennett remain the MST supervisor? How would the ongoing supervision he provided, then, differ from the supervision Laura would be providing to Leah? In addition, group supervision may offer counsellors additional support from fellow counsellors, but may not provide the individualised training necessary, particularly when certain counsellors struggle with mastering specific skills. Furthermore, confidentiality in group supervision requires more careful attention than in individual supervision, although the use of additional means of communication (e.g., telephone consultation, live teleconferencing) also extends the parameters of confidentiality.

Carter (2005) described the use of a technology-mediated managed learning environment for the supervision of student teachers enrolled in practicum in Australia. Digital cameras allowed the university-based supervisor to view and collect 'visual data of classroom events' (p. 487) but it is not clear how supervisory feedback was provided to the student teachers. Varied forms of technology clearly have the capacity to expand the nature of supervisory practice, particularly for the purpose of disseminating or transferring EBP from training room to therapy room. Clinicians with expertise in certain EBPs are able to provide supervision from a distance, thus augmenting or even replacing onsite supervision. Although technology affords innumerable possibilities for the supervision of EBP, ethical issues (e.g., confidentiality) must always be considered and evidence supporting technology-mediated distance supervision for supervisee skills enhancement and client wellbeing is still lacking.

Supervisor Qualifications and Competence

A fourth ethical issue in the supervision of EBPs pertains to supervisor competence. As discussed earlier, supervisors of EBPs such as MST, DBT, and MI need to have a certain level of proficiency as MST, DBT, or MI counsellors. However, skill level as a *supervisor* of an EBP remains unclear. What skills are necessary for a supervisor beyond those of counsellor proficiency in an EBP? Henggeler et al. (2002) described the MST *Supervisor Adherence Measure* (SAM), a means for therapists to assess MST supervisor skills on three factors: (a) the extent to which supervision emphasised the primary underpinnings of MST, (b) the extent to which the supervisor attempted to build the MST-related competencies of therapists and (c) the supervisor's knowledge and skill in MST and EBP intervention modalities. Their investigation of 12 MST supervisors who provided supervision to 74 MST therapists working with 285 youth and their families determined that only MST supervisors' knowledge of MST principles (one of the three factors of the SAM) predicted only two of three MST therapist skills: ability to collaborate with families and assess family progress. These findings raise questions about MST supervisor skills *as a supervisor*, and that simply being knowledgeable in MST principles does not make one an effective MST supervisor. It may be that supervision training and practice in only one model of supervision, and a model developed solely from a specific model of therapy, may actually restrict supervisory competencies and stifle further supervisor development.

Falender and Shafranske (2007) included the practice of self-assessment and a commitment to evidence-based practice among their 12 recommendations for implementing competency-based supervision. Determining supervisor competence, however, will remain problematic in the absence of empirical support.

Evaluation

Evaluation has been referred to as 'one of the key definitional features of clinical supervision' (Watkins, 1997, p. 611), which Bernard and Goodyear (2009) prioritised as 'the nucleus of clinical supervision' (p. 20). They listed 'evaluative' as the first of three characteristics of the supervisory relationship, and Holloway (1995) listed 'monitoring/evaluating' as the first of five functions of the supervisor. Evaluation is therefore considered an inherent feature of supervision and a function of the supervisor that cannot be avoided.

In the supervision of EBP, however, what is being evaluated and who gets to evaluate? Henggeler et al. (2002) described the *Therapist Adherence Measure* (TAM) specific to MST and designed to be completed by clients (i.e., family members with whom the MST therapist is working). It assesses three MST therapist skill areas: (a) ability to establish agreement with families on problems to address and collaborate with families to address these problems, (b) ability to change family interactions and (c) ability to follow-through on treatment progress. Supervisors could assess supervisee technical performance (i.e., ability to implement MST interventions) with each family unit the supervisee is responsible for, but such an evaluation is limited to clinical competence rather than professional competence, a distinction that Morgan and Sprenkle (2007) discussed. It also limited to client perspectives of therapist proficiency and thus does not include supervisor assessment. The exclusive reliance on the TAM may therefore not provide a complete picture of an MST therapist's competence as a mental health professional.

In the supervision of EBPs, we recommend that therapists be evaluated clinically as well as professionally. By this we mean that a supervisee's ability to adhere to a specific treatment protocol (i.e., perform specified technical skills) should only be part of the evaluation. A more comprehensive evaluation should also be considered, such as Fall and Sutton's (2004) 102-item *Supervisee Performance Assessment Instrument*. In addition to assessing supervisee intervention skills, this instrument evaluates supervisees on their conceptualisation skills, personalisation skills, professional behaviour and supervision skills. Supervisees would thereby benefit from more extensive feedback.

Ethics in Action: Developing and Maintaining Written Supervision Contracts

There are clearly ethical issues in any type of supervision conducted. The supervision of evidence-based practices (EBPs) has introduced new ethical issues to the practice of supervision or, more accurately, has generated additional and alternative perspectives about ethical practice not encountered in training supervision.

To maintain ethical practice in the supervision of EBPs, we recommend the use of a written supervision contract. Hewson (1999) described contracting in supervision as possibly 'the most important task engaged in by supervisor and supervisee' (p. 81) and Storm (1997) referred to the contract as the 'blueprint' for the supervision relationship. Falender and

Shafranske (2007) proposed that the development of a supervisory agreement or contract signifies competency-based supervision. Contracting for supervision also appears consistent with Gonsalvez, Oades and Freestone's (2002) objectives approach to supervision (i.e., formulating supervisor and supervisee objectives) and parallels the ethical standards (Codes 2.3.2. and 2.4.3.) of the Australian Counselling Association (2008) that counsellors contract with clients for counselling.

Establishing a written supervision contract is critical in any supervisory arrangement but is particularly necessary in the culture of accountability that EBPs represent. Specifically, a written supervision contract clarifies the services to be provided, the roles and responsibilities of all parties involved, the purpose and length of supervision and the supervisory procedures (e.g., frequency, format), including evaluation. Documenting, in writing, at the beginning of a supervisory arrangement these and other elements of supervision and then reviewing adherence to the contract at certain periods of time could be one measure of supervision effectiveness. Contracting for supervision can also be viewed as a quality assurance measure, thereby applying a value of EBPs to the practice of supervision. One way that the use of a contract may exemplify quality is in its function of opening up lines of communication. Nelson and Friedlander (2001) reported that most conflict occurs due to opposing expectations between supervisor and supervisee about what should take place in the supervision relationship (e.g., confusion over who was in charge, who would be evaluating). In light of this, Thomas (2007) suggested that the use of a written supervision contract could serve to curtail misunderstandings or at least lessen the extent or intensity of conflict between the supervisor and supervisee.

Although several examples of written supervision agreements exist (e.g., Haynes, Corey, & Moulton, 2003; Sutter, McPherson, & Geeseman, 2002), we are most familiar with and have routinely used the format we designed several years ago (Osborn & Davis, 1996). A current example can be found at http://chdsw.educ.kent.edu/supcontract and provides a template for a written agreement, beginning with the section that outlines the purpose, goals and objectives of supervision. The next section describes the context of supervision services and includes when and how often supervision will take place, as well as the method the supervisor will use to monitor the supervisee's performance (e.g., live supervision). The third section clarifies how the supervisee will be evaluated and refers to both formative and summative evaluations. We recommend that when the supervisor reviews the initial contract with supervisees in the first supervision session, each supervisee receives a copy of the actual evaluation form that the supervisor will use when conducting evaluations. In MST supervision, this may be the *Therapist Adherence Measure*. With Motivational

Interviewing, this may include the *Motivational Interviewing Treatment Integrity* (MITI 3.0) instrument (Moyers, Martin, Manuel, Miller, & Ernst, 2007) or the *Motivational Interviewing Skill Code* (MISC 2.1; Miller, Moyers, Ernst, & Amrhein, 2008). The remaining three sections of the written supervision contract are separate listings of the supervisor's and supervisee's duties and responsibilities (including some supervisee learning objectives), procedural considerations (e.g., emergency procedures and contact, record-keeping, process for addressing supervisor–supervisee disagreement), and the supervisor's competencies or scope of practice.

In the supervision of EBPs, a written supervision contract can serve to clarify the exact purpose and nature of supervision, the length and frequency of supervisory contact, the duties and responsibilities of the assigned supervisor and what is expected of the supervisee. In the case of Dr Bennett, Laura and Leah, a written supervision contract could delineate both Dr Bennett's and Laura's supervisory responsibilities. It could also explain when individual supervision would be indicated, what protocol to follow in crisis and other emergency situations, who at Horizons or Ignite would be consulted in the event of differences of opinion or outright conflict and any expectations of professional competence in addition to skill or technical proficiency. The method of determining supervisee skills and competence should be included in the contract (e.g., live observation, supervisee self-report, client report), as well as a description of the format of supervision (e.g., group, telephone contact). In the case of Dr Bennett, Laura and Leah, we would recommend that one written supervision contract be drafted that all three persons would contribute to and eventually sign off their approval. Rather than having separate contracts for each supervisory dyad, one contract for all three would help to foster cohesion and collaboration and would also be consistent with the standard group supervision format of MST.

We believe the development and incorporation of a written contract in clinical supervision promotes ethical practice. It can be considered a tangible example of ethical principles in action. From our own use of a contract with supervisees, we believe its intent is to embody the five ethical principles outlined in the Preamble of the American Psychological Association's (2002) *Ethical Principles of Psychologists and Code of Conduct*: beneficence and nonmaleficence, fidelity and responsibility (e.g., establishing relationships of trust), integrity (e.g., promoting accuracy and honesty), justice or fairness and respect for people's rights and dignity. The use of a contract may also signify the supervisor's commitment to competency-based supervision, as defined by Falender and Shafranske (2007).

Conclusion

Targeted and skill-specific supervision is a type of supervision rendered when counsellors are delivering an evidence-based practice (EBP). It is a relatively new type of supervision that has been a required component of clinical trials testing EBPs. Although its primary purpose is to ensure counsellor adherence or fidelity to the therapeutic approach, this type of supervision must also consider the professional competence of supervisees, especially if supervision is ongoing, as in dialectical behaviour therapy.

Ethical issues common in other types of supervision (e.g., training supervision) are also present in the supervision of EBPs. However, the nature, purpose and format of EBP supervision highlight certain ethical issues not encountered in other types of supervision. To promote ethical practice, we recommend the use of a written supervision contract, which serves as a quality assurance measure consistent with the culture of accountability associated with EBPs.

Educational Questions and Activities

Six questions/activities that could be pondered in a workshop or class session:

1. Many approaches that are recognised as evidence-based practices (EBPs) began as innovative approaches, practices that diverged from what were considered at one time to be 'standards of care'. The primary purpose of supervising a clinician in an EBP is to ensure the clinician adheres to the principles and (standard) practices of the EBP. Although regarded as 'quality control', how might this type of supervision be controlling and restrict or constrain clinician (and supervisory) innovation? How might such a practice run counter to the innovative origins of that EBP?

2. Four types of supervision are discussed in this chapter: (a) training supervision, (b) remedial supervision, (c) ongoing supervision and peer consultation and (d) targeted and skill-specific supervision.

   (a) Of these types, which one would you say carries with it (by virtue of its practice) the greatest number of ethical implications? That is, which supervision type inherently has the most ethical considerations for a supervisor to contend with or manage? What are these ethical issues? Provide an example of each issue based on your supervisory experience (as a supervisor or supervisee).

   (b) Of these four supervision types, which one would you say you are most suited for as a supervisor? Which one would you most prefer to provide? Explain your response.

3. Two evidence-based practices mentioned in this chapter conduct supervision in a group format as standard supervisory practice: multisystemic therapy (MST) and dialectical behaviour therapy (DBT). Compared to individual supervision, what would you consider to be the benefits of conducting supervision in a group format and what might be the shortcomings?

(a) How might group supervision/peer consultation be a practice consistent with the principles and practices of these two EBPs? If individual supervision were to be added to MST and DBT as standard practice, what would be the benefit?

(b) Which of these two formats (group or individual supervision) might be more amenable to addressing and resolving ethical issues that arise in clinical practice?

4. Consider Morgan and Sprenkle's (2007) contention that an emphasis of supervision is on clinical competence or professional competence or a combination. How might supervision of a clinician implementing an evidence-based practice focus on the supervisee's clinical competence and professional competence? How would you propose providing both targeted/skill-specific supervision (for the purpose of achieving clinical competence) and holistic/ongoing supervision (for the purpose of achieving professional competence)? Describe how you would attempt to conduct supervision as a combination or synthesis of these two foci. What do you believe would constitute the minimal skill level in the clinical domain that you are supervising?

5. Five ethical issues related to the supervision of evidence-based practice are discussed: (a) purpose of supervision, (b) managing multiple relationships and interpersonal dynamics, (c) format of supervision, (d) supervisor qualifications and competence and (e) evaluation. Which issue has more prominence or significance in your experience as a supervisee or practice as a supervisor? Which ones are you most challenged by? Explain.

6. As part of a group exercise, solicit or identify three persons from a larger group gathering (e.g., classroom or workshop) who are willing to assume the role of Leah, Laura and Dr Bennett, the three persons described in the case. After reviewing the case, have the three of these persons sit at the front of the room or in the middle of the larger group gathering (a 'fishbowl' exercise) and allow each person in this supervisory triad to describe his or her role, as well as his or her experience as a member of this supervisory triad (about 5 minutes each). Allow them to describe their role and experiences without interruption (e.g., 'As Leah, I'm the one brand new to Horizons and so Laura and I have only

recently met'). Now select one of the five ethical issues presented and, in the context of the case described, invite Leah, Laura and Dr Bennett to discuss as a group how they would address this issue in their work together (allow about 20 minutes). Once their discussion with one another has concluded, invite persons in the larger gathering to comment on the ethical issue described and how it might be resolved, asking each of the three members of the supervisory triad to respond.

Selected Internet Resources

- Australian Counselling Association. (2008). *Code of conduct.* Retrieved January 22, 2008, from http://www.theaca.net.au
  Addresses current standards of practice in the counselling profession within Australia.

- *Association for Counselor Education and Supervision* (2008). Retrieved November 11, 2008, from http://www.acesonline.net/
  The flagship organisation in the United States addresses best practices in the specialisation of counselling and clinical supervision practices.

- Sexton, T.L. (2008). *ERIC Educational Reports, Evidence-Based Counseling: Implications for Counseling Practice, Preparation, and Professionalism.* Retrieved November 11, 2008, from http://findarticles.com/p/articles/mi_pric/is_199900/ai_2465534000
  Dr Sexton, a prolific scholar in the area of Evidence-Based Counselling Practices, offers a sound template for clinicians to follow in their efforts to conduct ethical services following evidence-based interventions.

- Fogel, J. (2008). *MedScape Today, Evidence-Based Psychotherapy Outcomes Assessment.* Retrieved November 11, 2008, from http://www.medscape.com/viewarticle/471654
  Dr Fogel addresses current outcome assessment modalities important to evidence-based psychotherapy.

References

American Psychological Association. (2002). *Ethical principles of psychologists and code of conduct.* Washington, DC: Author.

APA Presidential Task Force on Evidence-Based Practice. (2006). Evidence-based practice in psychology. *American Psychologist, 61,* 271–285.

Australian Counselling Association. (2008). *Code of conduct.* Brisbane, Australia: Author. Retrieved January 22, 2009, from http://www.theaca.net.au

Australian Counselling Association. (2009). *Professional supervision.* Brisbane, Australia: Author. Retrieved January 22, 2009, from http://www.theaca.net.au

Bernard, J.M., & Goodyear, R.K. (2009). *Fundamentals of clinical supervision* (4th ed.). Upper Saddle River, NJ: Pearson Education.

Binder, J.L., & Strupp, H.H. (1997). Supervision of psychodynamic psychotherapies. In C.E. Watkins (Ed.), *Handbook of psychotherapy supervision* (pp. 44–62). New York: John Wiley.

Bohart, A.C. (2005). Evidence-based psychotherapy means evidence-informed, not evidence-driven. *Journal of Contemporary Psychotherapy, 35,* 39–53.

Borders, L.D. (1991). A systematic approach to peer group supervision. *Journal of Counseling & Development, 69,* 248–252.

British Association for Counselling and Psychotherapy. (2007). *Ethical framework for good practice in counselling and psychotherapy.* Leicestershire, England: Author. Retrieved August 30, 2008, from http://www.bacp.co.uk

Carter, D. (2005). Distributed practicum supervision in a managed learning environment (MLE). *Teachers and Teaching: Theory and Practice, 11,* 481–497.

Cobia, D.C., & Pipes, R.B. (2002). Mandated supervision: An intervention for disciplined professionals. *Journal of Counseling & Development, 80,* 140–144.

Cormier, S., Nurius, P.S., & Osborn, C.J. (2009). *Interviewing and change strategies for helpers: Fundamental skills and cognitive behavioural interventions* (6th ed.). Belmont, CA: Brooks/Cole-Cengage.

Falender, C.A., & Shafranske, E.P. (2007). Competence in competency-based supervision practice: Construct and application. *Professional Psychology: Research and Practice, 38,* 232–240.

Fall, M., & Sutton, Jr., J.M. (2004). *Clinical supervision: A handbook for practitioners.* Boston: Pearson Education.

Fruzzetti, A.E., Waltz, J.A., & Linehan, M.M. (1997). Supervision in dialectical behavior therapy. In C.E. Watkins, Jr. (Ed.), *Handbook of psychotherapy supervision* (pp. 84–100). New York: Wiley.

Gambrill, E., & Gibbs, L. (2002). Making practice decisions: Is what's good for the goose good for the gander? *Ethical Human Sciences and Services, 4,* 31–46.

Gonsalvez, C.J., Oades, L.G., & Freestone, J. (2002). The objectives approach to clinical supervision: Towards integration and empirical evaluation. *Australian Psychologist, 37,* 68–77.

Gottlieb, M.C., Robinson, K., & Younggren, J.N. (2007). Multiple relations in supervision: Guidance for administrators, supervisors, and students. *Professional Psychology: Research and Practice, 38,* 241–247.

Gould, L.J., & Bradley, L.J. (2001). Evaluation in supervision. In L.J. Bradley & N. Ladany (Eds.), *Counselor supervision: Principles, process, and practice* (pp. 271–303). Philadelphia, PA: Brunner-Routledge/Taylor & Francis.

Granello, D.H., Kindsvatter, A., Granello, P.F., Underfer-Babalis, J., & Hartwig Moorhead, H.J. (2008). Multiple perspectives in supervision: Using a peer consultation model to enhance supervisor development. *Counselor Education and Supervision, 48,* 32–47.

Haynes, R., Corey, G., & Moulton, P. (2003). *Clinical supervision in the helping professions: A practical guide.* Pacific Grove, CA: Brooks/Cole-Thomson Learning.

Heaven, C., Clegg, J., & Maguire, P. (2006). Transfer of communication skills training from workshop to workplace: The impact of clinical supervision. *Patient Education and Counseling, 60,* 313–325.

Henggeler, S.W., & Borduin, C.M. (1990). *Family therapy and beyond: A multisystemic approach to treating the behavior problems of children and adolescents.* Pacific Grove, CA: Brooks/Cole.

Henggeler, S.W., & Schoenwald, S.K. (1998). *Multisystemic therapy supervisory manual: Promoting quality assurance at the clinical level.* Charleston, SC: MST Institute.

Henggeler, S.W., Schoenwald, S.K., Liao, J.G., Letourneau, E.J., & Edwards, D.L. (2002). Transporting efficacious treatments to field settings: The link between supervisory practices and therapist fidelity in MST programs. *Journal of Clinical Child Psychology, 31,* 155–167.

Hettema, J., Steele, J., & Miller, W.R. (2005). Motivational interviewing. *Annual Review of Clinical Psychology, 1,* 91–111.

Hewson, J. (1999). Training supervisors to contract in supervision. In E. Holloway & M. Carroll (Eds.), *Training counselling supervisors: Strategies, methods and techniques* (pp. 67–91). London: SAGE.

Holloway, E. (1995). *Clinical supervision: A systems approach.* Thousand Oaks, CA: Sage.

Ladany, N., Ellis, M.V., & Friedlander, M.L. (1999). The supervisory working alliance, trainee self-efficacy, and satisfaction. *Journal of Counseling & Development, 77,* 447–455.

Linehan, M.M. (1993). *Cognitive–behavioral treatment of borderline personality disorder.* New York: Guilford.

Linehan, M.M., Comtois, K.A., Murray, A.M., Brown, M.Z., Gallop, R.J., Heard, H.L., et al. (2006). Two-year randomized controlled trial and follow-up of dialectical behavior therapy vs. therapy by experts for suicidal behaviors and borderline personality disorder. *Archives of General Psychiatry, 63,* 757–766.

Lynch, T.R., Trost, W.T., Salsman, N., & Linehan, M.M. (2007). Dialectical behavior therapy for borderline personality disorder. *Annual Review of Clinical Psychology, 3,* 181–205.

McAuliffe, D., & Sudbery, J. (2005). Who do I tell? Support and consultation in cases of ethical conflict. *Journal of Social Work, 5,* 21–43.

Miller, W.R., Moyers, T.B., Ernst, D., & Amrhein, P. (2008). *Manual for the motivational interviewing skill code (MISC,* Version 2.1). Retrieved September 5, 2008, from http://casaa.unm.edu/download/misc.pdf

Miller, W.R., & Rollnick, S. (2002). *Motivational interviewing: Preparing people for change* (2nd ed.). New York: Guilford.

Miller, W.R., Yahne, C.E., Moyers, T.B., Martinez, J., & Pirritano, M. (2004). A randomized trial of methods to help clinicians learn motivational interviewing. *Journal of Consulting and Clinical Psychology, 72,* 1050–1062.

Milne, D. (2007). An empirical definition of clinical supervision. *British Journal of Clinical Psychology, 46,* 437–447.

Morgan, M.M., & Sprenkle, D.H. (2007). Toward a common-factors approach to supervision. *Journal of Marital and Family Therapy, 33,* 1–17.

Moyers, T.B., Martin, T., Manuel, J.K., Miller, W.R., & Ernst, D. (2007). *Revised Global Scales: Motivational Interviewing Treatment Integrity* (MITI), 3.0. Retrieved September 5, 2008, from http://casaa.unm.edu/download/miti3.pdf

Nelson, M.L., Barnes, K.L., Evans, A.L., & Triggiano, P.J. (2008). Working with conflict in clinical supervision: Wise supervisors' perspectives. *Journal of Counseling Psychology, 55,* 172–184.

Nelson, M.L., & Friedlander, M.L. (2001). A close look at conflictual supervisory relationships: The trainee's perspectives. *Journal of Counseling Psychology, 48,* 384–395.

Norrie, J., Eggleston, E., & Ringer, M. (2003). Quality parameters of supervision in a correctional context. *New Zealand Journal of Psychology, 32,* 76–83.

Osborn, C.J., & Davis, T.E. (1996). The supervision contract: Making it perfectly clear. *The Clinical Supervisor, 14*(2), 121–134.

Pretorius, W.M. (2006). Cognitive behavioural therapy supervision: Recommended practice. *Behavioural and Cognitive Psychotherapy, 34,* 413–420.

Psychotherapy and Counselling Federation of Australia (PACFA, 2009). *Renewal requirements for the PACFA register.* Melbourne, Australia: Author. Retrieved May 20, 2009, from http://www.pacfa.org.au/nationalregister/cid/5/parent/0/t/nationalregister/l/layout

Rapisarda, C.A., & Britton, P.J. (2007). Sanctioned supervision: Voices from the experts. *Journal of Mental Health Counseling, 29,* 81–92.

Reamer, F.G. (2006). Nontraditional and unorthodox interventions in social work: Ethical and legal implications. *Families in Society, 87,* 191–197.

Robyak, J.E., Goodyear, R.K., & Prange, M. (1987). Effects of supervisors' sex, focus, and experience on preferences for interpersonal power bases. *Counselor Education and Supervision, 26,* 299–309.

Schoener, E.P., Madeja, C.L., Henderson, M.J., Ondersma, S.J., & Janisse, J.J. (2006). Effects of motivational interviewing training on mental health therapist behavior. *Drug and Alcohol Dependence, 82,* 269–275.

Smith, J.L., Amrhein, P.C., Brooks, A.C., Carpenter, K.M., Levin, D., Schreiber, E.A., et al. (2007). Providing live supervision via teleconferencing improves acquisition of motivational interviewing skills after workshop attendance. *American Journal of Drug and Alcohol Abuse, 33,* 163–168.

Storm, C.L. (1997). The blueprint for supervision relationships: Contracts. In T.C. Todd & C.L. Storm (Eds.), *The complete systemic supervisor: Context, philosophy, and pragmatics* (pp. 272–282). Boston: Allyn and Bacon.

Strong, S.R., & Matross, R.P. (1973). Change processes in counseling and psychotherapy. *Journal of Counseling Psychology, 20,* 25–37.

Sutter, E., McPherson, R.H., & Geeseman, R. (2002). Contracting for supervision. *Professional Psychology: Research and Practice, 33,* 495–498.

Thomas, J.T. (2007). Informed consent through contracting for supervision: Minimizing risks, enhancing benefits. *Professional Psychology: Research and Practice, 38,* 221–231.

Watkins, C.E. (1997). Some concluding thoughts about psychotherapy supervision. In C.E. Watkins (Ed.), *Handbook of psychotherapy supervision* (pp. 603–616). New York: John Wiley.

chapter five

Recent Supervision Scholarship

Nadine Pelling

Clinical Supervision: An Applied Activity and Research Focus

Clinical supervision is generally an applied area of psychology, counselling, social work and nursing. Supervisors use skills to provide feedback
and help support and develop novice practitioners in a manner that
increases their competence when working with clients. Indeed, the majority of this textbook outlines the ethics, methods, models and interventions
one can use in applied supervisory interactions. However, there is another
aspect to clinical supervision that is less often reviewed. This aspect
involves research.

The typical model of training used in psychology in many countries,
and other related areas, is that of the scientist–practitioner (Pelling, 2004).
According to this model clinicians are expected to be both competent
basic researchers as well as practitioners so that when in practice clinicians
can apply the latest scholarly knowledge to their work to benefit clients, as
well as work in a self-reflective manner, continuously examining their
actions and their results with clients.

Unfortunately, as many have noted, there is a divide between scientists
and clinicians and among researchers between qualitative and quantitative
methodologies (Pelling, 2000). Many clinicians are not actively engaged
in the production or ingestion of research. Indeed, clinicians have been
known to remark that published research tends to not apply to their work
and, in essence, gives them metaphoric indigestion.

What is the current state of supervision scholarship? What is being
published in articles on supervision, from where is the scholarship originating and what methods are being used in supervision scholarship? To
answer these questions a series of short literature searches were conducted.

It was hoped that the literature searches would provide a glimpse of the current supervision scholarship. Please note that the following is not meant to be and is not an annotated bibliography on the scholarship in supervision, but instead a brief content analysis of the scholarship on supervision produced by two brief literature searches.

Method

Two brief literature searches were conducted in order to examine the current state of supervision scholarship. First, a search was conducted in May 2008 covering all published articles (not books or book chapters or book reviews) from the start of 2000 onwards. Second, in October 2008 another search from January 2008 onwards was conducted. Key search words included supervision, clinical or counselling/counseling. All searches were computer-based and used standard databases in the counselling and psychological fields including ERIC, PsychLit, and PsychInfo.

Relevant publications were then printed on paper and the abstracts and/or articles collected electronically were examined for country of origin of author, basic methodology employed or if the paper was a review/editorial, and general supervision research subtopic including psychology, counselling and medicine.

Results

Article publications were found in a diversity of journals. For instance, *Professional Psychology: Research & Practice, Computers in Human Behavior* and *Australian Psychiatry* were all represented. Additionally, solo, joint and teams of authors consisting of eight or more authors contributed to the groups of published manuscripts obtained in the conducted searches. While a few publications originated from Scandinavia, as well as Israel and elsewhere, these are not represented on the following tables for simplicity as the majority of publications came from Australia, New Zealand, Hong Kong, the United States , Canada, and the United Kingdom.

Table 5.1 shows scholarship type and general topic by country published since January 2000 to May 2008. Table 5.2 shows the scholarship type and general topic by country published since January 2008 to October 2008.

It is clear from both these tables that, for the last 8 years and recently over the last 10 months, discussion or review papers are the most popular type of scholarship in clinical supervision (39% and 49% respectively). Generally, such publications include models for the use of supervision or the outlining of various topics in supervision. For instance, Aten, Strain and Gillespie (2008) outline the transtheoretical model of supervision in their recently published journal article. Quantitative research articles were

TABLE 5.1

Clinical Supervision Scholarship Type and General Topic by Country Published Since January 2000 to May 2008

		Country						
		Australia	NZ	Hong Kong	US	Canada	UK	Total
Scholarship type	Quantitative	5	1	2	1		2	11
	Qualitative	1	1		2	1		5
	Discussion or review paper	2	4	1	8		2	17
	Unable to determine from abstract	3	1	5	1			10
	Total	11	7	8	12	1	4	43
Scholarship topic	Psychology	1		3	9		3	16
	Counselling	5	4	4	2		1	16
	Medical (psychiatry, nursing, medical practitioner training)	5	3	1				10
	Other (psychotherapy, group, school psychology, music therapy)				1	1		2
	Totals	11	7	8	12	1	4	44

Note: Categories are not necessarily mutually exclusive (i.e., some mixed method research exists and is counted in both quantitative and qualitative sections).

also popular accounting for 25% and 31% of the literature reviewed, respectively. Examples of this type of published research included Riva and Erickson Cornish's (2008) examination of group supervision practices as psychology predoctoral internship programs.

In the two time periods reviewed the majority of articles on supervision were published via authors based in Australia and the United States; Australian-based authors accounting for 25% and 10% of the supervision articles in the two time periods and 27% and 76% of authors were based in the United States during the two time periods. The publications included Gonsalvez and McLeod's (2008) article on a science-informed practice of clinical supervision in the Australian context and an article on the perspectives of wise supervisors when working with conflict in clinical supervision from a Wisconsin group of authors (Nelson, Barnes, Evans, & Triggiano, 2008).

For both literature search time periods, psychology and counselling literature dominated with 36% and 29% of the literature relating to psychology and 37% and 31% relating to counselling. Other areas of supervision were also included such as nursing supervision and music therapy supervision but to a lesser extent.

TABLE 5.2

Clinical Supervision Scholarship Type and General Topic by Country Published Since January 2008 to October 2008

		Country						
		Australia	NZ	Hong Kong	US	Canada	UK	Total
Scholarship type	Quantitative	2			18		2	22
	Qualitative		1		11	1	1	14
	Discussion or review paper	5		1	26		3	35
	Unable to determine from abstract							
	Total	7	1	1	55	1	6	71
Scholarship topic	Psychology	7			11	1	1	20
	Counselling		1		18		3	22
	Medical (psychiatry, nursing, medical practitioner training)			1	7		2	10
	Other (psychotherapy, group, school psychology, music therapy)				17			17
	Totals	7	1	1	53	1	6	69

Note: Categories are not necessarily mutually exclusive (i.e., some mixed method research exists and is counted in both quantitative and qualitative sections).

Discussion

It is no surprise that a largely applied area such as clinical supervision would engender a large amount of scholarship that is applied (model based/review material) in nature versus research-based scholarship. However, if supervisory practices are to be grounded in research more quantitative, qualitative and mixed model research versus commentary is in order. Similarly, more quantitative versus qualitative or case studies of supervision were published. It is possible that the supervisory arena could benefit from an increase in a diversity of methodology that may be more relevant to practitioners (i.e., qualitative and case study presentations).

It was also not a revelation that the majority of publications were based on research conducted in the United States, given the large population of that country and high number of active researchers. Nevertheless, the large number of publications from Australia was unexpected. The fact that the *Australian Psychologist* published a special section on clinical supervision in 2008 (Gonsalvez, 2008) may in part explain this finding.

Given that the databases searched were generally within areas of psychology, education and counselling it is not surprising that counselling and psychology were highly represented topics relating to clinical supervision. As a result, it is possible that if medical or legal databases were specifically searched then different results regarding applied/clinical supervision would result.

This brief overview of recent supervision scholarship has its limits in that it is simply meant as a concise overview, a snapshot in time that is likely to change as academic knowledge and training continues to move forward. Additionally, electronic database searches do have their limits. First, there are some delays as to when certain articles are published and then available on the databases. Second, not all journals are indexed by all databases. For instance, a recent quantitative examination of supervisory development undertaken by the current author is not yet available in some databases because of the time-lag between publishing and indexing (Pelling, 2008).

Concluding Statement

A few general points can be recommended based on this recent supervision scholarship snapshot. First, more research and less editorialising needs to occur and research should include quantitative and qualitative methodologies, and case studies. Second, for collaborative efforts American and Australian researchers should seek out those in countries where little supervision research is being conducted. It would be great to see some additional cross-cultural/international research on clinical supervision being published that can help broaden the researchers' and readers' perspectives. Similar collaborations could be made with those in non-psychology or counselling-related fields involved with supervision, such as medicine and nursing. Finally, we must remember that as scientist–practitioners we not only supervise applied work via clinical supervision but also produce research via research supervision. The research supervision field appears wide open to many research possibilities relating to the relationship, process and productivity variables.

Educational Questions and Activities

1. What is the typical model used in psychology training?
   (a) scientist–practitioner.
2. Why do some believe that clinicians should also be competent basic researchers?
   (a) so that the latest scholarly knowledge can influence applied work and so that clinicians can work in a self-reflective manner with clients.
3. What divide has historically existed among researchers?
   (a) methodology, that is, quantitative versus qualitative methods.

4. What is the most popular type of scholarship in clinical supervision?
   (a) discussion or review papers, including the presentation of models for use in supervision.

5. What country accounts for most of the publications found in the searches conducted?
   (a) the United States.

6. What does the author recommend regarding supervision scholarship?
   (a) that more research and less editorialising be published.
   (b) that research supervision is a wide open area for exploration.
   (c) that collaboration across countries and professional groups relating to supervision occur.

Selected Internet Resources

- Association for Counselor Education and Counseling Supervision. (2006). *Counselor Education and Supervision.* Retrieved June 5, 2009, from http://chdsw.educ.kent.edu/ces/
- Association for Counselor Education and Counseling Supervision. (2006). *News and information.* Retrieved June 5, 2009, from http://www.acesonline.net/

Selected Reference for Further Reading

Falender, C.A., & Shafranske, E.P. (2008). *Casebook for clinical supervision: A competency-based approach.* Washington, DC: American Psychological Association.

References

Aten, J., Strain, J., & Gillespie, R. (2008). A transtheoretical model of clinical supervision. *Training and Education in Professional Psychology, 2*(1), 1–9.

Gonsalvez, C. (2008). Introduction to the special section on clinical supervision. *Australian Psychologist, 42*(2), 76–78.

Gonsalvez, C., & McLeod, H. (2008). Toward the science-informed practice of clinical supervision: The Australian context. *Australian Psychologist, 43*(2), 79–87.

Nelson, M., Barnes, K., Evans, A., & Triggiano, P. (2008). Working with conflict in clinical supervision: Wise supervisors' perspectives. *Journal of Counseling Psychology, 55*(2), 172–184.

Pelling, N. (2000). Scientists versus practitioners: A growing dichotomy in need of integration. *Counselling Psychology Review, 15*(4), 3–7.

Pelling, N. (2004). Counselling psychology: Diversity and commonalities across the western world. *Counselling Psychology Quarterly, 17*(3), 239–245.

Pelling, N. (2008). The relationship of supervisory experience, counseling experience, and training in supervision to supervisory identity development. *International Journal for the Advancement of Counselling, 30*(4), 235–248.

Riva, M., & Erickson Cornish, J. (2008). Group supervision practices at psychology predoctoral internship programs: 15 years later. *Training and Education in Professional Psychology, 2*(1), 18–25.

Approaches

The 'Approaches' section, comprised of four chapters, will enable both trainees and supervisors to re-examine the important role of the working alliance in facilitating change through supervisory encounters, while furthermore exploring the major models and processes used to enhance learning. Chapter 6 addresses psychodynamic, cognitive–behavioural and developmental models for supervision and then examines case studies to feature the practical components of the theories. Chapter 7 offers an alternate nonapproach-bound way to supervise, which has evidence for enhancing clinical outcomes in brief interventions. A model is provided that respects the interpersonal process of therapy as a critical construct through which all interventions could be offered. Chapter 8 reviews findings from a range of studies that suggest supervision is a very powerful process with the potential for both enhancing and inhibiting the growth of supervisees. In this light, it gives remarkable attention to the processes and interventions that can be used to support the learning of supervisees. Chapter 9 introduces supervisees' worst imagined client case scenarios and then systematically explores these fears regarding client work so that we can experience the reality of others having similar fears which has an anxiety reducing impact.

Chapter Overview

CHAPTER 6

'Models of Supervision: From Theory to Practice' by Bert Biggs, Matt Bambling and Zoe Pearce heralds an impressive style of writing that clearly and methodically presents each of the major models of supervision, and associated components, and then follows up each with interesting practical examples that elucidate the concepts. The chapter is one the reader will review several times because of the concentration of terms and notions, but will be thankful to do so as it will significantly enhance both clinical interventions and the process of supervision. The enumerated 'secrets that supervisors and trainees keep from each other' is a list that will easily stimulate quality dialogue in supervision, and aid enormously in the development of ultimately collegial relationships with supervisees.

Chapter Themes

In this chapter you will explore the following themes:

• the psychodynamic model of supervision
• the behavioural and cognitive models of supervision
• the developmental model of supervision.

CHAPTER 7

'Alliance Supervision to Enhance Client Outcomes' by Matt Bambling provides a very interesting and timely model for supervision that addresses brief therapy, clinical outcomes, empirically research and non-approach bound concepts; all themes that have experienced popular backing in recent decades. Bambling's innovative model is explained in some detail, and has a significant orientation toward examining and developing the interpersonal and alliance related factors in supervision. This writing stands as one of the few research-focused chapters in the text, hence is not only a welcome addition but an opportune reminder of the scientist–practitioner model clinicians adopt as they work. As with other chapters, the case examples are additive to the reader's understanding of concepts and processes that are also well explicated.

Chapter Themes

In this chapter you will explore the following themes:

- why focus on alliance?
- three-stage alliance supervision
- stage 1 of TSAS: Early engagement
- case example: State one of TSAS, negotiating task, bond and goal to maximise early engagement
- TSAS focused supervision insights
- stage 2 of TSAS: Developmental features of alliance
- case example: A type one alliance issue
- TSAS supervision insights
- integrating stages 1 and 2 of TSAS
- case example, type two alliance; integrating bond, task and goal into type-based alliance thinking; a context for intervention
- TSAS supervision insights
- stage 3 of TSAS: Rupture management
- stage 3 of TSAS: Rupture management and integrating stages 1 and 2
- TSAS supervision insights.

CHAPTER 8

'Processes and Interventions to Facilitate Supervisees' Learning' by Keithia Wilson and Alf Lizzio comprehensively addresses one of the most basic yet significant questions asked of supervision, that is, 'How does it impact learning?' This chapter identifies that if we are clear about what we ultimately want from the process, and we know how best we learn, as well being cognisant of the power of reflective practice, there is a greater likelihood of the supervisory experience being powerful and positive for all involved. Central to the development of this writing is the focus on the supervisory relationship as a critical variable that impacts supervisee growth and development. Wilson and Lizzio's chapter is replete with many challenging questions and numerous helpful suggestions that will enable the reader to systematically grasp, in due course, the more effective ways of facilitating learning in meaningful ways.

Chapter Themes

In this chapter you will explore the following themes:

- establishing an effective working alliance
- what learning goals shall we pursue?
- what approach to learning suits our circumstances?
- what type of relationship do we wish to have?
- what management processes do we wish to establish?
- supervisor reflection
- supervisee reflection
- initial contracting
- ongoing review
- supervisory meta-competencies
- processes for constructive feedback
- forms of participation and voice
- facilitating reflective practice
- specific supervisory methodologies
- case studies
- observation
- role play
- a contextual model for role play.

CHAPTER 9

'Addressing Supervisee Fears in Supervision' by Nadine Pelling is a short chapter but one the reader will readily related to and benefit from. All clinicians have some fear as they conduct their professional role. Here the worst case scenario idea is explored with the most frequently raised issues, and thankfully some ways of responding are also included, as the reader is simultaneously reassured and validated.

Chapter Themes

In this chapter you will explore the following themes:

- 'Tell me your fears'
- worst client case scenario categories
- harm to client/client in great pain
- difficult clients
- danger to therapist
- ethical responsibilities
- questioning therapist competence
- general activities for increasing knowledge, self/other awareness, and skill.

chapter six

Models of Supervision: From Theory to Practice

Herbert Biggs, Matthew Bambling and Zoe Pearce

This chapter will address psychodynamic, cognitive–behavioural and developmental models in supervision by initially considering the historical underpinnings of each and then examining in turn some of the key processes that are evident in the supervisory relationships. Case studies are included where appropriate to highlight the application of theory to practice and several processes are fully elaborated over all models to enable a contemporary view of style and substance in the supervision context.

The Psychodynamic Model of Supervision

Psychodynamic supervision is grounded in Freud's psychoanalytic theory.[1] As such, many of the processes and relationships that are addressed in psychoanalytic psychotherapy are also present in the psychodynamic supervisory relationship. This section will first consider the historical underpinnings of psychodynamic supervision and some of the key processes that are prevalent in the psychodynamic supervisory relationship. The extent to which the supervisory relationship can be considered similar to the therapeutic relationship has been the focus of substantial debate and will therefore also be briefly discussed.

Historical Background

Historically, psychodynamic supervision owes its beginnings to Freud's psychoanalytic model of psychotherapy. Indeed, Freud is often labelled as the first psychotherapeutic supervisor (Bernard & Goodyear, 2004) with informal supervision sessions designed to educate analysts and discuss each other's work. Riess and Herman (2008) describe this as the 'master–

apprentice' model of supervision, and one can imagine Freud firmly positioned as the master, holding court to a gathering of inspired apprentices.

By the 1920s, formal training standards were introduced by the International Psychoanalytic Society. The standard set required analysts to participate in their own personal analysis and to participate in supervision, referred to as 'control analysis' (Ekstein & Wallerstein, 1976). In this approach, the supervising analyst was responsible for performing both the role of supervisor and personal analyst for the trainee psychoanalyst. Not surprisingly, it was not long before some psychoanalysts began to question the wisdom of having these dual roles in place. By the 1930s the substantial debate that surrounded this issue resulted in a professional division. The Budapest School continued with the practice of using supervision as both an instructional tool and a means for personal analysis, whereas the Institute in Vienna argued that both roles could not be fulfilled by the one person and mandated psychoanalysts seek personal analysis as separate from the supervisory relationship (Bernard & Goodyear, 2004). The Hungarian argument promoted supervision as an extension or continuation of personal analysis, where supervision would address both transference from therapy and countertransference from supervision. On the other hand, the German approach argued the two should remain separate because supervision was designed to teach and the analyst's personal problems and issues needed to be raised in a different forum, during personal analysis. Therefore, psychodynamic supervision can be thought of as providing the historical foundation for the classic controversy that is still apparent today (Carroll, 2007): how do you distinguish between therapy and supervision?

Psychodynamic Supervision Processes

Andersson (2008) suggests the key element of psychodynamic supervision is to explore the supervisee's conscious and unconscious reactions to clients and the process of therapy. Many of the processes that are drawn upon in a psychodynamic supervision session will seem familiar to therapists from a number of orientations, as they are concepts that have been adopted quite widely. Terms such as 'alliance', 'parallel processes' and 'transference' have all derived from early psychoanalytic theory. A few of the key psychodynamic processes often utilised and reflected upon in supervision will be discussed.

Working Alliance

With early links to psychoanalytic theory (e.g., Greenson, 1967; Sterba, 1934), the supervisory working alliance closely mirrors that of the client–therapist therapeutic alliance. Now widely considered to be pantheoretical, and conceptualised best by Bordin (1983), the supervisory working alliance is

> ... that sector of the overall relationship between the participants in which supervisors act purposefully to influence trainees through their use of technical knowledge and skill and in which trainees act willingly to display their acquisition of that knowledge and skill. (Efstation, Patton, & Kardash, 1990, p. 323)

The working alliance is a collaborative relationship where the personal and interpersonal qualities of both the supervisee and supervisor are used to formulate a relationship based around trust and security, not unlike Bowlby's (1973/1998) attachment paradigm.

Progressing towards a successful working alliance involves addressing three aspects of supervision: the supervision bond, mutually understood goals of supervision and agreed tasks of supervision (Bordin, 1983). The supervision bond develops as the relationship grows with trust, caring, empathy and liking increasing over time. Goals of supervision often include the acquisition of technical skills and knowledge, improved understanding of self and others, developing comfort with process issues in therapy and overcoming obstacles that may impact on a therapist's progress with a client. The tasks of supervision will be the actions agreed upon by supervisor and supervisee that assist with achieving the supervision goals. When these three components are strong and mutually satisfying, an effective working alliance is in place.

Substantial research has investigated the predictors and outcomes of a successful working alliance (see Bernard & Goodyear, 2004 for a comprehensive review). Self-disclosure in supervisees is greater in supervisory relationships where the quality of the alliance is rated as strong compared to when quality is considered poor (Webb & Wheeler, 1998). The working alliance also impacts on elements of the therapist's work, with greater rapport and a stronger alliance related to greater job satisfaction compared to less rapport and poorer alliance (Mena & Bailey, 2007). Recent research tends to suggest that a strong working alliance between supervisor and supervisee is important for buffering the impact of traumatic work environments and reducing the risk of vicarious traumatisation (Dunkley & Whelan, 2006). The working alliance has also been linked to therapist ratings of self-efficacy, although the results appear to be confusing. Ladany and colleagues (Ladany, Ellis, & Friedlander, 1999) suggest the strength of the working alliance does not appear to have a strong impact on therapist ratings of self-efficacy, but a more recent study by Lent et al. (2006) suggests otherwise. In any event, a strong working alliance between supervisor and supervisee can contribute positively to supervisee development.

Parallel Processes

Another term used frequently across models of supervision, but that also developed out of psychoanalytic theory, is the notion of the parallel process. Friedlander, Siegel and Brenock (1989) defined this concept as involving behaviour where supervisees will 'unconsciously present themselves to their supervisors as their clients have presented to them. The process reverses when the supervisee adopts attitudes and behaviours of the supervisor in relating to the client' (p. 149). Therefore the supervision dyad begins to mirror the therapy dyad in a meaningful and instructional manner. If a therapist experiences a problem in supervision when discussing a particular client, this can represent an unconscious expression of a client's problem in therapy (Andersson, 2008; Ekstein & Wallerstein, 1976).

Parallel processes in psychodynamic supervision involve bringing that which is unconscious into the conscious so that it can be reflected upon, discussed and resolved. Often the first sign that a parallel process is evolving is unusual or atypical behaviour in the therapist during supervision sessions (Deering, 1994). Once the supervisor has drawn attention to the existence of this parallel process, the therapist may appear less confused or more able to understand the feelings they were experiencing.

Case Example: Parallel Process.

Isabella is a trainee psychotherapist who has been having supervision sessions with Helen, a psychodynamic supervisor, for almost a year. In her latest supervision session, Isabella began discussing a recent therapy session with a new client, Ray, a troubled and angry adolescent who presents as sullen and disengaged during sessions. He regularly tests the therapeutic boundaries and Isabella's patience. When Isabella presents this case to Helen she unconsciously re-enacts Ray's in-session behaviour during her supervision session, questioning Helen's words and making statements that test her relationship with Helen. The 'mood' of her therapy sessions with Ray is mirrored during this supervision session with Helen. Helen is able to recognise the parallel process that Isabella is unconsciously adopting and uses her role as supervisor to illustrate how Isabella might want to proceed in her sessions with Ray and how she may best handle his behaviour. In effect, Helen models to Isabella an appropriate course of action to take in future sessions with Ray. By questioning Isabella's assumptions and feelings about Ray's behaviour, both explicitly and implicitly, Helen slowly draws out Isabella's unconscious beliefs and motivations surrounding Ray's therapy. She then openly voices her observations and she and Isabella finish the session by reflecting on the parallel process that occurred. The next time Isabella sees Ray she presents herself to Ray much as Helen did during supervision, adopting Helen's supervisory manner and approach and using it in the therapy session.

Isabella's behaviour during supervision illustrates what Deering (1994) refers to as an upward parallel process. Isabella's subsequent therapeutic approach with Ray could be classified as a downward parallel process. In this case, the downward process was therapeutic and directed towards improving client outcome. Not all downward parallel processes may be so positive. Deering (1994) provides the example of a supervisor pushing their supervisee towards the achievement of a goal too quickly and the supervisee responding by placing similar pressure on their client.

Transference and Countertransference

Another essential element of psychodynamic supervision is the processing of transference and countertransference experiences. Transference refers to the client's unconscious feelings and behaviour directed towards the therapist that stem from the client's background and early experiences (Andersson, 2008). Countertransference refers to the feelings and impulses a therapist experiences as a result of interacting with a particular client (Ladany, Friedlander, & Nelson, 2005; Rosenthal, 1999) that may result either from the client's behaviour (objective countertransference), or from the therapist's background (subjective countertransference). Thus the psychodynamic supervision triangle of client, therapist and supervisor has the potential to influence two relationships — the supervisory relationship and the clinical relationship (Beck, Sarnat, & Barenstein, 2008).

During supervision the psychodynamic supervisor will encourage their supervisee to process and reflect on the transferences and countertransferences that occur as a function of the therapeutic and supervisory relationships.

> When disturbing states of mind are transmitted from client to supervisee, they are often subsequently enacted with the supervisor rather than verbally described to him or her. By attending to the supervisee's countertransference experience and to the supervisory relationship, such states become accessible for processing. (Beck et al., 2008, p. 69).

While there is a tremendous amount of theoretical writing and narrative case studies describing the usefulness of transference and countertransference as a supervisory process, there is not a great deal of empirical literature on the topic. Zaslavsky, Nunes, Eizirik and Nurse (2005) explored supervisory countertransference and concluded that countertransference became more direct and objective as the supervisory relationship continued, and the supervisors in their study (at an institution accredited by the International Psychoanalytical Association) see it as quite important to hold up the distinction between supervision and personal analysis for trainee analysts.

Case Example : Countertransference

Joan is in her mid-30s and is a trainee psychoanalyst who has been separated from her husband for almost 3 years. She is raising her daughter as a single parent while beginning her career as an analyst. She has been undertaking her own personal analysis since her divorce and is proud of the fact that she is commencing a new career, single-handedly raising her daughter and is financially independent of her ex-husband. One of Joan's regular clients is Sammie, who started seeing Joan following her own relationship breakdown 12 months earlier. She presents as someone who is helpless and unsure of her place in the world, who cannot see herself coping without a partner in her life, and who has repeatedly expressed a desire to reconnect with her ex-husband. She is reliant on her ex-husband for financial support and remains unmotivated to find employment or 're-enter' the world.

During supervision, Joan tells her supervisor, Robert, about Sammie's latest behaviour and she feels she has stalled in her sessions with Sammie. Joan describes Sammie as unmotivated and unwilling to change. After some careful questioning by Robert, Joan expresses a frustration with what she sees as Sammie's laziness and believes Sammie is taking the easy way out of her problems. Joan is critical of Sammie's reliance on her ex-husband for support and believes that Sammie is capable of achieving quite a lot if she puts her mind to it.

Robert must tread carefully here for he recognises that Joan's reaction to Sammie's behaviour is tied up not only in Joan's frustration with Sammie's perceived unwillingness to change (objective transference) but also in Joan's beliefs about what women can achieve and her own experience as a successful single parent (subjective transference). Robert prompts Joan to reflect on her reactions to Sammie's motivations and defence mechanisms, and points out the obvious countertransferences that Joan appears to be expressing. He helps Joan to recognise how her own beliefs have coloured her perceptions of Sammie's behaviour and encourages Joan to discuss these beliefs and their historical development with her analyst at their next session. He and Joan then go on to discuss Sammie's behaviour and formulate a plan for how to genuinely explore with Sammie her goals for life and therapy.

This example illustrates the delicate boundaries that psychodynamic supervisors must navigate as a part of the supervisory relationship. Indeed, even very early psychoanalytic theorists (e.g., Searles, 1955) distinguish between 'disturbing experiences with the patient [that are] reframed as crucial data, diagnostic of the patient's problems, rather than as intrusions that should be relegated to the therapist's personal therapy' (Sarnat, 1992, p. 389). Thus we see the aforementioned divide occurring between those analysts who believe supervision can include personal therapy, and those who see supervision as quite distinct from the analyst's own personal therapy.

Teach or Treat?

The historical foundations of psychodynamic supervision mean that many of the practices used in this supervisory approach parallel those used in the provision of psychodynamic psychotherapy so it is hardly surprising that therapy and supervision are often confused. It is beyond the scope of this chapter to engage in lengthy discussion of this issue, however it is important to acknowledge the distinction. Wheeler (2007) argues that 'a balance needs to be struck that enables exploration and support, but avoids supervision becoming therapy' (p. 247). Freud might have seen himself as both master analyst and supervisor for his trainee analysts, but the contemporary ethical view is to encourage the supervisee to seek personal analysis outside the supervisory relationship. This is not to say that countertransference is avoided in supervision, but that the focus of processing countertransferences is to use them as an instructional, education tool rather than a personally therapeutic process (Sarnat, 1992).

When considering the distinction between psychodynamic supervision as therapy and supervision as supervision, it is important to consider some of the key differences between the two, differences that see the analyst and supervisor performing very different roles. As Hyman (2008) discusses, unlike therapy, supervision is not confidential especially if conducted within a training course/university. In addition, the supervisor is responsible for addressing issues such as poor progress, lack of ethical behaviour and poor record-keeping that may need to be addressed with an institutional supervisor. The supervisor may also need to address supervisee behaviour, such as lateness or missed appointments, in a manner that is different to how a therapist deals with the same behaviour in a client. A final important distinction is that supervisors evaluate their supervisees, whereas psychodynamic psychotherapists rarely formally evaluate their clients in the same manner.

Seeking personal analysis appears to be beneficial to analysts on a number of levels. In addition to providing the opportunity to work through transference and countertransference processes and discussing the therapist's own defence mechanisms, it seems that analysts undertaking their own personal therapy outside the supervisory relationship make for better therapists. An interesting study by Coleman (2002) surveyed a sample of community clinicians and trainees and found that analysts who undergo their own personal therapy are given higher ratings of empathy and warmth compared to those therapists not currently seeking personal therapy. Not only does the therapist benefit from therapy, but it appears the therapist's clients can too.

Conclusion

Psychodynamic supervision has developed considerably since Freud's master–apprentice model of psychoanalytic supervision. Contemporary approaches argue in favour of distinguishing between supervision as an instructional tool versus supervision as a therapeutic tool. Many of the processes that occur in supervision, however, form the basic tenets of psychoanalytic psychotherapy. For example, the notion of the working alliance stems from discussions of the therapeutic alliance; downward parallel processes can impact on a client just as strongly as they impact on a therapist; reflection on transferences and countertransferences have become as much a part of supervision as they are a hallmark of discussions about psychoanalytic therapy sessions. While it is important to remember that psychodynamic supervision cannot replace individual personal therapy, quality supervision invariably involves more than just the technical presentation and teaching of skills. Psychodynamic supervision forms a type of secure base from within which the trainee analyst can explore their feelings and impulses and, as such, psychodynamic supervision is most effective when it embraces a therapist's experiences, feelings and reactions towards both client and supervisor, and the supervisor's similar experiences, feelings and reactions.

The Behavioural and Cognitive Models of Supervision
Historical Background

Historically, therapy and counselling texts have separated behavioural and cognitive theory and methods. In more recent times, however, there has been a therapeutic and praxis rapprochement whereby those interested in behavioural change have developed a more cognitive orientation, and cognitive theorists and practitioners have integrated behavioural techniques as part of a broader treatment suite.

Behavioural therapy's aetiology is heavily influenced by the work of Pavlov, Watson and Skinner and their premise that our behaviour is determined by what happens to us as a result of our behaviour. The concept of reinforcement is critical. If we are reinforced for our behaviour, then most likely we will continue to engage in that behaviour. If we are ignored or punished, the behaviour is likely to abate or cease. In this classic view of behaviourism, internal processes and cognitions are given little emphasis. The focus was on direct and observable behaviour. Behavioural therapy, as summarised by Mischel (1971) has three common features:

- Behaviour therapies attempt to modify problematic behaviours.
- Like the social behaviour theories that guide them, behaviour therapies emphasise the individuals' current behaviours rather than the historical origins of the problems.

• There is a belief in a general assumption that undesired behaviour can be understood and changed using the same learning principles that govern desired behaviour.

These features underpin three other important principles that form part of the scientific basis of behaviour therapy and an empirical approach to the modification of human functioning:

• It is based on the results of empirical research using rigorous scientific methodology.

• It applies behaviour change principles that have been demonstrated by basic research

• Its clinical and applied approaches must continually meet benchmark scientific standards.

Bandura (1989) emphasised that the client should be deeply involved in the choice and direction of treatment and moved behaviourism toward behavioural humanism. His concept of self-efficacy emphasised individual rights and collaboration in the counselling and treatment process, by emphasising that individuals develop best when they have control of their own destiny. This view and following important work by Meichenbaum (1991), which emphasised person–environment interaction, gave focus to a view of behaviour being reciprocally influenced by thoughts, feelings, physiological processes and the consequences of behaviour. There was a de-emphasis of the centre of control being in the external environment, and a shift to a centre stage role for the client. The fusion of these approaches has produced a cognitive–behavioural therapy and counselling approach (CBT), which has become a potent dynamic in counselling and psychotherapy.

Cognitive and Behavioural Fundamentals

The cognitive contribution to CBT has been heavily influenced by the work of Albert Ellis. His model of rational–emotive therapy (RET) was a pioneering method of CBT (Ellis, 1983). Fundamental principles include unconditional acceptance of all clients, encouragement to clients to think rationally and be in touch with their emotions, and a strong emphasis on follow-up activity by the client after the counselling session. This 'home-work' seeks to have clients apply ideas from the counselling sessions to their daily lives as important to the change process. A process result is to aim for the client to decide on an action for logical reasons that are also satisfactory emotionally — hence the term rational–emotive. The individual must both think and feel that a decision is correct. RET endeavours to correct thought patterns and minimise irrational ideas, while simultaneously attempting to change dysfunctional feelings and behaviours. An important mnemonic coined by Ellis conveniently shapes the process:

A the objective facts, events, behaviours that an individual encounters

B the person's belief about A

C the emotional consequences, or how a person acts and feels about A

D disputing irrational beliefs and thinking

E the effect of disputation in D on the client

F new feelings and emotions associated with the situation.

An analogous technique identifying faulty thought patterns was pioneered by Beck (1991). An eradication of harmful automatic thoughts, an examination of current thinking processes and an eventual development of new forms of cognition characterise the constructs. The following steps summarise the process:

- recognising maladaptive thinking and ideation
- noting repeating patterns of ideation that tend to be ineffective
- distancing and decentring help clients remove themselves from the immediate fear, thought or problem so that they can think about it from a distance
- changing the rules of thinking.

Both theories and therapeutic approaches place the client as a principal agent of change, who is challenged by the 'here and now' imperative and where solutions are not necessarily found by delving into past history.

The behavioural contribution to CBT has been heavily influenced by the work of Pavlov, Watson and Skinner, as previously noted. Ivey, Ivey and Simek-Morgan (2007) describe some of the key behavioural change procedures.

Pinpointing behaviour. Move from general observations (e.g., 'this hyperactive child is difficult to control') to noting precise observable behaviours, such as the number of times the child interrupts the teacher or the number of times the child leaves the chair.

Positive reinforcement. The provision of rewards for desired behaviour. Use of learning theory concepts such as extinction, shaping, and intermittent reinforcement to elicit and maintain desired behaviour.

Charting. Charting or diary entry of the number of occurrences of important behaviours before, during, and after treatment. Assists in observing whether a behaviour is maintained after treatment and whether a new strategy should be tried.

Relaxation training. Client mastery of simple relaxation techniques, allow further exploration to solve more complex issues.

Biofeedback and self-regulation. Instrumentation is now readily available for biofeedback to assist in a variety of client tension patterns.

Systematic desensitisation. Consists of three primary steps. (1) Training is systematic deep muscle relaxation, (2) construction of anxiety hierarchies and (3) matching specific objects of anxiety from the hierarchy with relation training.

Modelling. Seeing and hearing directly, either live or via film or digital media, brings home a message more clearly and directly than advice or description.

Social skills training. Skills training often involves the following cognitive–behavioural components: (a) rapport/structuring; cognitive and emotional preparation for the instruction, (b) cognitive presentation and cueing; explanation and rationale for acquisition of the skill, (c) modelling; role plays, digital media, demonstrations enacted, (d) practice; mastery of the skill to a high level through practice, (e) generalisation; movement of the skill from the training session to in vivo application.

Assertiveness training. A balance of learning to stand up for individual rights (overt behaviour) and simultaneously consider the thoughts and feelings of others (client cognitions).

Stress inoculation and management. Training for: (a) a cognitive understanding of the role of stress in an individual's life, (b) specific coping skills and (c) working with thoughts and emotions attendant to the stress situation to motivate remedial action.

Supervision

Supervision plays an essential role in the benchmarking and quality assurance of practitioners during initial training and throughout a professional career. What then are the elements of good supervision and what can be expected from their adoption by the therapist? Pretorius (2006) asserts the primary goal of CBT supervision is to help the therapist adopt the philosophy of CBT as the basic approach for changing clients' cognitions, emotions and behaviours to facilitate improvement or recovery. A secondary goal is to teach the therapist specific skills or techniques. There are striking similarities between both goals — both are systematic, goal-directed, structured, time-limited, collaborative, person-focused, confidential and active. Both emphasise mutual trust, openness, practice, experience, change facilitation, building on existing strengths and skills and response to feedback.

Perris (1993) argues that CBT supervision tends to follow a relatively didactic model. Leise and Beck (1997) and Leise and Alford (1998) suggest the following structure for each CBT session: checking in, setting the agenda, bridging from the previous supervision session, enquiring about previously supervised cases, reviewing homework, prioritising of agenda items, discussing an individual recorded case, using direct instruction and guided discovery, using standardised supervision instruments, assigning new relevant homework and eliciting feedback from the supervisee. This framework has been overlaid by Armstrong, Twaddle and Freeston (2003) who identify and describe four interacting levels for the CBT supervision framework. The first level, *primary inputs*, includes the context in which the supervision occurs, the clients' impact on supervision, and the selectivity with which the supervisee reports therapy — a subject to which we will return later in this chapter. The second level, *parameters*, outlines the nature and development of the supervisory project. The third level, *dynamic focus*, examines the changing emphasis on case conceptualisation, technique and the therapeutic relationship. The fourth level, *learning process*, is an experiential process of learning with stages outlined for supervision to proceed to achieve new knowledge, skill and application.

Most commentators agree that the nature and quality of the relationship between supervisor and supervisee is paramount to successful supervision, but there is no universal agreement as to how this can be achieved. For example Dobson and Shaw (1993) suggest that the three principal activities of cognitive therapists and supervisors are, in descending order, relationship activities, case conceptualisation and learning techniques. However, in a survey of UK cognitive–behavioural psychotherapists, Townend, Iannetta and Freeston (2002) confirm that 16 topics were discussed during supervision and were, in descending order of frequency: case formulation, cognitive analysis, cognitive interventions, behavioural interventions, three systems analysis, functional analysis, application of techniques, emotional responsibility, goal setting, therapeutic bond, client safety, homework, ethical issues, evaluation methods, therapist safety, and exclusion criteria. In the evidence of the latter study, it has to be assumed that relationship activities are occurring in a less overt way, if at all, than in the conceptualisation of Dobson and Shaw.

An insightful and frank set of observations by Ladany (2004) helps gain some understanding of an elusive and perhaps fruitless search for a supervision template in the cognitive and behavioural therapy environment. Ladany commences by stating 'There is a theory which states that if ever anyone discovers exactly what the Universe is for and why it is here, it will instantly disappear and be replaced by something even more bizarre and inexplicable' (p. 1). He follows by noting from the beginning of his psychotherapy training how he was struck by how fabulously incompetent were those he deemed 'supervisors', that it was not until he received the title of supervisor himself that he learnt how fabulously incompetent he also could be. Ladany presents his investigations into psychotherapy supervision research by posing a series of four questions.

If nothing else what should a supervisor do? Drawing on his own experience of supervision, Ladany notes the few superb supervisors who shaped him demonstrated great skilfulness at developing a strong supervisory alliance, along with providing a good mix of challenge and support that allowed him to grow as a therapist-in-training. He recommends that supervisors attend to the development of a strong supervisory alliance using and generalising their psychotherapy skills (e.g., empathy, clarification). The alliance, developing as it does most readily in the early relationship, should be considered as grounded in the supervisory work. That is, attend more to the alliance when the relationship is developing or when there is a rupture in the alliance, and attend to it less when a supervisor's technical skills are needed to focus more on the trainee's development.

What are some of the worst things a supervisor can do? First, ignore the supervisory working alliance, which only creates a weak foundation on which to facilitate change in the trainee. Second, use developmental cookie-cutters to treat trainees. It seems likely there are trainee and supervisor factors that account for more of the variance in how a trainee will respond to supervision and among them are trainee tolerance for ambiguity, experience with the specific client base, general clinical experience, past effective supervision experiences, conceptualisation ability, and supervisor personality and ability factors. Third, approach supervision with the belief that supervisor ethics are for wimps. Ladany and colleagues (Ladany, Lehrman-Waterman et al., 1999) proposed supervisor ethical guidelines and then determined how well practicing supervisors adhered to them. The guidelines were an amalgam of several well-published professional body guidelines. This work yielded 18 ethical categories relevant to supervisors. Fifty-one per cent of the respondents reported their supervisors violated at least one of these guidelines. Why? Many supervisors never received training to become a supervisor and, in addition, many supervisors may judge the 'critical feedback' role as being counterintuitive to the nonjudgmental and supportive roles typically adopted in supervision.

Do not tell trainees how they will be evaluated and then evaluate them capriciously. Ladany notes that a variety of studies point to the difficulty supervisors have in providing evaluations of trainee performance. There is little evidence that it is done well, with subjective and qualitative measures lacking rigour and quantitative measures having poor psychometric properties (Ellis & Ladany, 1997). Ladany and Muse-Burke (2001) suggest that for any evaluation approach a series of components needs to be considered. Among them are the mode of therapy (e.g., individual, group, family or couples), the domain of supervisee behaviours (e.g., psychotherapy or supervision), the area of competence (e.g., psychotherapy techniques, theoretical conceptualisation, assessment), methods (e.g., trainee self-report, case notes, audiotape, live supervision), proportion of caseload (e.g., all clients, subgroup of clients, one client), and evaluator (e.g., supervisor, clients, peers, objective raters). Although not all of these parameters could or should be considered in any given evaluation approach, the value of any approach can be determined based on how well each of these components are incorporated.

Demonstrate you are racist, sexist, or homophobic both overtly and subtly. Ladany noted often witnessing how supervisors could act overtly bigoted when he was a trainee, but in other venues they came across as champions of multiculturalism. His research findings indicated clearly that self-reported multicultural competencies are not related to demonstrated multicultural competencies. The development of the Heuristic Model of Nonoppressive Interpersonal Development codes individuals into one of two groups; a socially oppressed group (SOG) — female, person of colour, gay/lesbian/bisexual, disabled, working-class); or a socially privileged group (SPG) — male, white, heterosexual, physically able, middle- to upper- class. Irrespective of group, individuals also move through similar phases of means of interpersonal functioning (MIF) — thoughts and feelings about oneself as well as the behaviours based on one's identification with a given demographic variable. The phases of MIF are adaptation, incongruence, exploration and integration. Individuals can be more advanced in terms of their MIF for one variable over another. For example, a supervisor in the adaptation phase in terms of gender identity, will likely minimise and dismiss a trainee's desire to consider gender issues in relation to client conceptualisation. To better understand the multiple identity interactions that occur in supervision, Ladany hypothesises four supervisor–supervisee interpersonal interaction types for each demographic variable: progressive, in which the supervisor is at a more advanced stage than the trainee; parallel-advanced, in which the supervisor and trainee are at comparable advanced MIF stages; parallel-delayed, in which the supervisor and trainee are at comparable delayed MIF stages; and regressive, in which the trainee is at a more advanced stage than the supervisor. Each of these interaction types has implications for trainee and client outcome. Specifically, the facilitation of trainee outcome is predicted to occur from most to least for the following types; parallel-advanced, progressive, parallel-delayed, and regressive.

What secrets do supervisors and trainees keep from each other? Ladany reports sets of both supervisor and supervisee non-disclosures. The following are noted as rarely disclosed:

Supervisee	*Supervisor*
• Negative reactions to their supervisors	• Negative reactions to counselling and professional performance
• Personal issues	• Supervisor personal issues
• Clinical mistakes	• Negative reactions to supervisee's supervision performance
• Evaluation concerns	
• General client observations	• Supervisee's personal issues
• Negative reactions to the client	• Negative supervisor self-efficacy
• Countertransference	• Dynamics at training site
• Client-counsellor attraction issues	• Supervisor's clinical and professional issues
• Positive reactions to the supervisor	• Supervisee appearance
	• Positive reactions to therapy and professional performance
• Supervision setting concerns	
• Supervisor appearance	• Attraction to supervisee
• Supervisee–supervisor attraction issues	• Reaction to supervisee's clients
• Positive reaction to the client	• Experience as a supervisor with other supervisees

The overall assessment on both sets of nondisclosures probably inform us more of issues of power differential deference, impression management, fear of political suicide and choice of client development over supervisee development. The reasons for nondisclosure will invariably be multidimensional and closely related to the strength of the working alliance. The best that could be said is that both supervisors and supervisees should be aware of what is generally omitted in order to realistically evaluate what can be profitably and developmentally disclosed in their own relationship. It involves judgment replete with all the elements of good supervision referred to earlier, namely mutual trust, openness, practice, experience, change facilitation, building on existing strengths and skills and response to feedback.

The behavioural and cognitive approaches share much of the supervision challenge with the other contemporary approaches discussed in this chapter. At the core of the matter, supervision is a dynamic that should be aimed at the most efficient and effective process to enable an intending therapist to both inculcate the philosophy of the technique and gain knowledge and skills in the application of the therapy.

The Developmental Model of Supervision

The developmental model is a unique approach to supervision as it is not bound to psychotherapy theory. The developmental model has its strongest conceptual links with educational theory. It has had considerable influence on the practice of supervision across all theoretical orientations, and has been subject to more empirical research than any other approach to supervision. Three areas will be addressed in this section: (1) defining the key assumptions and principles of developmental supervision, specifically the Integrated Developmental Model of Supervision (IDM); (2) demonstrating how IDM supervision is used in practice and (3) examining the research to assess the efficacy of the developmental approach.

Developmental supervision defines good supervision as occurring when supervisors assess supervisee experience-based skill factors and use these to structure a learning environment that meets individual supervisee learning goals. In the most basic terms, the developmental model purports that experience level is the key factor that should mediate supervisory structure and supervisee learning needs.

The Integrated Developmental Model of Supervision

There are a number of developmental models of supervision that share key assumptions regarding the structuring of learning environment based on supervisee experience level. For the purposes of this discussion the focus will be on the integrated developmental model (IDM) as informed by the work of Stoltenberg, McNeill and Delworth (1998). Essentially IDM describes a process where the supervisor modifies the structure of supervisory activity on a continual basis to match the growing clinical experience of the supervisee. The importance of altering supervisory structure to match growing supervisee competency cannot be overemphasised as it provides the method by which more advanced skills are developed (Hansen & Barker, 1964; Hogan, 1964; Littrell, Lee-Borden, & Lorenz, 1979; Loganbill, Hardy, & Delworth, 1982; Stoltenberg, 1981; Stoltenberg & Delworth, 1987). IDM supervisory structure is conceptualised as a series of experience-related predefined levels through which the emerging therapist must progress to gain clinical competence with defined supervisor behaviours for each level of progression (Littrell et al., 1979; Loganbill et al., 1982; Stoltenberg, 1981).

Supervision that is structured and directive is hypothesised as optimal for beginning supervisees, whereas supervision that is collegial and consultative is optimal for advanced supervisees. In practical terms the supervisor makes an assessment of experience level and competency of the supervisee and prescriptively matches supervisory activity and teaching strategies in accordance with the appropriate developmental level. The model is relatively structured and prescriptive and the capacity for a supervisee to prioritise his or her own learning goals with a supervisor is limited (see Tables 6.1 and 6.2.)

Applying IDM Overriding Structure to Competency Domains

The supervisor goals are to facilitate the IDM overriding structures — motivation, autonomy and awareness — as these are the desired internal supervisee characteristics that allow the supervisee to engage with the domain categories (Table 6.1). These domain categories may be considered competencies that will be achieved to differing degrees at each developmental level and mastered through progress to higher levels (Table 6.2). Motivation, autonomy and awareness are mediated by the interpersonal and structural environment of supervision. Initially, the supervisor develops a purposeful supervisor–supervisee relationship, which enables communication, trust and creates a shared understanding of roles, responsibilities and boundaries of supervision. Emphasis is then placed on clarifying expectations, developing goals in clinical work and professional development and how work will be evaluated, for example, observation of videotaped work. The supervisor may at this stage assess the level of the model that suits the supervisee and structure the learning environment accordingly.

The supervisor will then observe supervisee practice in domain-related areas such as interpersonal skills, clinical skills, case management skills, the client–therapist relationship, achievement of standards and use of models and theory. The supervisor then assesses these observations to evaluate the specific skill and professional development needs of the supervisee, which is provided as feedback. The supervision meeting serves as the primary mode of providing feedback and skills training, communication, problem-solving and the opportunity for the supervisor to model the required target skills. Importantly, the supervisor follows up all agreed leaning and

TABLE 6.1

Levels of Supervisee Development: Assessment Domains (Stoltenberg & Delworth 1987)

Overriding structures	Specific domains
Self- and other awareness	Intervention Assessment techniques Interpersonal Assessment
Motivation	Client conceptualisation Individual differences Theoretical orientation
Autonomy	Treatment plans and goals Professional ethics

TABLE 6.2
Levels of Supervisee Development: IDM Supervision Levels (Stoltenberg & Delworth 1987)

Experience level	Supervisee characteristics	Supervisory environment
Level 1 Motivation Autonomy Awareness	*Relationship building and goal setting* Focused on: • own anxiety • dependence on external authority • motivation to learn techniques • imitative approach • limited self-awareness and conceptual or categorical thinking In transition towards level 2: become anxious regarding new approaches and have unrealistic expectations	*Trust builder and contractor* Structure to manage anxiety Training in domain competencies is: • prescriptive • instruction • supportive • interpretative • modelling approaches • skills training • feedback on strengths and weaknesses
Level 2 Motivation Autonomy Awareness	*Affective issues and skills deficits* Focused on: • dependency–autonomy conflict • fluctuating motivation • greater understanding of client, confusion and/or defensiveness In transition towards level 3: increased desire to personalise orientation, conditional autonomy, understands limitations, beginning awareness of self in client work	*Counsellor and teacher* Training in domain competencies is: • through providing less structure • through modelling greater autonomy • encouraging higher levels of involvement • support (particularly for difficult issues) • communication of ambivalence • in providing difference perspectives • through poor focus on process issues
Level 3 Motivation Autonomy Awareness	*Confidence in expertise* Focused on: • emotional impact on self • confidence in ability • autonomy • motivation to understand strengths and weaknesses • professional identity focus • personal responsibility • a high degree of empathy and understanding In transition to level 4: will demonstrate stability of operation across all domains.	*Colleague* Training in domain competencies is: • through mutual sharing • involvement as peer • by exemplification • by confrontation and challenging interventions with client • with conceptualisation • through dealing with affective reactions • through observation • by engaging in more complex cases

TABLE 6.2 (continued)
Levels of Supervisee Development: IDM Supervision Levels (Stoltenberg & Delworth 1987)

Experience level	Supervisee characteristics	Supervisory environment
Level 4 Motivation Autonomy Awareness	*Self-responsibility and autonomy* Master counsellor Focused on: • moving conceptually and behaviourally move across domains • how professional identity is stable across domains • personal understanding across domains • awareness of impact of personal on professional work	*Consultant* Training in domain competencies is achieved: • by being collegial • by allowing the supervisee to provide more structure • with more focus on personal and professional integration • by clinical integration • by being personally confronting • be beying change-oriented to prevent stagnation • through high process and experience of case focus

treatment planning tasks with the supervisee, ensuring they provide the appropriate training and the agreed client plans have been implemented.

A Typical Developmental Supervision Scenario and Experience-Level Related Structure

Trevor was supervising Jennifer on her first clinical placement. Jennifer was anxious as she had not seen many clients before and was unsure she could deal with the type of problems clients might present. Trevor spent some time getting to know her and developing a positive working relationship. He talked with Jennifer about her previous therapy experience, her studies, understanding of the therapeutic process and client change as well as her personal fears and doubts. Thinking in IDM terms, Trevor realised she was a beginning level therapist and would need a high level of direction and structure in supervision (Level 1). This assessment was confirmed after Trevor viewed her first videotaped therapy session. Trevor assessed that supervisory activity should focus on teaching Jennifer case conceptualisation, to formulate and implement treatment plans (domain competencies) and to manage her anxiety and fears about conducting therapy.

Trevor, in negotiation with Jennifer, formulated a set of learning goals for supervision based around Level 1 goals. Jennifer agreed with these goals and wanted to include her own goal to learn how to recognise and work with process issues in therapy such as defences, resistance and transference. Trevor noted that these were more advanced skills and probably related to issues of ambivalence regarding competency and autonomy and dependence that might be played out in supervision when Jennifer progressed to Level 2. Trevor said that he would provide her with instruction in recognising these issues in supervision when appropriate, but the main focus of supervision would relate to the agreed learning goals (as her learning needs related more to Level 1 issues). Trevor explained that these core learning goals were foundational good therapy and their mastery would provide a base to build more advanced skills. He assured Jennifer that there would be plenty of time to explore process issues as she became more confident with the basics of treatment. Supervision was conducted in a formal and structured way, with Jennifer presenting her cases in supervision from detailed notes and occasional videotapes of therapy. The supervisory discussion focused on the agreed goals. Soon Trevor was confident that Jennifer was developing competency in foundational skills and was well on the way to achieving Level 1 learning goals. As Jennifer's confidence increased Trevor decided to use a few supervision strategies based on Level 2. He raised issues regarding the dynamics of therapy and interpreted client behaviour to help Jennifer understand therapeutic process. Trevor noticed Jennifer was beginning to explore her own emerging autonomy as a therapist sharing her views and ideas about therapeutic process.

Trevor also began to expect Jennifer to process her own reactions to client work in supervision. Trevor noticed that even though Jennifer was progressing well in developing skills and achieving learning goals, the focus of supervision was still educational. Jennifer easily felt unsure of herself and Trevor often had to provide support and encouragement aimed at helping her manage her anxiety about not recognising therapeutic issues or not being a perfect therapist. Trevor realised that even though Jennifer was doing some work in supervision consistent with Level 2, her needs for supervision structure were still related to Level 1 and she was in a transition between levels. He also realised that this experience of supervision would be formative to Jennifer's emerging professional identity as a therapist.

Trevor noted after 6 months of weekly supervision that Jennifer had increased in confidence in therapy and could conceptualise the important issues of a case and formulate and implement basic treatment plans. Trevor and Jennifer felt that the initial learning goals were achieved and developed new goals that focused more on treatment dynamics and process issues in therapy, as well as more advanced treatment skills and interventions. Trevor reduced the level of structure of supervision and provided direct training only as needed and began to encourage Jennifer's autonomy by developing her own hypotheses and testing these out in therapy. Jennifer responded by becoming more autonomous in supervision, occasionally asserting herself regarding preferences for supervisory activity and structure and expressing more confidence in client work. At other times Jennifer appeared somewhat ambivalent about the reduction in supervision structure and her emerging autonomy. Trevor recognised that Jennifer was well established in Level 2 of the developmental process and making good progress.

About the same time, the service employed a graduate therapist in a senior position. Liz was a very experienced therapist, having graduated from a clinical doctoral program. As principal staff supervisor, Trevor met with Liz and quickly assessed she was likely competent across all domains, did not need a structured learning environment, and could set her own agendas in supervision to meet her goals. Trevor conducted supervision with Liz in a very collegial way, giving a great deal of autonomy, allowing her to structure the supervision according to her needs in accordance with Level 4 of the developmental model. His assessment of her skills was confirmed when he observed her first contracted video of a client session, where she demonstrated a high level of skill in all domain competencies. He noticed that in supervision Liz did not often discuss case conceptualisation and treatment planning, but rather focused on her own reactions to the case and deep insights into client dynamics and process of treatment, as well as issues relating to her own ongoing professional development.

Research and the Developmental Model

The case examples above demonstrate the commonsense appeal of IDM that supervisee experience level should determine the structure of the supervisory environment and assessment of learning needs. Does the evidence support this proposition? The answer is not as straightforward as it might seem. Research into what constitutes optimal supervisory structure has provided results that in some cases are contradictory and in others difficult to interpret. The assumption of a relationship between experience and supervision structure has been criticised by a number of researchers. Holloway (1987), Roehlke, (1984) and Ellis, Ladany, Krengel and Schult (1997) concluded there was little evidence to establish any developmental processes in supervision or that any supervisee learning needs were related to experience level and that developmental theory is prescriptive and therefore cannot accommodate other factors that might mediate supervisee learning needs. However, when the evidence is examined in detail, important conclusions can be made.

The Changing Needs of the Supervisee

Worthington (1987) found that beginning level supervisees preferred structure and direction by their supervisor and experienced supervisees preferred less structure and direction. While providing some support for experience level being the key mediating variable in supervision, an unexpected finding was that some supervisee-preferred supervisory behaviour was not consistent with experience level. Experience level might mediate case conceptualisation; experienced supervisees focus on transference and countertransference, self-efficacy and self-awareness when conceptualising cases; whereas new therapists focus on the technical skills necessary to conceptualise cases. No effect was found for intermediate or transitional levels of the model in any study (Borders & Leddick, 1988; Holloway & Wampold, 1986; Holloway, 1987, 1992; Winter & Holloway, 1992; Worthington & Stern, 1985). Interestingly, any effect for developmental level was lost when situational factors were evident, such as when a supervisee engaged a new supervisor or dealing with a crisis situation. In these instances the need for structure and support was present in supervision regardless of experience level (Krause & Allen, 1988; Miars, et al. 1983; Wiley & Ray, 1986). Supervisors are also able to recognise variation in the needs of beginning and advanced level supervisees (Krause & Allen, 1988; Miars, et al. 1983; Wiley & Ray, 1986; Holloway, 1987, 1992).

These studies demonstrate some support for the view that the experience level of the supervisee can influence supervisory structure, but only between novice and experienced supervisees. No effect is evident for intermediate experience levels on supervisory structure; nor do these studies demonstrate how experience level can mediate the transition of the therapist through intermediate stages of supervision. Further, these studies identify variance in the needs of supervisees for structure that cannot be explained by experience level alone.

The Effect of Supervisee Characteristics

An alternative argument suggests that it is the characteristics of a supervisee, such as facilitative skills (Carlozzi, Campbell, & Ward, 1982), cognitive style (Holloway & Wampold, 1986; Winter & Holloway, 1992) and level of ego development as defined by attitudes and rigidity of thinking (Borders, Fong, & Cron, 1988) that determine the preference for structure in supervision. These characteristics might exert an influence on supervision that is independent of experience level.

The evidence appears somewhat contradictory with support for both experience level and individual characteristics as defining supervisee preferences for structure in supervision and little relationship with supervisee skill level. These disparate positions can be reconciled by a novel study (Tracey & Sherry, 1993) that suggests experience level and individual characteristics of supervisees interact to structure the supervisory environment.

A number of findings regarding the IDM from the literature appear reasonably robust:

• Research only demonstrates an effect on supervisee preference for supervisory structure between lowest and highest levels of experience.

• There is no evidence, as predicted by developmental theory, that supervisees progress through intermediate levels of supervisory structure based on increasing experience level.

• The relationship between experience level and skill development is not strong.

There is reasonably strong evidence that several additional factors may mediate the experience–supervisory structure of supervision. These factors are:

ipt[{3].ication>

.>

)al">

- Individual supervisee characteristics and situational factors in supervision strongly influence the relationship between experience level and structure in supervision.
- In some cases, individual characteristics exert more influence on the structural preference of supervisees for supervisory environment than experience level alone.

The evidence suggests IDM supervision might be a more effective model if the structure of supervision is adapted to include the needs created by supervisee characteristics, in addition to experience level. In fact, supervisors should assess and prioritise individual characteristics of supervisees and situational factors when considering the best learning structure–experience level combination for the supervisory environment.

Conclusion

From its earliest foundations in psychoanalytic psychotherapy to contemporary approaches like IDM, supervision in the helping professions remains dynamic and multifaceted. Despite the often vast differences between these three approaches to supervision, it is worth noting all endorse a strong supervisory alliance as fundamental to the success of supervision. Psychodynamic supervision utilises processes not out of place in a cognitive–behavioural supervision session; IDM is equally as reliant on supervisee characteristics and environmental factors as is psychodynamic supervision. Another characteristic shared by all three approaches to supervision is the relative dearth of empirical evidence investigating the efficacy of each supervisory approach. While each approach has attracted research into the processes that take place during the supervision session, thus providing evidence of the mediated components of each model, there is little evidence testing the overall impact of any one complete model of supervision. Whether this reflects a reliance on an eclectic approach to supervision, whether it reflects difficulty identifying and articulating markers of efficacy in supervision, or whether if reflects a lack of agreement surrounding who supervision ultimately benefits the most (client or supervisee), the stage is set for a greater research focus in the area of psychotherapeutic supervision.

Educational Questions and Activities

1. In groups discuss the following:
   (a) Define the key principles of psychodynamic, CBT and IDM models of supervision?
   (b) How do they differ in theoretical assumptions, processes and techniques?

    (c) What is the contribution of each approach to supervisee skill development?

    (d) Which approach do you like best and why?

    (e) Can these approaches be integrated into your supervision practice? Provide a rationale?

2. What does a psychodynamic supervisor do in supervision?

    (a) teaches treatment planning skills and therapeutic techniques

    (b) develops a positive supervisory alliance with their supervisee

    (c) assesses supervisee skill and experience and structures the learning environment accordingly

    (d) helps the supervisee understand the interpersonal processes and intrapsychic issues that occur in therapy

    (e) both b and d

    Answer: (e)

3. Why do Psychodynamic, CBT and IDM supervision prioritise the importance of a good working relationship between supervisor and supervisee?

    (a) All approaches assume that a positive working relationship will assist in achieving supervisory learning goals.

    (b) Supervisors want their supervisee's to have a good experience working with them.

    (c) It is important to feel good when in supervision.

    (d) A good supervisory alliance makes it possible to give honest feedback to each other.

    Answer: (a)

4. If your supervisee reports they are not making progress in therapy with a client what should you do from a CBT supervision perspective?

    (a) revisit the treatment plan and provide more skilful techniques

    (b) examine the interpersonal dynamics of the case

    (c) decide how to address supervision session learning outcomes based on the developmental level of the supervisee

    (d) examine how the supervisee really feels about working with their case

    Answer: (a)

5. There is little evidence of efficacy for psychodynamic, CBT or IDM supervision. Consider the following:

    (a) What is the real value of supervision?

    (b) How do you know if supervision works?

    (c) How should supervision be evaluated?

    (d) Who is supervision ultimately for, the supervisee or the client?

Selected References for Further Reading

Bambling M., & King R., (2000). Supervision and the development of counsellor competency. *Psychotherapy in Australia, 6*(4), 58–63.

Holloway, E., (1996). Supervision: Its contributions to treatment efficacy. In J. Talbott (Ed.), *Yearbook of Psychiatry & Applied Mental Health, 4,* 134–135.

Stoltenberg, C.D., & Delworth, U. (1987). *Supervising counsellors and therapists: A developmental approach.* San Francisco: Jossey-Bass.

Endnote

1 For the purposes of this brief overview, the authors use the term 'psychodynamic' to encompass all related contemporary psychoanalytic theories, whereas 'psychoanalytic' is used to represent only Freudian theory.

References

Andersson, L. (2008). Psychodynamic supervision in a group setting: Benefits and limitations. *Psychotherapy in Australia, 14,* 36–41.

Armstrong, P., Twaddle, V., & Freeston, M. (2003). *Supervision: Integrating practical skills with a conceptual framework.* Unpublished manuscript, Newcastle Centre for Cognitive and Behavioural Therapy, Newcastle, UK.

Bandura, A. (1989). Human agency in social cognitive theory. *American Psychologist, 37,* 122–147.

Beck, A. (1991). Cognitive therapy: A 30-year retrospective. *American Psychologist, 46,* 368–375.

Beck, J.S., Sarnat, J.E., & Barenstein, V. (2008). Psychotherapy-based approaches to supervision. In C.A. Falender & E.P. Shafranske (Eds.), *Casebook for clinical supervision: A competency-based approach* (pp. 57–96). Washington, DC: American Psychological Association.

Bernard, J.M., & Goodyear, R.K. (2004). *Fundamentals of clinical supervision* (3rd ed.). Boston: Pearson Education.

Borders, L., Fong, M., & Cron, E. (1988) In session cognitions of a counselling student: A case study. *Counselor Education and Supervision, 17,* 7–12.

Borders, L.D., & Leddick, G.R. (1988). A nationwide survey of supervision training. *Counselor Education & Supervision, 27,* 271–283.

Bordin, E.S. (1983). Supervision in counseling: II. Contemporary models of supervision: A working alliance based model of supervision. *The Counseling Psychologist, 11,* 35–42.

Bowlby, J. (1973/1998). *Attachment and loss: Vol. 2. Separation: Anxiety and anger.* London: Pimlico.

Carlozzi, A., Campbell, N., & Ward, G. (1982) Dogmatism and externality in locus of control as related to counsellor training skill in facilitative responding. *Counsellor Education and Supervision, 21,* 227–236.

Carroll, M. (2007). *Counselling supervision: Theory, skills and practice.* London: Sage.

Coleman, D. (2002). Personal therapy: A catalyst to relational awareness. *Irish Journal of Psychology, 23,* 73–85.

Deering, C.G. (1994). Parallel process in the supervision of child psychotherapy. *American Journal of Psychotherapy, 48,* 102–110.

Dobson, K.S., & Shaw, B.F. (1993). The training of cognitive therapists: What have we learned from treatment manuals? *Psychotherapy, 30,* 573–577.

Dunkley, J., & Whelan, T.A. (2006). Vicarious traumatisation in telephone counsellors: Internal and external influences. *British Journal of Guidance & Counselling, 34,* 451–469.

Efstation, J.F., Patton, M.J., & Kardash, C.M. (1990). Measuring the working alliance in counselor supervision. *Journal of Counseling Psychology, 37,* 322–329.

Ekstein, R., & Wallerstein, R.S. (1976). *The teaching and learning of psychotherapy.* New York: International.

Ellis, A. (1983). The origins of rational-emotive therapy (RET). *Voices, 18,* 29–33.

Ellis, M.V., & Ladany, N. (1997). Inferences concerning supervisees and clients in clinical supervision: An integrative review. In C.E. Watkins (Ed.), *Handbook of psychotherapy supervision* (pp. 567–607). New York: Wiley.

Ellis, M., Ladany,N., Krengel, M., & Schult, D. (1997). Clinical supervision research from 1981 to 1993: A methodological critique. *Journal of Counseling Psychology, 43,* 35–50.

Friedlander, M.L., Siegel, S.M., & Brenock, K. (1989). Parallel process in counseling and supervision: A case study. *Journal of Counseling Psychology, 36,* 149–157.

Greenson, R. (1967). *The technique and practice of psychoanalysis.* New York: International Universities Press.

Hansen, J., & Barker, E. (1964) Experiencing and the supervisory relationship. *Journal of Counselling Psychology, 11,* 107–111.

Hogan, R.A. (1964). Issues and approaches in supervision. *Psychotherapy: Theory, Research and Practice, 1,* 139–141.

Holloway, E., (1992) Supervision: a way of teaching and learning. In Brown, S., & Lent, R. (Eds.) *Handbook of Counselling Psychology.* New Jersey: John Wiley & Sons.

Holloway, E., (1987) Developmental models of supervision: its development? *Professional Psychology: Research and Practice, 19,* 138–140.

Holloway, E., & Wampold, B. (1986) Relation between conceptual level and counselling related tasks. A meta-analysis. *Journal of Counselling Psychology, 33,* 310–319.

Hyman, M. (2008). Psychoanalytic supervision. In A.K. Hess, K.D. Hess, & T.H. Hess (Eds.), *Psychotherapy supervision: Theory, Research, And Practice* (2nd ed., pp. 97–113). Hoboken, NJ: John Wiley & Sons.

Ivey A.E., Ivey, M.B., & Simek-Morgan, L. (2007). *Counselling and psychotherapy: A multicultural perspective.* Boston: Pearson.

Krause, A., & Allen, G. (1988) Perceptions of counselor supervision: An examination of Stoltenberg's model from the perspectives of supervisor and supervisee. *Journal of Counselling Psychology, 35,* 77–80.

Ladany, N. (2004). Psychotherapy supervision: What lies underneath? *Psychotherapy Research, 14,* 1–19.

Ladany, N., Ellis, M.V., & Friedlander, M.L. (1999). The supervisory working alliance, trainee self-efficacy, and satisfaction. *Journal of Counseling & Development, 77*, 447–455.

Ladany, N., Friedlander, M.L., & Nelson, M L. (2005). *Critical events in psychotherapy supervision: An interpersonal approach.* Washington, DC: American Psychological Association.

Ladany, N. Lehrman-Waterman, D.E., Molinaro, M., & Wolgast, B. (1999). Psychotherapy supervisor ethical practices: Adherence to guidelines, the supervisory working alliance, ands supervisee satisfaction. *The Counselling Psychologist, 27*, 443–475.

Ladany, N., & Muse-Burke, J.L. (2001). Understanding and conducting supervision research. In L.J. Bradley & N. Ladany (Eds.), *Counselor supervision: Principles, process, & practice* (3rd ed., pp. 304–329). Philadelphia: Brunner-Routledge.

Leise, B.S., & Alford, B.A. (1998). Recent advances in cognitive therapy supervision. *Journal of Cognitive Therapy: An International Quarterly, 12*, 91–94

Leise, B.S., & Beck, J.S. (1997). Cognitive therapy supervision. In C.E. Watkins (Ed.), *Handbook of psychotherapy supervision* (pp. 113–133). Hoboken, NJ: John Wiley & Sons.

Lent, R.W., Hoffman, M.A., Hill, C.E., Treistman, D., Mount, M., & Singley, D. (2006). Client-specific counselor self-efficacy in novice counselors: Relation to perceptions of session quality. *Journal of Counseling Psychology, 53*, 453–463.

Littrell, J., & Lee-Borden, N., & Lorenz, J. (1979). A developmental framework for counselling supervision. *Counsellor Education and Supervision, 19*, 129–136.

Loganbill, C., Hardy, E., & Delworth, U. (1982) Supervision: A conceptual model. *The Counselling Psychologist, 10*, 3–42.

Meichenbaum, D. (1991). Evolution of cognitive behaviour therapy. In J. Zeig (Ed.), *The evolution of psychotherapy II.* New York: Brunner/Mazel.

Mena, K.C., & Bailey, J.D. (2007). The effects of the supervisory working alliance on worker outcomes. *Journal of Social Service Research, 34*, 55–65.

Miars, R., Tracey, T., Ray, P., Cornfeld, J., O'Farrell, M., & Gelson, C. (1983) Variation in supervision process across trainee experience levels. *Journal of Counselling Psychology, 30*, 403–412.

Mischel, W. (1971). *Introduction to personality.* New York: Holt, Reinhart and Winston.

Perris, C. (1993). Stumbling blocks in the supervision of cognitive psychotherapy. *Journal of Clinical Psychology and Psychotherapy, 1*, 29–43.

Pretorius, W.M. (2006). Cognitive behavioural therapy supervision: Recommended practice. *Behavioural and Cognitive Psychotherapy, 34*, 413–420

Riess, H., & Herman, J.B. (2008). Teaching the teachers: A model course for psychodynamic psychotherapy supervisors. *Academic Psychiatry, 32*, 259–264.

Rosenthal, L. (1999). Group supervision of groups: A modern analytic perspective. *International Journal of Psychotherapy, 49*, 197–213.

Sarnat, J.E. (1992). Supervision in relationship: Resolving the teach–treat controversy in psychoanalytic supervision. *Psychoanalytic Psychology, 9*, 387–403.

Searles, H. (1955). The informational value of the supervisor's emotional experiences. *Psychiatry, 18,* 135–146.

Sterba, R. (1934). The fate of the ego in analytic therapy. *International Journal of Psychoanalysis, 15,* 117–126.

Stoltenberg, C. (1981) Approaching supervision from a developmental perspective: The counsellor complexity model. *Journal of Counselling Psychology, 28,* 59–65.

Stoltenberg, C.D., & Delworth, U. (1987). *Supervising counsellors and therapists: A developmental approach.* San Francisco: Jossey-Bass.

Stoltenberg, C., McNeill, B., & Delworth, U. (1998). *IDM supervision: An integrated developmental model for supervising counselors and therapists.* San Francisco: Jossey-Bass.

Townend, M., Iannetta, L., & Freeston, M.H. (2002). Clinical supervision in practice: A survey of UK cognitive–behavioural psychotherapists accredited by the BABCP. *Behavioural and Cognitive Psychotherapy, 30,* 485–500.

Tracey, T., & Sherry, P. (1993) Complementary interaction over time in successful and less successful supervision. *Professional Psychology: Research and Practice, 24,* 304–311.

Webb, A., & Wheeler, S. (1998). How honest do counsellors dare to be in the supervisory relationship? An exploratory study. *British Journal of Guidance & Counselling, 26,* 509–524.

Wheeler, S. (2007). What shall we do with the wounded healer? The supervisor's dilemma. *Psychodynamic Practice: Individuals, Groups and Organisations, 13,* 245–256.

Wiley, M., & Ray, P. (1986). Counselling supervision by developmental level. *Journal of Counselling Psychology, 33,* 439–445.

Winter, M., & Holloway, E. (1992). Relation of trainee experience, conceptual level and supervisory approach to selection of audiotaped counselling passages. *The Clinical Supervisor, 9,* 2 87–103.

Worthington, E. (1987). Changes in supervision as counsellors and supervisors gain experience: A review. *Professional Psychology: Research and Practice, 18,* 189–209.

Worthington, E., & Stern, A. (1985). The effects of supervisor and supervisee degree level and gender on the supervisory relationship. *Journal of Counselling Psychology, 32,* 252–262.

Zaslavsky, J., Nunes, M., Eizirik, C., & Nurse, G. (2005). Approaching countertransference in psychoanalytical supervision: A qualitative investigation. *International Journal of Psychoanalysis, 86,* 1099–1131.

—|—|—|—|—|—

chapter seven

Alliance Supervision to Enhance Client Outcomes

Matthew Bambling

Overview

Clinical supervision has traditionally been considered an important part of the training and professional development of therapists, being rated highly in the experience of trainees as well as practitioners in the field (Orlinsky, Botermans, & Ronnestad, 2001; Steven, Goodyear, & Robertson, 1998). However, the evidence base for any supervision approach improving outcomes with clients is lacking (Bambling & King, 2000). In this chapter, an alternate nonapproach-bound model of supervision is presented that has preliminary evidence for enhancing client outcomes in brief psychological treatment. The focus of this Three-Stage Alliance Supervision (TSAS) prioritises the interpersonal process of counselling as an independent factor, as well as the core construct through which all technical interventions should be given. Below is an introduction to the supervision model used in the first empirical investigation of supervision and client outcome (Bambling, King, Raue, Schweitzer, & Lambert 2006). While this chapter does not constitute the supervision manual it will provide the reader with sufficient knowledge to adopt an alliance focus in their supervision practice.

Introduction

There are many approaches to supervision, some embedded in models of counselling such as psychodynamic or cognitive–behavioural, or independent of therapy model such as a developmental approach. Bernard and Goodyear (1992) found that therapists assessed supervision as an indispensable training activity that increased both self- and therapeutic awareness. Further, therapists have rated supervision highly as an educational procedure that develops treatment skills and professional competency (Steven, Goodyear, & Robertson, 1998). Supervision is usually considered an important posttraining professional activity and is not restricted to the graduate training setting. During supervision, a supervisor and therapist may systematically examine case-specific treatment and process issues as a method of enhancing both therapist awareness and skills necessary to manage the complexities of client work. Within the practice of psychotherapy and counselling, there is the expectation that supervision might enhance the clinical impact of therapeutic intervention. Therefore, a supervised therapist might reasonably expect to achieve greater clinical outcomes in client work than an unsupervised therapist (Steven et al., 1998).

The proposition that supervision is a procedure that can enhance client outcome was an assumption based on its historical importance in the training and practice of psychotherapy. However, the evidence for how supervision might influence the process of therapy towards positive client outcome has been nearly nonexistent, until recently (Bambling et al., 2006; Bambling & King, 2000). Empirical research into supervision typically focused on supervisory alliance, therapist approach, confidence and core skills, rather than on clearly defined client outcomes such as client symptom reduction (Bambling & King, 2000; Ellis, Dell & Good, 1998; Ladany, Ellis, & Fridlander, 1999). The best test of supervision would be to focus on enhancing an outcome-mediating construct such as the working alliance between client and therapist.

Why Focus on Alliance?

The working alliance represented a usable supervision construct because it is a relational process and involves specific interpersonal skills in therapy. The working alliance is measurable and has a robust relationship with symptom improvement and quality of therapeutic work (Horvath & Bedi, 2002; Martin, Garske, & Davis, 2000). Therefore, the effect of supervision might be found in working alliance scores in the treatment of depression, which is particularly sensitive to alliance in client symptom reduction.

To test this proposition further a three-stage model of alliance supervision (TSAS) was developed that could be operationalised through two accepted supervision methods, skill and process focuses in brief therapy (Bambling et al., 2006). TSAS was tested in a randomised treatment trial of the treatment of depression using eight sessions of problem-solving therapy with 103 clients. Skill and process foci were derived from two dominant traditions in psychotherapy supervision however, the focus was on alliance more so then technique of therapy. In one approach, the supervisor focused on the development of therapist skills thought to enhance alliance based on the CBT tradition (alliance skill focus). In the other, the supervisor focused on therapist awareness of and sensitivity to the therapeutic relationship based on the psychodynamic tradition (alliance process focus).

As demonstrated in Figures 7.1 and 7.2, supervision significantly enhanced working alliance, $f(2) = 54.91$, $p < .01$, and symptom outcome, $f(2) = 13.73$, $p < .01$, for therapists delivering the standardised problem-solving therapy compared with therapists delivering the same treatment without supervision. Of interest is that skill and process focus did not create differential effects, both focuses were similar in effect ($MD = 8.36$, $SE = 4.62$, $p = .221$). The finding of no effect for supervision approach means it is likely that the effectiveness of TSAS rests in common supervision mechanisms. Clients receiving the supervised problem-solving therapy were more likely to complete the full treatment compared to the no supervision control, $\chi^2 (2, n = 103) = 23.83$, $p < .01$. Treatment retention is an important outcome factor as failure to complete therapy means no treatment effect.

The most interesting and unexpected finding of this research was that the supervision had an effect from the first session of therapy. In the supervision conditions, therapists met with supervisors prior to their first treatment session and were given some basic training in the TSAS model to be used in supervision with either skills or process procedures. Simply

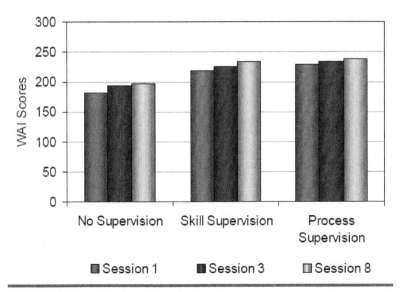

FIGURE 7.1
Working alliance scores by supervision condition.

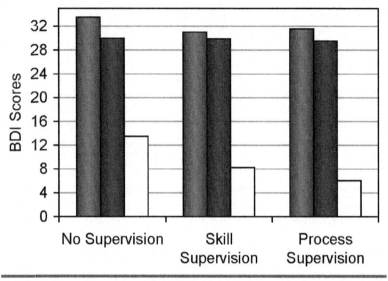

FIGURE 7.2
Symptom response BDI scores by supervision condition.

being aware of the alliance model presented in this chapter seemed to give therapists an advantage over their colleagues in the control conditions. It is likely that those therapists in the control condition were more focused on the technical delivery of the standardised problem-solving therapy, whereas the supervised therapists prioritised relational interventions. This first session finding suggests a training effect for the TSAS supervision manual when used with therapists. Indeed, the model is now used as part of the therapist training curriculum at two prominent Queensland (Australia) universities. The TSAS model is presented below without the skill and process procedures, which will be available in the full treatment manual at a later date.

Three-Stage Alliance Supervision
Introduction
The Three-Stage Model of Alliance Supervision (TSAS) presented here is exactly as used in the randomised clinical trial to test supervision and client outcome (Bambling et al., 2006). The TSAS model was developed by integrating some of the psychotherapy theoretical and empirical constructs of Bordin (1980, 1983), Luborsky, Singer and Luborsky, (1975), and Safran et al., (1990). In this chapter, the TSAS model is described in an applied form with case examples that highlight the application of the

model. Client and therapist names and some details in the clinical examples have been changed to ensure confidentiality.

TSAS is designed to provide procedures for supervisors to assist therapists to recognise and manage the working alliance in therapy. Therefore, this model has a strong educational focus that relies on supervisor capacity to teach and model the principles of alliance management to supervisees. To assist supervisees achieve TSAS learning outcomes a priority is given to developing a positive supervisory alliance with supervisees. A strong supervisory alliance has been shown to enhance:

- supervisee engagement in the supervision process
- preparedness to collaborate with the supervisor in the tasks and goals of supervision
- capacity to learn skills (Lambert & Ogles 1997)
- capacity to model supervisor skills (Schacht, Howe, & Berman, 1989)
- capacity to use learned skills in client work (Bambling & King 2000; Pierce & Schauble 1971; Steven et al., 1998).

Therefore, if supervisors aim to use TSAS principles to maximise supervisee perception of the supervisory alliance, learning outcomes may be enhanced and the behaviours experienced, observed and learned in supervision will be more likely applied to client work.

TSAS

TSAS combines three approaches that may be considered pantheoretical. The first stage of this model is adapted from the work of Bordin (1980) — being bond, task and goals of therapy — and is conceptualised as a series of collaborative tasks. The bond, task and goal components of alliance are particularly relevant to early engagement in therapy. The second stage is adapted from the work of Luborsky et al. (1975). The alliance is conceptualised as having features that may be considered developmental and occurs as two types. The first alliance type, referred to as type 1, relates to the therapeutic bond and early collaboration. The second alliance type, referred to as type 2, relates to the work stage of therapy. From the TSAS perspective, alliance types provide a framework to understand therapeutic process and appropriateness of interventions. The third stage of the TSAS model is adapted from research into alliance rupture management to provide a set of techniques for addressing or avoiding alliance problems (Safran, Muran, & Samstag, 1994). Therefore, the working alliance is conceptualised as a process requiring active therapist management that is explicitly and implicitly negotiated between client and therapist. This explicit and implicit negotiation provides a procedure for therapists to match alliance behaviours to client idiosyncratic preferences for alliance behaviour to enhance client perception of working alliance in therapy (Bambling & King 2001).

STAGE ONE OF TSAS: EARLY ENGAGEMENT

Bordin (1976a, 1976b, 1980, 1989) proposed a definition of the working alliance that contains three component behaviours. This position emphasised the client's positive attachment and collaboration with the therapist against self-defeating thoughts and behaviour. The bond, task and goal components require little modification for use as a supervision construct. The concept of the bond represents the system of positive attachment between the client and therapist and includes the development of trust, acceptance and confidence. The key questions a client asks when developing the bond component is 'Will I be safe and can I work with this therapist?' The therapeutic bond may be defined as the mutual liking, respect and trust between the client and therapist; it is characterised by therapist genuineness, warmth and understanding, and by client confidence in the therapist. Skills that may demonstrate the quality of the bond can be: tone of voice, degree of comfort towards a client discussing difficult issues, therapist nondefensiveness, therapist empathy and the value both participants each place on the other's contribution (Bordin, 1976a, 1976b, 1980, 1989). The primary means of assessing the bond in TSAS is to assist the supervisee assess how the client views the bond by understanding their feelings about each other in therapy.

Tasks are global therapeutic strategies or methods that refer to counselling behaviours, interventions and cognitions that form the counselling process. Supervision offered from the TSAS approach focuses on ensuring that the techniques of the therapy or the strategies developed make sense to the client as an appropriate means of working with their problems. When clients define the tasks as relevant, there is greater acceptance and responsibility for undertaking therapeutic tasks in treatment. The key question a client may ask in therapy regarding the task component is, 'Do I believe that the way my therapist works with me is the correct way to deal with my problems?' It is useful to assist supervisees to understand task functions by thinking about the client perception of techniques: Does it make sense to the client? Does the client understand the rationale for the treatment technique? Does the client agree? Further, therapist roles are attached to implementing tasks. When therapists use a strategy of exploration they adopt the role of facilitator as they help clients to increase awareness of their own thoughts, feelings, values and needs. Where therapists use a strategy of confrontation or direction, they adopt the role of an expert. Most importantly, active negotiation of the appropriateness of treatment techniques and therapist role, and how these apply to the type of problem the client presents, is likely to build consensus about the usefulness of therapy to achieve desired goals. The task component of alliance can be assessed in TSAS according to how responsive the supervisee appears to client reaction and acceptance of the technique of therapy. For agreement to be present regarding the task component of alliance, techniques and ensuing therapist roles should be seen as important, appropriate and clearly understood by both participants.

Goals represent the agreed outcomes and priorities of therapeutic work between the client and therapist. Both must see goals of the session and long-term therapeutic goals as meaningful and relevant. Goals must also be seen as relevant and consistent to interventions or the task component of therapy. Goals may include decrease in symptoms, improvement in interpersonal skills or relationships, awareness of conflicts, development of new ways of thinking and behaving. Often, goals are not made explicit; rather, they are inferred from the topic or focus of the session. The key questions a client may ask when defining the goal component of alliance in therapy are 'To what degree is my therapist clear about my priorities for change and do we share those priorities?' In TSAS, supervisees should be assisted to become aware of client-explicit and implicit goals through actively negotiating these early in therapy through the use of strategic questions and feedback. Goals in therapy can be assessed as the extent to which both participants see the goals of therapy as important, appropriate and clear. Disagreement may be demonstrated through the supervisee/ therapist prioritising different goals to those of the client during a session.

Supervisors should give priority to ensuring that therapists negotiate the bond, task and goal components early in therapy with the client, as it will set realistic expectations and build consensus regarding the therapy. More importantly, consensus ensures the supervisee/therapist is clear regarding what the client is seeking from treatment. A common cause of early poor alliance is unrealistic or unclear expectations by the client. If there is not adequate clarity then supervisee/therapists may find they are working at odds with their client. An additional benefit of early negotiation of task and goal components of the alliance is that it may assist in the development of the bond. Bordin (1980) demonstrated that some attention to the task and goal component in the first session can aid the bond component to develop (see example below). The bond component may be challenging to negotiate in some cases due to client attachment and trust issues. In all cases, it is recommended that attempts be made to actively negotiate the bond in a collaborative non-threatening manner, regardless of individual client attachment and trust issues. For example, in most cases it is important to address early concerns about counselling and negotiate early therapeutic boundaries, and give some attention to task and goals. For clients who may have greater difficulty with developing a bond, some extra attention may be given to issues of confidentiality, addressing client anxiety, not imposing unwanted work or direction, working within client's immediate priorities, demonstrating empathy without being overly intimate and clarifying client expectations of the counselling relationship (Bambling & King, 2001). The bond, task and goal component are the primary early engagement strategy in TSAS model. However, they remain useful strategies to use throughout therapy as a method of continually negotiating therapy and developing a system of mutual feedback that will assist in keeping therapy matched to client preference.

Case Example: Stage 1 of TSAS

Negotiating task, bond and goal to maximise early engagement in therapy in a case of a 25-year-old male presenting with a major depressive episode.

John was a therapist at a community mental health service who was conducting a first session with Mike. Mike had attended a prior intake interview where he was diagnosed with a major depressive episode.

John: What brings you here to see me today?

Mike: I have been feeling very bad, kind of depressed, so many things have been going wrong.

John: Sounds like you have a lot on your plate; can you tell me what has been happening to make you feel depressed?

Mike: I have been feeling so depressed, I am having trouble getting out of bed, I am worried about my job, my relationship, you know it reminds me of when I was a kid and my father never had regular work, I feel insecure about everything now.

John: There are a lot of things here. How long have you been feeling so bad?

Mike: Since work started downsizing ... about a month, I think. I have to work more hours now, but I am really worried that this job will finish, you know my girlfriend and I are thinking about buying a house.

John: I can see why you are feeling depressed at this time. Okay, I will tell you a bit about the way I work here and see if working with me interests you. The approach I use makes an assumption that there is a link between the problems you are having and your feelings of depression. What do you think?

Mike: Well yeah, that seems kind of logical.

John: Okay then, in that case would you agree that if we could work on some of the problems you mentioned it might be likely to improve the way you feel?

Mike: Yeah, I think it could.

John: How we work with depression here is for you and I to work out what we can do about your problems as a team. However, the therapy is for your benefit and therefore you get to identify what you want to work on and the most realistic plan of getting you from where you are now a bit closer to where you would like to be. So we mostly work in the here and now of what is going on for you and apply a systematic approach to solve problems. We normally provide around six sessions here if needed. How does that sound?

Mike: Yeah that would be good, as I want to sort this stuff out and feel confident again.

John: Okay, you can be sure that therapy is confidential and I won't release any information about our work without your express permission or instruction. I am interested if you have any concerns about counselling or if there are things I should know that will help our work, or help me avoid making you uncomfortable?

Mike: Privacy worries me a bit so I am glad it is confidential. The way we will work together sounds fine. I haven't had counselling before, so don't really know what to expect … I am not sure how comfortable I will feel about talking about personal stuff. Maybe I need to test things out a bit as we go?

John: Sounds very reasonable, how about I check with you from time to time to see if we are on track or not moving too quickly? I would like you to feel free to let me know if things are not progressing the way you would like or you are not happy about anything we are doing. That is the best way we can ensure that this process will be of most use to you.

Mike: Sounds good.

John: Okay, perhaps we can identify which problems are most pressing and which problem is worrying you the most today out of all the problems you told me about. You mentioned your job, right?

Mike: Well actually, my biggest worry today is my relationship, my mood is really grating on my girlfriend … she must be getting sick of it.

John: So out of all the problems you mentioned if we worked on your relationship concerns today, would that be your choice?

Mike: Yeah, that would be great.

TSAS Focused Supervision Insights

In this first session scenario with Mike, John asked orientating questions to get a general sense of Mike's problems and general interest in change and goals for counselling. John then specifically addressed task issues with Mike by explaining the approach used in collaborative language, basic rationale and length of treatment to develop consensus and interest in proceeding. Some general attention was then given to bond issues by explaining confidentiality and asking Mike about his concerns. John responded to Mike's concerns by negotiating a feedback process.

Finally, goals were made more explicit for the purposes of the session. John's notion of what Mike wanted to work on was not correct. Mike had prioritised a different session goal to what the therapist assessed as a priority, his relationship with his girlfriend. John willingly accommodated and negotiated Mike's goal for the first session discussion. John had actively negotiated the bond, task and goal aspects of alliance to best match them to Mike's immediate needs and perceptions. Mike was likely to have experienced John as being sensitive and in tune with his needs as well as feeling understood. In this scenario, early engagement was maximised by use of bond, task and goal behaviours and a strong early alliance would be likely formed.

STAGE TWO OF TSAS: DEVELOPMENTAL FEATURES OF ALLIANCE

Luborsky et al. (1975) defined working alliance as dynamic and as occurring in phases. Two types of alliances were identified and the strength of both these alliance categories was related to positive treatment outcome (Luborsky et al., 1975). The beginning stage of therapy is marked by type one alliance that is based on the client experiencing the therapist as supportive and helpful. Type two alliance, the work stage of therapy, is typical of later phases of treatment. Type two provides a sense of working together, shared responsibility and collaboration in achieving treatment goals. Assisting supervisees to identify alliance type in therapy provides a basis for matching therapeutic interventions to the alliance that may minimise strains and ruptures. The following two examples demonstrate how to use these ideas in the supervisory context

Case Example: A Type 1 Alliance Issue

Jim was an experienced therapist at a university clinic and had seen Tom, a very depressed student for the second session. Tom was not improving and complained of feeling worse and stated that he was experiencing a strong desire to bring a gun to the university and go on a shooting spree and then kill himself. Tom then said to Jim, 'but this information is between you and me, and I don't want you to tell anyone what I am thinking about doing'.

TSAS Supervision Insights

In this situation, Jim felt that Tom had engaged in a therapeutic process as he had returned for a second session and was talking to about his concerns and possible actions. However, evaluating the therapy from the perspective of alliance type, Tom had not begun therapeutic work. Tom was unsure if he could work with Jim or if therapy could help him and was looking for some indication of boundaries and containment to begin to define the bond, task and goals of therapeutic work. If therapy were to succeed in this extreme example, before any therapeutic work could occur, type one issues must be addressed. Jim would need to demonstrate to Tom that he was able to deal with his difficulties and extremes. Jim decided that he should let Tom know that he took his threats seriously and describe clearly what measures he would take to ensure both Tom's and others' safety and then negotiate a therapeutic contact in the form of a contract and management plan between sessions.

Case Example: Integrating Stages 1 and 2 of TSAS

Type two alliance — integrating bond, task and goal into type-based alliance thinking: a context for intervention.

Jennifer was seeing Mark, a client who was depressed, and she began to wonder if his depression was secondary to a narcissistic personality disorder. Mark would complain that his wife and children did not respect him or do what he said. It was clear to Jennifer that Mark was aggressive and dominating with his wife and children and felt very underappreciated. Whenever Jennifer tried to discus the impact of Mark's behaviour on his family he would become angry and accuse her of not understanding or respecting him. Jennifer would become scared and withdraw.

TSAS Supervision Insights

In supervision Jennifer discussed this apparent therapeutic impasse. Examining this case from an alliance perspective revealed several issues. Firstly, a bond had developed, or type one alliance was achieved. Mark kept his appointments and would take the trouble to dress nicely, so contact with Jennifer was important to him. There was some idea of a goal as Mark was committed to dealing with family problems. However, type two, the work stage of therapy, had not yet developed, there was no understanding or agreement between Mark and Jennifer regarding how his goal would be achieved. The block to moving to type two alliance in therapy was that the task component of alliance had not been adequately negotiated with Mark.

Using Jennifer's insights about Mark's narcissism it was clear he experienced confronting questions as insults and as siding with his perception of disrespectful family members. It was clear that if therapy was to be effective then this impasse had to be confronted. However, given Mark's sensitivities, confrontation needed to be couched in an alliance-appropriate form as not to rupture the relationship and risk termination. Jennifer decided she would confront Mark using collaborative and supportive language as not to injure his narcissism and match her intervention to alliance type one. Jennifer felt this intervention would invite Mark to engage in the work stage (type two) by negotiating how the communication and feedback tasks of therapy should be conducted around difficult issues.

In the following session Jennifer told Mark that she wanted to raise an issue with him because she both respected him (using Mark's language as a reference point) and valued their work together. Jennifer said she was concerned that if she did not raise this issue it would affect their mutual work on his goal of sorting out family issues. Jennifer told Mark that sometimes she would react to what he said and would like to honestly respond to him but held back because she was concerned that he would become angry and upset with her and may discontinue counselling. She said she knew that because respect was important to him he would not like this to be the case and would want to negotiate how she could talk to him more honestly and openly. Mark expressed concern and said he wanted honest responses but knew he could get angry easily. Jennifer and Mark contracted a process for communicating and feedback. In the next supervision session Jennifer reported that the intervention was successful and she had also noticed greater engagement and Mark had begun to do work in therapy indicating that type two alliance was developing.

STAGE THREE OF TSAS: RUPTURE MANAGEMENT

A considerable body of research suggests that in successful therapy it is relatively common for the working alliance to go through a series of ruptures and repairs, or become strained (Horvath & Symonds, 1991; Safran Crocker, McMain, & Munay, 1990; Safran, Muran, Wallner, & Samstag, 1992). Strains and ruptures are often the result of clients dealing with problematic issues and difficult patterns of behaviour. If therapy is to be successful then alliance rupture must be repaired. Unrepaired alliance ruptures are related to treatment dropout (Safran, Muran, Samstag, & Winston, 2002). The quality of early alliance is particularly important to later successful rupture management as it assists clients to deal with the strains of therapeutic work. The ability of a therapist to directly intervene to address problems in the therapeutic relationship is a key intervention that has been shown to repair ruptures, improve working alliance and reduce early treatment termination (Safran et al., 1992). The final stage of the TSAS model focuses on managing strains and ruptures through assisting supervisees to focus on conflictual or potentially problematic relationship patterns in therapy. Interventions are then created to correct alliance ruptures to improve overall client engagement and total quality of alliance in therapy.

STAGE 3 OF TSAS: RUPTURE MANAGEMENT AND INTEGRATING STAGE 1 AND 2

Case Example: The Third Stage of the TSAS Model

Integrating rupture management with alliance type and bond, task and goal aspects of alliance.

Mary was a therapist who was seeing Wendy, a 45-year-old woman who was depressed. Wendy lived an isolated life and found intimacy difficult and struggled with the early working alliance. Wendy identified some goals for change in the first session relating to her relationships with adult siblings, yet spent the following three sessions talking about her family of origin experiences. Eventually, Mary felt that Wendy should start working on these issues according to her expressed goals. A subtle conflict developed between them regarding the goals and tasks of therapy. Wendy did not appear interested in the therapeutic interventions Mary provided or the strategies used in counselling to achieve stated goals. Eventually, Wendy implied she would terminate therapy as she was not getting anything out of treatment, at which point Mary sought supervision.

TSAS Supervision Insights

Wendy's difficulties with interpersonal relationships made it difficult for Mary to identify alliance development. Mary had doubts whether Wendy was doing any work in therapy. However, Wendy had in fact progressed to the type two work stage alliance. From an alliance point of view the difficulty was that Mary was working with a set of goals originally contracted with Wendy. Wendy had implicitly changed her goals over a number of sessions, stating to Mary that she was finding the exploration of family-of-origin issues for the first time in her life very useful. The tendency for Wendy to evoke power issues in others resulted in loss of empathy, reducing awareness of the alliance rupture or need to repair the alliance. A serious alliance rupture had occurred that involved bond, task and goal issues and dropout was likely without intervention. Mary decided to confront the relational issues directly to address the alliance rupture and renegotiate the bond, task and goals of therapy. Wendy missed her next session and Mary made a follow-up telephone call. Mary told Wendy she had thought about their prior session and she was concerned that she was off track with Wendy's needs and not giving her the freedom to explore issues that were important to her. Mary renegotiated the tasks and goals of the therapeutic work with Wendy. Wendy was clearly pleased and returned to therapy. Mary found that as communication had improved there was opportunity to give and receive feedback that assisted her to keep therapy matched to Wendy's needs and preferences. In this case Mary had identified an alliance rupture and intervened directly to repair the rupture. Addressing relational problems by validating and accommodating Wendy's view of the therapy and renegotiating the task and goals also had a positive impact on the bond. Mary reported that Wendy seemed to connect more with her after alliance was repaired and there was a sense of greater energy in the type two, the work stage of alliance.

Conclusion

TSAS provides an intuitively appealing simple model that supervisors can integrate into their practice that has demonstrated efficacy. As TSAS is founded in a pantheoretical framework it should be possible for supervisors of all approaches to integrate it into their practice. The significant effects found for a pre-treatment session of TSAS suggests that this mode of supervision provides an important educational experience for supervisees, assisting them to develop sensitivity to the alliance. In summary, the TSAS supervisor assists the supervisee to understand, establish, manage and repair the working alliance with their client during treatment. TSAS supervisors prioritise developing a positive supervisory alliance with their supervisee and actively model working alliance principles and provide feedback as key learning strategies.

TSAS is the first supervision model to have proved to be an effective agent to enhance client outcome through directly impacting on the quality of therapist work. However, the message of TSAS is that it is not the specific techniques of supervision but rather the focus of supervision that has an impact, which suggests that there is much yet to be learned about how supervision influences client outcome. Therefore, this new evidence for supervision in brief therapy should be regarded as preliminary and clearly more research is needed to better understand the mechanisms by which supervision achieves benefits for clients.

Educational Questions and Activities

1. What are the key principles of TSAS?
   (a) understanding therapeutic process from an alliance perspective.
   (b) a focus on treatment techniques.
   (c) managing the working alliance with clients in therapy.
   (d) dealing with client resistance in therapy
   (e) a and c
   (f) all of the above.
   Answer (e)

2. What does a TSAS-oriented supervisor do in supervision?
   (a) models TSAS skills for their supervisee
   (b) develops a positive supervisory alliance with their supervisee
   (c) teaches the TSAS model to supervisees
   (d) provides regular evaluation and feedback to supervisees

(e) a and c

(f) all of the above.

Answer (f)

3. Why might a focus on working alliance be more important than a focus on delivering the techniques of therapy in supervision?

   (a) Working alliance between client and therapist predicts treatment outcome whereas therapy technique does not.

   (b) Working alliance as rated by clients mediates their response to therapy regardless of treatment approach.

   (c) Working alliance as rated by clients predicts engagement and retention in counselling.

   (d) all of the above

   Answer (d)

4. If your supervisee reports they are stuck in therapy with a client what should you do from a TSAS perspective?

   (a) revisit the treatment plan

   (b) confront the client about the impasse

   (c) provide more skilful techniques to address the impasse

   (d) examine the issues existing in the working relationship between therapist and client

   Answer (d)

5. What are the three components that constitute the TSAS model?

   (a) bond, task, goal; stages of alliance; managing strains and ruptures in the working alliance

   (b) education, learning goals, and experience level

   (c) understanding defences, transference and the unconscious processes in therapy

   (d) developing individualised treatment plans, teaching therapeutic skills and measuring symptom reduction.

   Answer (a)

References

Bambling, M., King, R., Raue, P., Schweitzer, R., & Lambert, W. (2006). Clinical supervision: Its impact on working alliance and outcome in the treatment of major depression. *Psychotherapy Research, 16*(3), 317–331.

Bambling, M., & King, R. (2001). Therapeutic alliance and clinical practice. *Psychotherapy in Australia, 8*(1), 38–47.

Bambling, M., & King, R., (2000). Supervision and the development of counsellor competency. *Psychotherapy in Australia, 6*(4), 58–63.

Bernard, J., & Goodyear, R. (1992). *Fundamentals of clinical supervision.* Boston: Allyn & Bacon.

Bordin, E. (1976a). *The working alliance; Basis for a general theory of psychotherapy.* Paper presented at the Annual Convention of the American Psychological Association, Washington, DC.

Bordin, E. (1976b). The generalizability of the psychoanalytic concept of the working alliance. *Psychotherapy: Theory Research and Practice, 16,* 252–260.

Bordin, E.S. (1980, June). *Of human bonds that bind or free.* Paper presented at the annual meeting of the Society for Psychotherapy Research, Pacific Grove, CA.

Bordin, E.S. (1983). A working alliance based model of supervision. *The Counseling Psychologist, 11*(1), 35–42.

Bordin, E.S. (1989, April). *Building therapeutic alliances; the base for integration.* Paper presented at the annual meeting of the Society for the Exploration of Psychotherapy Integration, Berkeley, CA.

Ellis, M., Dell, D., & Good, G. (1988). Counselor trainees' perceptions of supervisor roles: Two studies testing the dimensionality of supervision. *Journal of Counseling Psychology, 35,* 315–334.

Horvath, A.O. (1991) *What do we know about the alliance and what do we still have to find out?* Paper presented at the annual meeting of the Society for Psychotherapy Research, Lyon, France.

Horvath, A., & Bedi, R. (2002). The alliance. In J.C. Norcross (Ed.), *Psychotherapy relationships that work* (pp. 37–69). Oxford: Oxford University.

Horvath A.O., & Symonds B.D. (1991). Relation between working alliance and outcome in psychotherapy: A meta-analysis. *Journal of Counseling Psychology 38*(2), 139–149.

Lambert, M., & Ogles, B. (1997). *The effectiveness of psychotherapy supervision.* In Watkins, C., Jr. (Ed.), *Handbook of psychotherapy supervision* (pp. 421–446). New York, John Wiley & Sons.

Ladany, N., Ellis, M., & Fridlander, M. (1999). The supervisory alliance, trainee self-efficacy, and satisfaction. *Journal of Counselling and Development, 77,* 447–455.

Luborsky, L., Singer, B., & Luborsky, L. (1975). Comparative studies of psychotherapies: Is it true that 'everybody has won and all must have prizes'? *Archives of General Psychiatry, 32,* 995–1008.

Martin D.J., Garske J.P., & Davis, M.K. (2000). Relation of the therapeutic alliance with outcome and other variables: A meta-analytic review. *Journal of Consulting and Clinical Psychology, 68*(3), 438–50.

Orlinsky, D., Botermans, J., & Ronnestad, M. (2001). Towards an empirically grounded model of psychotherapy training: Four thousand therapists rate influences on their development. *Australian Psychologist, 36,* 139–149.

Pierce, M., & Schauble, G. (1971). Graduate training of facilitative counsellors: The effects of individual supervision. *Journal of Counselling Psychology, 17,* 210–215.

Safran, J., Crocker, P., McMain, S., & Munay, P. (1990).Therapeutic alliance rupture as a therapy event for empirical investigation. *Psychotherapy, 27,* 154–164.

Safran, J., Muran, J., & Samstag, L. (1994). Resolving therapeutic ruptures: A task analytic investigation. In A.O. Horvath & L.S. Greenberg (Eds.), *The working alliance: Theory, research, and practice.* New York: Wiley.

Safran, J., Muran, C., Samstag, S., & Winston, A. (2002, June). *A comparative treatment study of potential treatment failures.* Paper presented at the Society for Psychotherapy Research annual meeting, Santa Barbara, CA.

Safran, J., Muran, J., Wallner, S., & Samstag, L. (1992, June). *A comparison of therapeutic alliance rupture resolution and nonresolution events.* Paper presented at the annual meeting of the Society for Psychotherapy Research, Berkeley, CA.

Schacht, J., Howe, E. Jr., & Berman, J. (1989). Supervisor facilitative conditions and effectiveness as perceived by thinking- and feeling-type supervisees. *Psychotherapy, 26,* 475–483.

Steven, D., Goodyear, R., & Robertson, P. (1998). Supervisor development: an exploratory study in changes in stance and emphasis. *Clinical Supervisor, 16*(2), 73–88.

chapter eight

Processes and Interventions to Facilitate Supervisees' Learning

Keithia Wilson and Alf Lizzio

This chapter seeks to answer the fundamental question: What supervisory processes and interventions can be used to support the learning of supervisees? Three types of interventions will be considered: contracting and relationship-building, supervisor metacompetencies for facilitating learning and specific supervisory learning activities.

Supervision is a complex intervention that is best conceptualised as an interpersonal exchange (Bernard & Goodyear, 2004). Thus, any meaningful consideration of supervisory interventions needs to be contextualised within the supervisory relationship. There is strong evidence to indicate that the quality of supervision in the formative stages of professional development has a longstanding effect on supervisees (Barnett, Doll, Younggren, & Rubin, 2007; Milne & Westerman, 2001), and findings from a range of studies indicate, collectively, that supervision is a powerful process with the potential for both enhancing, as well as stunting the growth of supervisees (Barnett, Cornish, Goodyear, & Lichtenberg, 2007; Gazzola & Theriault, 2007a, 2007b). The empirical evidence indicates that the quality of the supervisory relationship is both a foundational intervention goal in its own right and enabling of more specific supervisory methods and interventions used (Kilminster & Jolly, 2000).

Given that the origins of supervision lie in the helping professions, it is not surprising that supervisory methods and processes have traditionally been conceptualised using counselling frameworks. However, the increasing generality of the process to a wider range of professions has facilitated the broadening of the construct from a counselling to an educational

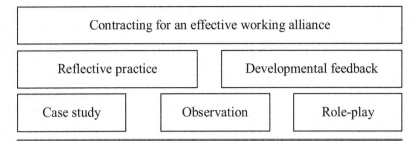

FIGURE 8.1
The structure of supervisory interventions.

orientation (Carroll, 1996; Lizzio & Wilson, 2002). This is leading to a greater emphasis on understanding professional supervision as a learning relationship (Lizzio, Stokes, & Wilson, 2005).

Facilitating supervisees' learning can be conceptualised as a scaffolded process (see Figure 8.1). At the most foundational level the process of contracting is used to establish a working alliance that optimises supervisees' development and self-regulation. The learning potential of the supervisor–supervisee alliance is then realised through the metaprocesses of critical reflection on the supervisees' practice and the provision of quality developmental feedback. These metaprocesses are inherent facets of the commonly used supervisory interventions of case study, observation and role-play.

Thus, this chapter is structured in three parts. The first part focuses on meta-process interventions, in particular contracting, that can contribute to a positive supervisory working alliance. The second part focuses on the learning processes (for instance, facilitation of reflective practice and the provision of constructive feedback), which underpin the effectiveness of the supervisory interventions. The third part focuses on the use of specific interventions (for example, case study, observation, role-plays) in supervision.

Establishing an Effective Working Alliance

The quality of the supervisory relationship is the basis for learning in supervision and makes a critical contribution to both positive processes and outcomes (McMahon & Simons, 2004; Worthen & McNeil, 1996). A strong supervisory working alliance, at best, prevents the development of supervisor–supervisee conflict, and at worst, mitigates supervisor–supervisee differences and difficulties (Bordin, 1993; Nelson, Barnes, Evans, & Triggiano, 2008). As Watkins (1997) eloquently states, the supervisory relationship is 'a necessary ingredient to the making, doing, and being of the supervision process itself and seemingly facilitates or potentiates whatever takes place within that process' (p. 4). Despite the importance of quality supervisory relationships, the experience of relationship difficulties is relatively common. Negative supervision experiences have been reported from a number of authors (e.g., Barnett et al., 2007; Ellis, 2001). For example, Galante (1998) found 47% of trainees in her study had experienced at least one ineffective supervisory relationship. Thus, at a metaprocess or macro level, a positive supervisory working alliance can be considered the most potent intervention for promoting effective personal and professional development in supervisees.

So, what are the qualities of an effective supervisory relationship? There is reasonable consensus that a trusting and collaborative relationship is a prerequisite for success, and that supervisors need to create a safe learning environment in which supervisees can openly discuss their work, raise concerns about their competence and personal limitations, and have permission and support to experiment with new strategies, techniques and behaviours (Barrett & Barber, 2005; Ellis, 1991; Ladany, Ellis, & Friedlander, 1999; Wulf & Nelson, 2000). Moreover, there is strong evidence to indicate that timing is important in the development of an effective supervisory relationship. The quality of supervision in the formative stages of professional development has been shown to have a longstanding effect on supervisees (Milne & Westerman, 2001). Thus, interventions that build a trusting, collaborative and safe working relationship at the outset of supervision are critical to learning success.

A potent early intervention for building an effective supervisory working alliance is contracting. The *content* purpose of contracting is to establish a clear working agreement regarding the goals, roles and processes of the supervisee–supervisor relationship. The failure to establish such shared expectations from the outset has been identified as a key source of conflict between supervisees and supervisors (Nelson et al., 2008). Beyond this, not surprisingly, more effective outcomes are reportedly achieved when supervisees are engaged as active partners (e.g., conjoint goal-setting, process review) in the supervisory process (Sheikh, Milne, & MacGregor, 2007) and have some input into and control over the supervisory process (Kilminster & Jolly, 2000). Thus the *process* purpose of contracting is to establish supervisees as empowered co-creators of the supervisory process. Some regulatory boards in North America, Europe and Australia require supervisors to outline their beliefs about and orientation to supervision (e.g., the supervision model that informs their practice, modalities typically employed). Such transparency can be thought of as a 'supervisor's epistemological declaration' (Liddel, 1988, p. 157) and the accountable disclosure of the professional and organisational elements within the supervision context (Magnuson,

Norem, & Wilcoxon, 2000). Thus the *ethical* purpose of contracting is to provide the supervisee with the basis for informed choice. There is also considerable literature that supports the importance of goal-setting in learning (Brookfield, 1986). For example, learning contracts have been demonstrated to result in stronger engagement with learning processes and more effective learning outcomes (Knowles, 1984). Thus the *educational* purpose of contracting is to optimise the relevance and effectiveness of supervisees' learning.

So what are the key areas of contracting in supervision? Contracting involves both supervisor and supervisee discussing the following types of questions:

• What learning goals shall we pursue?
• What approach to learning suits our circumstances?
• What type of relationship do we wish to have?
• What management processes do we wish to establish?

We propose that a capacity to formulate and set explicit and meaningful goals is not only a key part of the contracting process, but also the foundation for a mutually empowering and systematic learning process for both supervisor and supervisee. Thus, the process of contracting is, in fact, the primary or meta-intervention in supervision. The core learning goal or capability that enables a professional to continue to develop and direct themselves outside the context of supervision is proposed as a capacity for self-management and self-regulated learning — a set of metaskills that enable more specific skills to be appropriately and strategically applied. Thus, used reflectively and interactively, these agenda-setting or contracting processes are, in essence, interventions to facilitate supervisee self-regulation.

What Learning Goals Shall We Pursue?

There is strong agreement that effective supervision is goal-focused and outcome-oriented (Kilminster & Jolly, 2000). A supervisor and supervisee having a 'shared map' or 'common language' about the range of goals and outcomes they might achieve together in supervision provides a number of benefits: facilitating the coordinated setting of goals, and making clearly discussable the developmental nature of supervision and the fact that priorities will necessarily change over time. There are a range of approaches to identifying learning goals (e.g., from structured checklists to open-ended discussions) and use will vary depending on personal preferences, career stage and the requirements of regulatory authorities. The following is one approach to conceptualising the potential domain of learning goals for supervision (Lizzio & Wilson, 2002):

- self-regulation: capacity to independently self-reflect on practice and learn from experience
- systemic competence: understanding and managing the context of professional practice, working relationships and organisational dynamics
- role efficacy: managing the expectations and requirements of one's formal role or position (e.g., work standards, practices and accountabilities)
- conceptual competence: conceptualising practice and explicating underlying principles that inform interventions
- ethical judgment: accountably addressing the issues and dilemmas stimulated by practice
- technical competence: mastery of the techniques and strategies for intervention and service delivery
- personal development: awareness and management of the personal aspects of professional practice.

What Approach to Learning Suits Our Circumstances?

There is a well-established distinction in the educational literature between didactic and collaborative/facilitative pedagogies (Smerdon, Burkam, & Lee, 1999). Didactic approaches involve a teacher-controlled process of knowledge transmission (Vaill, 1996) and emphasise the learner's need for instruction, support and guidance in decision-making (Corno & Snow, 1986). Facilitative approaches involve the learner's active involvement (Jarvela & Salovaara, 2004) and emphasise an interactive reflection on the learner's experience. Thus, for example, in the context of professional supervision, a supervisor providing advice on how to address a specific issue could be said to be employing a didactic approach. In the same situation if the supervisor helped the supervisee develop their own judgment on the issue they would be exemplifying a facilitative approach.

Our research conducted with graduates undertaking mandated professional supervision to gain registration as psychologists found that supervisors' approaches to supervision were similarly understood by supervisees in terms of facilitative and didactic approaches to learning (Lizzio et al., 2005). Importantly, supervisors' use of a facilitative approach reduced supervisees' anxiety and resistance and increased their sense of professional self-regulation. Similarly, Couchon and Bernard (1984) found that, in supervision sessions conducted before a counselling session, supervisors tended to be more directive and prescriptive with supervisees, but that little of this was able to be translated into practice by the supervisee. In contrast, however, a supervisor's behaviour was more facilitative following a counselling session, with resulting high levels of transfer of learning by the supervisee into their counselling practice. These findings do not suggest that supervisors should not engage in direct instruction where appropriate, but rather that 'teaching' should be delivered within a broader facilitative approach.

In addressing the question of 'what approach to learning best suits our circumstances?' the supervisor and supervisee might usefully discuss:

The *process of learning* in supervision

- When and how might the supervisor use facilitative and reflective methods of learning?
- When and how might the supervisor use teaching or information transmission methods?

The *content of learning* in supervision

- To what extent might the supervisor focus on theory?
- To what extent might the supervisor focus on practical techniques?

What Type of Relationship Do We Wish to Have?

The relational style of a supervisor has been defined as the distinctive and consistent manner of engaging with supervisees and implementing the process of supervision (Fernando & Hulse-Killacky, 2005; Kennard, Stewart, & Gluck, 1987). There is strong empirical support for the conceptualisation of the supervisory relationship as comprising the three relationship factors of support, challenge and openness (Lizzio, Wilson, & Que, in press). *Support* can be operationalised as the extent to which the supervisee feels adequate and affirmed as a result of their interactions with their supervisor. *Challenge* can be operationalised as the extent to which the supervisee feels challenged and stretched as a result of their interactions with their supervisor. *Openness* can be operationalised as the extent to which the supervisee feels their supervisor relates to them openly and nondefensively in regard to their background, limitations and opinions.

Achieving an optimal balance of support and challenge is essential to effective supervisee and client outcomes. This has been identified not only as one of the most frequent sources of conflict in supervision, but also as one that can be readily resolved (Moskowitz & Rupert, 1983). Overall, a supervisor's goal is to provide sufficient challenge to stimulate growth and development, with enough support to enable the supervisee to adequately respond to the learning opportunity without retreating.

Research into high-quality supervision has identified a key aspect of openness as the supervisor's willingness to surface and discuss potential or actual issues and to actively problem-solve them. Thus, openness has been related to effective conflict management in supervision (Nelson & Friedlander, 2001).

In addressing the question 'what type of relationship might we wish to have?' supervisor and supervisee might usefully discuss:

- What type and level of support might be valued? What forms of support might be counterproductive?
- What type and level of challenge might be valued? What forms of challenge might be counterproductive?
- What type and level of supervisor openness or disclosure might be appropriate?

What Management Processes Do We Wish to Establish?

There are also a range of practical management processes that need to be explicated as part of the working supervisory contract.

- Purpose: To what extent is supervision for purposes of professional development and/or monitoring of quality and accountability?
- Boundary management: What boundaries conditions (e.g., confidentiality, dual relationships) need to be discussed?
- Preparation: What level or type of preparation is expected between sessions?
- Feedback: How will the supervisory process be reviewed and evaluated?

Both supervisors and supervisees might use the contracting framework to inform critical self-reflection about their current and preferred approaches.

Supervisor Reflection

- What is your current approach to contracting? How systematically and explicitly do you use contracting as an intervention process?
- Which intervention domains (e.g., learning goals, learning processes, relationship profile and, management procedures) are under- or overemphasised in your practice?
- How do you use contracting to facilitate supervisees' capacity for self-regulation?
- Do you have a supervisory resumé or position that summarises your approach to supervision?

Supervisee Reflection

- To what extent are you willing to share responsibility for the management of the supervisory process?

- What are your needs and preferences across the various intervention domains (e.g., learning goals, relationships)?
- What conditions will optimise your learning in supervision?

Initial Contracting

- How might you as a supervisor educate about and empower your supervisee in the contracting process?
- How might you as a supervisee educate and empower yourself in the contracting process?
- What type of 'working agreement' do you both wish to have?

Ongoing Review

- How might you as a supervisor educate your supervisees about the developmental nature of supervision, and the fact that their priorities will necessarily change over time as their confidence and skills develop?
- How might you as a supervisee take responsibility for letting your supervisor know when you would like to discuss possible changes to ways of working?
- What ongoing processes might be used to review personal development and goal achievement in individual sessions and in supervision overall?

Supervisory Metacompetencies

There are a number of well-established supervisory methodologies to develop supervisees' capability (e.g., case studies, role-plays, observation of practice). While these will be discussed in a subsequent section of this chapter, it is firstly important to understand that their effective use is underpinned by two supervisory metacompetencies: providing supervisees with constructive feedback and facilitating supervisees' reflection of their practice. The central role of these metacompetencies is well acknowledged in the supervision literature (Hill, Stahl, & Roffman, 2007; Lambert & Arnold, 1987; Milne & James, 2000).

Processes for Constructive Feedback

Effective supervisors have been found to not only establish a nonthreatening and supportive learning environment, but relatedly to provide constructive feedback to their supervisees (Kilminster & Jolly, 2000). There is evidence to suggest that while the provision of feedback is generally perceived positively by trainees (Holmwood, 1993; Kadushin, 1992), critical and negative feedback from supervisors has been associated with increased anxiety and decreased sense of self-efficacy by supervisees (Larson & Daniels, 1998). Clearly, the quality of supervisor feedback would seem to be a key mediator of supervisees' ability to learn from experience.

At the level of general strategy there is a fair degree of consensus that feedback perceived to be effective evidences two key features. Firstly, effective feedback should provide specific information regarding the perceived gap between current and perceived performance (Butler, 1993; DeNisi & Kluger, 2000). Secondly, effective feedback should allow the recipient to participate or be actively involved. De Nisi and Kluger (2000) argue feedback that causes the recipient to focus less on the task and more on the self (a dynamic termed meta-task processing) is more likely to attenuate or reduce performance. The idea here is that focusing on self- or identity-related issues (e.g., 'What will my supervisor think of me?' 'What is going to happen to me at work if I do not perform well?' or 'Am I cut out to do this work?') occupy cognitive resources that could otherwise be used to improve task performance. Providing opportunities for supervisees to 'have a voice' has been found to mitigate self-oriented or meta-task processing when receiving negative or developmental feedback (Lind & Tyler, 1988; Lizzio, Wilson, & McKay, 2008).

Forms of Participation and Voice

While supervisee participation is clearly beneficial to the feedback process, it can be operationalised in different ways. The various forms of bilateral participation employed include: value-expressive or process control (the opportunity to express versions of events or rebut alternative versions; Greenberg, 1986); outcome control (the chance to contribute to the final decision or evaluation); general involvement (equitable proportion of airtime; Cawley, Keeping & Levy, 1998), and self-appraisal (opportunities to self-assess prior to external feedback; Kanfer, Sawyer, Earley, & Lind, 1987). While all of these modes of participation have been found to enhance the effectiveness of feedback, it is expressive participation (the opportunity for the recipient to present their personal viewpoints or reactions to feedback) that consistently evidences the stronger association with positive evaluations (Cawley et al., 1998).

The timing and nature of opportunities for supervisees' voice or participation are important considerations in the construction of a feedback intervention. Findings to date indicate that both inviting a supervisee to react or respond to feedback — a process of facilitating 'voice' subsequent to supervisor feedback (i.e., 'I'm interested to hear your opinions of what I've said?'), and providing opportunities for self-appraisal — a process of facilitating 'voice' prior to the supervisor feedback (i.e., 'Are there any issues from your point of view that would be useful for us to discuss?') (Lizzio, Wilson & McKay, 2008; Skarlicki & Folger, 1997) are effective strategies for reducing supervisee reactance. However, an invitation to respond to supervisor feedback is perceived most positively by supervisees, perhaps because this strategy provides opportunities for 'feedback correctability' (Skarlicki & Folger, 1997) and, on a symbolic level, may provide a stronger signal about the valuing of supervisees.

The optimal protocol for giving feedback has been found to combine a sequence of strategies: invitation to self-appraise positive feedback, developmental feedback and invitation to respond to the feedback. This strategy is consistently evaluated as more effective and as less risky (reducing supervisees' feelings of confusion and anxiety; Lizzio et al., 2008). This evidence-based protocol for providing constructive developmental feedback is presented below:

1. Invite and facilitate the supervisee to self-review using open-ended questions (e.g., 'How do you think you went with …?')

2. Express appreciation for their efforts (e.g., 'You really tried to …') acknowledge their achievements (e.g., 'You were able to …') & show awareness of the context (e.g., levels of complexity or difficulty; e.g., 'What I thought was particularly challenging was …')

3. Provide data based feedback on 'performance gaps'
   • be timely (give the feedback close to the event),
   • be specific and concrete,
   • provide data-based examples,
   • indicate the consequences of the behaviour/strategy/technique used for the client/system/supervisee.

4. Invite their response to your feedback and discuss their reactions (in terms of ability, motivation, opportunity, learning; e.g., 'I very much want to get your perspective on this. What is your first reaction?')

5. Invite their ideas for practice improvement or change (e.g., 'What do you think might be useful …')

6. Provide comment on their ideas, adding in any additional ideas you may have as the supervisor.

7. Invite their response to your ideas.

8. Collaboratively plan the supervisee's practice development and future learning (achievement, improvement, enabling)

9. Briefly review the feedback process for the supervisee's perceptions of fairness, effectiveness (e.g., 'I would value your feedback on this feedback process …')

10. Invite follow-up on the feedback at the next contact/session (e.g., 'Would it be useful to revisit this at a later date to see if …?')

Facilitating Reflective Practice

Supervisees commonly report that the greatest impetus for their change or learning comes from actual events or critical incidents that are outside of their control, experience and understanding (Kilminster & Jolly, 2000). Clearly, frameworks and interventions that are able to facilitate the extraction of 'learning from experience' and the development of 'confidence from crisis' are foundational components of a supervisor's repertoire. Not surprisingly, 'reflection on practice' has been proposed as the defining focus of supervisory practice (Booley, 1997; Fish & Twinn, 1997; Fisher, 1996; Paterson, 1994), and more recently we have seen the emergence of systematic training programs to develop reflective practice as a core learning mechanism in supervision (Sheikh et al., 2007).

Simply framed, supervisors are involved in assisting supervisees to learn from their experience. A practical understanding of experiential learning is central to the success of this enterprise. The experiential learning model is widely acknowledged as particularly appropriate for adult learning contexts such as supervision (Milne & Westerman, 2001). There is both theoretical argument (Hager, 1999) and empirical evidence (Kember & Leung, 2005; Lizzio & Wilson, 2004) to indicate that didactic strategies rarely contribute to generative or metacognitive learning outcomes. The tacit nature of key aspects of professional knowledge (Sternberg & Horvath, 1999) means that they are more likely to be developed through reflection on action (Marsick & Watkins, 1996). In this sense, metacognitive skill is developed though the process of reflecting on performance in context.

We argue that one of the fundamental goals of supervision should be developing the capacity for professional judgment: the ability to confidently act in 'no right answer' (Schon, 1983), or 'unfamiliar and changing' circumstances (Stephenson & Weil, 1992). In this regard it is important to distinguish the learning goals of 'developing competence' (a capacity to routinely apply previously acquired knowledge) and 'developing capability' (a capacity to generatively question the assumptions that inform current practice) (Stephenson, 1998). These goals respectively reflect Argyris and Schon's (1974) classic distinction between the processes of single and double loop learning.

The act of reflection, in itself, does not necessarily engender learning. Supervisors need to be able to scaffold supervisees' efforts at reflection to create a zone of proximal development (the gap between the quality of unassisted reflection and what can be potentially achieved with guidance or structure) (Vygotsky, 1978) is particularly relevant in this context. Supervisees' critical thinking will be enhanced if they are purposely engaged and supported in three related practices: examining their assumptions, considering evidence from multiple perspectives and taking responsibility for making a considered conclusion based on their reflections (King & Kitchener, 2004).

The ways in which people make sense of, or represent the world (their mental models, personal theories, guiding values, theories in use; Senge, 1990) is the primary focus or content of these reflective processes. As Dall'Alba and Sandberg (1996) demonstrate, the way in which practitioners understand professional practice (e.g., their underlying ideas and schemas about what they should be trying to achieve as a professional in a particular situation) is the basis for how they perform. In Argyris and Schon's (1974) terms, peoples' 'governing values' drive their 'action strategies'.

Thus, in essence, the process of problematisation or critical reflection involves making previous tacit aspects of situational appraisal (taken-for-granted beliefs and assumptions) explicit and subject to conscious scrutiny (Claxton, 1999). The guiding tenet is that awareness of assumptions is key to effectiveness. Untested assumptions (e.g., what we might construe others' motives to be in a situation), by definition, have a greater probability of contributing to ineffective outcomes. In this sense, effectiveness is a function of the degree of match or congruence between our espoused theory (what we think or say we believe and do) and our theory in use (what we actually believe and do) (Argyris & Schon, 1974). As Dall'Alba (2004) argues, it is the exploration of assumptions that facilitates a richer description of the interdependency of professionals and their practice.

A simple shared framework can be particularly helpful in facilitating critical reflective dialogue between supervisor and supervisee. The reflective practice cycle (see Figure 8.2) can be used to aid supervisees engage in structured planning or prospective analysis (*What might I do in this situation?*) or retrospective reflection (*What did I do in this situation?*). The framework can be used to scaffold reflection from *multiple points of entry*. Thus, for example, a supervisee might commence a discussion by reporting their intentions (*What they want to achieve*). The supervisor can help the supervisee explore their thinking by inviting either backward reflection (*e.g., What diagnosis are these intentions based on? What data informs your diagnosis?*) or forward reflection (e.g., *What might you actually do? What might be likely consequences?*).

The framework is particularly useful for helping supervisees reflect on potential gaps or discontinuities in their practice. The most common forms of these are:

- What is the level of congruence between what I observe (data or evidence) and the meaning I make (diagnosis)?
- To what extent does the data support my conclusions?

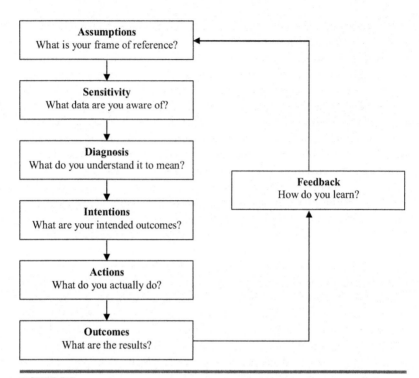

FIGURE 8.2
The reflective practice cycle in supervision.

- What is the difference between what I planned to do (intentions) and what I actually did (actions)? How do I explain this?
- What is the match between the outcomes I expected from my actions (intended consequences) and what actually resulted (unintended consequences)?

Specific Supervisory Methodologies

In this section we review three well-established methodologies for evaluating and enhancing supervisees' practice: case studies, observation of practice and role plays or modelling (Hill et al., 2007). Each of these methodologies emphasises different learning modes: case discussion, involving feedback and theorising can be seen as employing more 'symbolic' processes; observation of practice, generally through videotaped sessions is more directly 'iconic'; and role-play and the use of learning exercises make use of 'enactive' processes (Milne & Westerman, 2001). The purposeful combination of these methodologies provides a means through which supervisees can translate and evolve their declarative knowledge (*knowing about something*) to procedural knowledge (*know how to do something*) and strategic knowledge (*knowing when and why to do something*; Furr & Carroll, 2003).

How might a supervisor know when and what methodology to use? Choice of methodology is determined by a number of factors relevant to both the supervisor and the supervisee. Borders and Leddick (1987) elaborate six considerations in matching method to context: the supervisee's learning goals, level of experience and developmental needs, and learning style; in combination with the supervisor's theoretical orientation, goals for the supervisee and personal goals for the supervisory experience. It is also important to note that their complementary nature means that these methodologies can be usefully combined in a particular supervision session. Thus, for example, a case study discussion or the processing of a videotaped session may evolve to include role-playing particular aspects of the counsellor/supervisee's intervention.

Case Studies

Case studies are most widely used for skill development and are the most popular format for individual and group supervision (Holloway & Johnston, 1985). The commonly espoused goals of this methodology are to develop supervisees' skills in case conceptualisation, diagnosis and intervention. It is generally recognised that while behavioural skills can be developed relatively quickly with supervision, skills in conceptualising cases and the ability to make treatment decisions develop more slowly and require the direct facilitation by a supervisor (Holloway & Neufeldt, 1995; Kilminster & Jolly, 2000). The case study method is well suited for this purpose.

There is some evidence regarding the factors that facilitate or inhibit the efficacy of the case study as a learning tool in supervision. Nolan, Hawkes, and Francis (1993) found both the development of an effective working alliance and supervisory process competence to be particularly important factors facilitating change in supervisee's thinking and behaviour. Case studies were experienced as more effective when supervisors adopted an outcome orientation (reflection with a specific purpose or outcome in mind), and actively facilitated the level and quality of data (e.g., making timely observations).

The case study method is typically initiated by the supervisee either through relatively informal verbal *self-report*, or the more formal presentation of *case/process notes*. The more preparation of a case study by the supervisee prior to the session, the more likely the process is to be of value. Written documentation is particularly helpful in that it provides a clear focus for discussion in the session and allows the supervisor to more readily assess the supervisee's level of cognitive processing and understanding of the case. In fact, Goldberg (1985) argues that the major value of the case study is that it allows the supervisor to work with the supervisee's current level of functioning. From a psychosocial perspective, placing control for the presentation of case material in the hands of the supervisee may reduce perceived threat levels and the possibility of their engaging in defensive self-presentation or meta-task processing with the supervisor. In this regard, case studies may be an optimal early intervention for novice supervisees who may feel threatened by more direct forms of supervision.

There are several available formats to guide supervisees in the structuring of process notes in preparation for a supervision session (e.g., Schwartz, 1981). The following protocol, adapted from Bernard and Goodyear (2004), is a fairly typical approach to reflecting on a counselling session:

1. What were your *goals and strategies* for this counselling session?

2. Did anything happen *during* the session that caused you to reconsider either your goals or your strategies? How did you resolve this?

3. What was the major focus or *theme* of the session?

4. What are your current *hypotheses?*

5. Describe the *interpersonal or relationship dynamics* between you and the client during the session?

6. What was achieved in the session? How *successful* was it from your own and the client's perspective?

7. What did you *learn* about yourself and the helping process from this session?

8. What are your *goals and strategies* for the next session?

9. What *questions* or concerns do you want to raise with your supervisor?

Beyond reflection of 'set pieces', such as planned interventions or scheduled sessions, unanticipated or critical incidents also provide important opportunities for learning and development in supervision. Incidents outside of the control and experience of the supervisee have been found to be powerful catalysts for change, provided they are processed effectively (Furr & Carroll, 2003), and there is both anecdotal and case study-based evidence to support the efficacy of critical incident-based methodologies when facilitated expertly (Davis, 2006).

Critical incidents, by definition, involve a 'series of imperfect choices made in the light of limited information and pressing concerns'. Thus a simple 'choice-point' format, somewhat akin to Schon's (1992) notion of 'manoeuvring in the swamp of practice' may be particularly helpful in capturing the dynamics of unstructured or emergent situations. The sequence of prompts is along the lines of:

- Where were you?
- What did you do?
- What were the immediate consequences? For you? For others?
- Why do you think you did what you did?
- What did other people think about what you did?
- What were the implications of the above?
- How sure are you that you now understand this situation?
- Have you experienced this type of situation previously?
- What do you think you have learnt?
- What do you consider that you still need to learn?

Beyond the higher-order structure of a case study, the style of dialogue between supervisor and supervisee is particularly crucial to the type of learning achieved. Given the goals of self-regulation and independent professional judgment, it should not be surprising that supervisors employ Socratic methods of inquiry with the aim for the supervisee to 'discover their truth' in the exchange with their supervisor and progressively learn to understand and trust his or her own cognitive and emotional personal process. These are noble aims, but the success of this method hinges on the capacity of the supervisor to question out of the supervisee's, rather than their own, theoretical and personal frame of reference (Glickauf-Hughes & Campbell, 1991).

While the case study methodology has a figural role in supervisee development, its effective use requires a particular sensitivity to context. First, Holloway (1988) cautions that the case study methodology may require complex cognitive processing beyond the capacity of some supervisees. This suggests the importance of judicious pace and depth of inquiry to minimise feelings of supervisee incompetence and allow the incremental development of conceptual complexity. Second, Bernard and Goodyear (1992) observe that case notes can provide a way for the supervisee to control, and thus limit, the type of information presented on their practice for supervisor reflection. Thus, some clinicians only recommend exclusive reliance on case study presentations with advanced supervisees (Goldberg, 1985). Finally, there is a widely endorsed view that, while the use of case notes is a valuable practice, it needs to be supplemented by other interventions, particularly more direct observation of practice (Kilminster & Jolly, 2000; Milne, Pilkington, Gracie, & James, 2003).

Finally, it is worth noting that the supervisory process itself can offer a 'living case study' or parallel process of the supervisee's functioning in similar contexts (Glickauf-Hughes & Campbell, 1991). The value of parallel process is based on the assumption that a supervisee's difficulties with learning in supervision can often reflect similar difficulties between the supervisee as counsellor and their client. In order to effectively process these dynamics, a supervisor needs to be both empathically connected with the supervisee and able to disengage from his or her own emotional reactions.

Observation

Observation is perhaps the only form of direct supervision of practice, and typically implemented via one of three forms: audiotapes, videotapes and live observation. The added benefit of this methodology beyond case notes is the wider range of available data on the supervisee's interpersonal, therapeutic and process skills. All three observational modes have been found to produce learning outcomes. There is no empirical evidence that videotape is superior to audiotape as a means of enhancing supervisee performance or skills and audiotape remains the most practical means of observation in supervision (Bernard & Goodyear 1992). The strategic combination of observation and structured feedback (e.g., the rehearsal of microcounselling skills supplemented by supervisory feedback from audio or videotaped sessions) has been demonstrated to produce, not only enhanced counsellor skills, but also improved clinical outcomes for clients such as attendance and resolution of problem behaviours (Blashki, Hickie, & Davenport, 2003). Contrary to popular opinion, observational methods are not associated with high levels of supervisee anxiety (Ellis, Krengel, & Beck, 2002).

Context setting (providing the supervisee with a rationale), planning (establishing a protocol for the review and selection of practice samples) and contracting (negotiating a mutually suitable process) are central to the effective use of observation as a learning methodology. As a general principle, because of the time-intensive nature of this methodology, more productive outcomes may result from sessions with an identified 'point of focus'. Bernard and Goodyear (1992) suggest that useful criteria for identifying points of focus from a supervisee's perspective include: the most *productive* or important part of the session, the part of the session in which they feel the most challenge or sense of struggle or confusion. In addition, supervisors may also choose to bring a supervisee's attention to parts of the session where there is apparent incongruence, or where dynamics appear potently therapeutic or unfortunately strained or where recurring themes are well illustrated.

Actively managing the presentation of a practice sample will facilitate both time efficiency and learning outcomes. Apart from the basic requirement of selecting a particular tape segment in advance of the session, the supervisee can set the context for the supervisor by: providing their reason for selecting this particular sample, briefly summarising relevant history ('session to date'), explaining their intentions or goals in the practice sample and asking for specific help.

Perhaps the most widely used methodology for processing videotapes is Interpersonal Process Recall (IPR; Kagan, 1980). The process of IPR has been well documented and is relatively simple. The supervisor and supervisee together watch a prerecorded video counselling session. Both supervisor and supervisee are empowered at any point to stop the tape to explore what is happening. The particular rationale underlying Kagan's (1976) process is the safe exploration of issues that seem to be unaddressed in the session, for example, a supervisee's frustration, confusion, uncertainty or incongruence. The supervisor responds in the enquirer role using open-ended questions to facilitate the supervisee's exploration towards some resolution (insight, understanding). The supervisor facilitates the supervisee to surface, explore and understand their internal processes in response to the client and the counselling session. The particular value of the IPR process is the potential to identify 'psychological barriers to communication' for supervisees as counsellors and therapists (Kagan, 1980). Given that this is a time-consulting process, preparation is critical to ensure that the most salient events or interactions are processed.

Role-Play

Experiential learning through role-play is a well-established method for training counsellors in both microcounselling skills and interventions (Wilson & Gallois, 1993) and can also be used as an effective means for developing diagnostic and conceptualisation skills (Lizzio, Wilson, & Gallois, 1993). There is evidence that while simple counselling skills can be learned didactically, more complex skills such as empathy and timing of confrontation require more complex teaching methodologies, especially role-play and modelling (Lambert & Arnold, 1987). There is strong empirical support for the efficacy of role-play in counselling and clinical training (Glickauf-Hughes & Campbell, 1991; Rabinowitz, 1997), with the strongest level of skill development occurring when combined with modelling (O'Toole, 1979; Teevan & Gabel, 1978). Early career practitioners, in particular, report role-play in combination with modelling and feedback as an effective learning mechanism in supervision (Rabinowitz, 1997).

A Contextual Model for Role-Play

The complexity of professional practice necessitates supervisors employing approaches to role-play that take account of the context of behaviour. The simple use of role-play to rehearse or shape behaviour (e.g., assertion) without enhancing awareness of its situational appropriateness or interpersonal consequences is mechanistic training, rather than genuine professional development. The following 7-Step model can be used in both individual and group supervision. For a detailed description see Lizzio et al. (1993).

1. Identifying the focus. The supervisor and supervisee briefly discuss the 'focal situation' or 'focal task' (the supervisee wanting to develop more functional responses to previous, current or anticipated situations). This 'background briefing' (the setting, the people involved, the supervisee's typical behaviour and feelings) sets the scene for the role-play. For example, a female supervisee (call her Anita) may select a situation where she feels that she 'goes out of her way' to support a male client and receives what she believes is unfair criticism from him on the effectiveness of her counselling. Anita apologises but feels hurt, angry and resentful.

2. Specifying tentative goals. The supervisee nominates his or her learning goals (What I want to do differently and how this might be helpful to me). In the present example, Anita may have the initial goal of defending herself from what she perceives as unfair criticism from her client. It is important to remember that initial goals must be set with a tentative spirit and will be reviewed after further situational analysis.

3. Enacting present behaviour. The supervisee role-plays his or her present behaviour (this is how I responded or am likely to respond in this situation). The purpose is to provide a sample of behaviour in context to inform a discussion about responses, likely reactions of others, assumptions, and the broader context. In the present example, Anita enacts her typical way of responding, while the supervisor, another person (if in a group supervision context) or an empty chair can take the role of the 'ungrateful client'.

4. Analysing the situation. The aim here is to produce a rich description of the dynamics of the situation so as to well inform new responses that have a good chance of being both effective (likely to work better than the current response) and feasible (likely to be enacted). A rich description of the situation is likely to include some consideration of:

• personal issues, including the supervisee's assumptions, self-statements, anxieties and interaction style

- interpersonal issues, including the nature and history of the relationship and typical patterns of interaction between the supervisee and others involved (e.g., manipulative strategies involving anger or guilt used by either person)

- situational or contextual issues, including the relevant social rules and goals in the situation, the perception of other people, the organisational culture, social supports the supervisee can use, the nature of the task, the influence of gender, culture or professional status.

Beyond simple discussion, the processes that can be used to heighten the supervisee's awareness and training relevant behaviours in this step are as varied as the supervisor's skills and creativity. Some commonly used strategies include feedback from the supervisor to the supervisee, self-analysis by the supervisee, and group reaction and feedback in a group supervision context. The supervisor's input at this stage can include any number of activities such as:

- inductive questioning eliciting the supervisee's perceptions of their choices and alternatives

- interrupted role-play, where the action is stopped at crucial points during the enactment of typical behaviour in the situation and the dynamics of the situation are interpreted with the supervisee

- group reaction and feedback, or eliciting the perceptions of other people in a supervision group about the situation, as a way of introducing and reinforcing new perspectives on the situation

- role reversal, in which the supervisee takes the role of the other person (e.g., client), either in imagination or actual behaviour and tries to see the world from that person's point of view. The process of role reversal is intended to develop skills in meta-perception (Argyle, Furnham, & Graham, 1981), sensitise supervisees to the impact of their behaviour on clients, and make them more aware of their obligations as opposed to their rights in the situation.

- modelling, in which the supervisor takes the role of the supervisee in the situation and models alternative strategies.

5. Reassessing goals. The outcome of a well-conducted situational analysis is that the supervisee is better able to formulate well-informed goals (What I think is going on here is ... The type of response that I would like to work towards is ... This will be helpful to all concerned because ...).

6. Developing the preferred strategy. The situation is role-played again with the supervisee attempting to enact their preferred strategy through a process of 'successive approximations' (behaviour rehearsal and feedback).

7. Planning for action. The session can be usefully concluded with a discussion of the challenges related to transfer of learning ('doing this for real') and processes for self-management or support.

Conclusion

This chapter has focused on the supervisory processes and interventions that can be used to support learning and development in supervision. We have argued that, because all supervision depends on the quality of the working relationship between supervisor and supervisee, contracting and relationship-building are necessary and foundational supervisory interventions. We framed clinical supervision as a learning relationship and proposed the supervisory metacompetencies of facilitating reflection and providing constructive feedback as underpinning the effectiveness of supervisory interventions. Finally, we considered how specific supervisory interventions (i.e., case study, observation, role-plays) contributed to learning outcomes.

Educational Questions and Activities

1. Describe, using the contracting framework presented, your preferred supervisory working relationship. You may do this from either the perspective of a supervisor or supervisee.
   - What learning goals do you wish to emphasise?
   - What approach to learning suits you?
   - What type of relationship do you wish to have?
   - What management processes are important for you?
2. Identify two situations:
   - where you felt that you received constructive feedback
   - where you felt that you received ineffective feedback.
   Can you identify:
   - what did you do that helped or hindered the feedback process?
   - what did others do that helped or hindered the feedback process?
   - how might your reflections be relevant to enhancing feedback processes in supervision?
3. Use the evidence-based protocol for giving developmental feedback to construct a feedback message to a supervisee.
4. Identify a critical incident or interaction and use the reflective practice cycle to critically review the choices you made.
5. Identify a critical incident or interaction and use the role-play model to develop new responses or strategies.

Selected Internet Resources

- Professional supervision for psychologists
  http://www.psychology.org.au/study/working/registration_boards
- Professional supervision for social workers
  http://www.aasw.asn.au
- Professional supervision for counsellors
  http://www.theaca.net.au
- Professional supervision for school counsellors
  htpp://www.agca.com.au/
- Professional supervision for rehabilitation counsellors
  htpp://www.rcaa.org.au

Selected References for Further Reading

Kilminster, S.M., & Jolly, B.C. (2000). Effective supervision in clinical practice settings: A literature review. *Medical Education, 34,* 827–840.

Lizzio, A., & Wilson, K. (2007). Developing critical professional judgment: The efficacy of a self-managed reflective process. *Studies in Continuing Education, 29*(3), 277–193.

McMahon, M., & Patton, W. (2002). *Supervision in the helping professions.* Sydney, Australia: Pearson.

References

Argyris, C., & Schon, D. (1974). *Theory in practice: Increasing professional effectiveness.* San Francisco: Jossey-Bass.

Argyle, M., Furnham, A., & Graham, J.A. (1981). *Social situations.* London: Cambridge University Press.

Barnett, J.E., Doll, B., Younggren, J.N., & Rubin, N.J. (2007). Clinical competence for practicing psychologists: Clearly a work in progress. *Professional Psychology: Research and Practice, 38*(5), 510–514.

Barnett, J.E., Erikson Cornish, J.A., Goodyear, R.K., & Lichtenberg, J.W. (2007). Commentaries on the ethical and effective practice of clinical supervision. *Professional Psychology: Research and Practice, 38*(1), 268–275.

Barrett, M.S., & Barber, J.P. (2005). A developmental approach to the supervision of therapists in training. *Journal of Contemporary Psychotherapy, 35,* 169–183.

Bernard, J.M., & Goodyear, R.K. (1992). *Fundamentals of clinical supervision* (2nd ed.). Boston: Allyn & Bacon.

Bernard, J.M., & Goodyear, R.K. (2004). *Fundamentals of clinical supervision* (3rd ed.). Boston: Allyn & Bacon.

Blashki, G., Hickie, I.B., & Davenport, T.A. (2003). Providing psychological treatments in general practice: how will it work? *Medical Journal of Australia, 179,* 23–25.

Booley, S. (1997). The supervisory role in the fostering of critical self-reflection capacity in social workers. *Social Work, 33*(2), 110–119.

Borders, L.D., & Leddick, G.R. (1987). *Handbook of counseling supervision.* Alexandria, VA: Association for Counselor Education and Supervision.

Bordin, E.S. (1993). A working alliance based model of supervision. *The Counseling Psychologist, 11*(1), 35–42.

Brookfield, S.D. (1986). *Understanding and facilitating adult learning.* San Francisco: Jossey-Bass Publishers.

Butler, R. (1993). Effects of task- and ego-achievement goals on information-seeking during task engagement. *Journal of Personality and Social Psychology, 65,* 18–31.

Cawley, B.D., Keeping, L.M., & Levy, P.E. (1998). Participation in the performance appraisal process and employee reaction: A meta-analytic review of field investigations. *Journal of Applied Psychology, 83,* 615–633.

Carroll, M. (1996). *Counseling supervision: Theory, skills and practice.* London: Cassell.

Claxton, G. (1999). *Wise up: The challenge of lifelong learning.* London: Bloomsbury.

Corno, L., & Snow, R.E. (1986). Adapting teaching to individual difference among learners. In M.C. Wittrock (Ed.), *Handbook of research on teaching* (pp. 605–629). New York: Macmillan.

Couchon, W.D., & Bernard, J.M. (1984). Effects of timing of supervision on supervisor and counsellor performance. *The Clinical Supervisor, 2,* 3–21.

Dall'Alba, G. (2004). Understanding professional practice: investigations before and after an educational program. *Studies in Higher Education, 29,* 679–692.

Dall'Alba, G., & Sandberg, J. (1996). Education for competence in professional practice. *Instructional Science, 24,* 411–437.

Davis, P.J. (2006). Critical incident technique: A learning intervention for organisational problem-solving. *Development and Learning in Organisations: An International Journal, 20,* 13–16.

DeNisi, A., & Kluger, A.N. (2000). Feedback effectiveness: Can 360-degree appraisals be improved? *Academy of Management Executive, 14,* 129–139.

Ellis, M.V. (1991). Critical incidents in clinical supervision and in supervisor supervision: Assessing supervisory issues. *Journal of Counseling Psychology, 38*(3), 342–349.

Ellis, M.V. (2001). Harmful supervision, a cause for alarm: Comment of Gray et al. (2001) and Nelson and Frielander (2001). *Professional Psychology: Research and Practice, 48,* 401–406.

Ellis, M.V., Krengel, M., & Beck, M. (2002). Testing self-focused attention theory in clinical supervision: Effects of supervisee anxiety and performance. *Journal of Counseling Psychology, 49,* 101–106.

Fernando, D.M., & Hulse-Killacky, D. (2005). The relationship of supervisory styles to satisfaction with supervision and the perceived self-efficacy of master's-level counseling students. *Counselor Education and Supervision, 44*(4), 293–304.

Fish, D., & Twinn, S. (1997). *Quality supervision in the healthcare professions. Principled approaches to practice.* Oxford: Butterworth-Heinemann.

Fisher, M. (1996). Using reflective practice in clinical supervision. *Professional Nursing, 11*(7), 443–444.

Furr, S.R., & Carroll, J.J. (2003). Critical incidents in student counselor development. *Journal of Counseling and Development, 81,* 483–489.

Galante, M. (1998) Trainees' and supervisors' perceptions of effective and ineffective supervisory relationships, *Dissertations Abstracts International, 49,* 933B.

Gazzola, N., & Theriault, A. (2007). Relational themes in counseling supervision: Broadening and narrowing processes. *Canadian Journal of Counseling, 41*(4), 228–243.

Glickauf-Hughes, C., & Campbell, L. (1991). Experiential supervision: applied techniques for a case presentation approach. *Psychotherapy, 28*(1), 625–635.

Goldberg, D.A. (1985). Process notes, audio, and video tape: Modes of presentation in psychotherapy training. *The Clinical Supervisor, 3,* 1–13.

Greenberg, J. (1986). Determinants of perceived fairness of performance evaluations. *Journal of Applied Psychology, 71,* 340–342.

Hager, P. (1999). Finding a good theory of workplace learning. In D. Boud & J. Garrick (Eds.), *Understanding learning at work* (pp. 65–82). London: Routledge.

Hill, C.E., Stahl, J., & Roffman, M. (2007). Training novice psychotherapists: Helping skills and beyond. *Psychotherapy: Theory, Research, Practice, Training, 44*(4), 364–370.

Holloway, E.L. (1988). Instruction beyond the facilitative conditions: A response to Biggs. *Counselor Education and Supervision, 27,* 252–258.

Holloway, E.L., & Johnston, R. (1985). Group supervision: Widely practiced but poorly understood. *Counsellor Education and Supervision, 24*(4), 232–240.

Holloway, E.L., & Neufeldt, S.A. (1995). Supervision: Its contributions to treatment efficacy. *Journal of Consulting and Clinical Psychology, 63*(2), 207–213.

Holmwood, C.B. (1993). The gentle art of feedback. *Australian Family Physician, 22*(10), 1811–1813.

Jarvela, S., & Salovaara, H. (2004). The interplay of motivational goals and cognitive strategies in a new pedagogical culture. *European Psychologist, 9,* 232–244.

Kadushin, A. (1992). Social work supervision: A research update, *The Clinical Supervisor, 2,* 9–27.

Kagan, N. (1976). *Influencing human interaction.* Washington, DC: American Association for Counseling and Development.

Kagan, N. (1980). Influencing human interaction — eighteen years with IPR. In A.K. Hess (Ed.), *Psychotherapy Supervision: Theory, research and practice* (pp. 262–286). New York: John Wiley.

Kanfer, R., Sawyer, J., Earley, P.C., & Lind, E.A. (1987). Fairness and participation in evaluation procedures: Effects on task attitudes and performance. *Social Justice Research, 1,* 235–249.

Kennard, B.D., Stewart, S.M., & Gluck, M.R. (1987). The supervision relationship: Variables contributing to positive verses negative experiences, *Professional Psychology: Research and Practice, 18,* 172–175.

Kember, D., & Leung, D.Y.P. (2005). The influence of active learning experiences on the development of graduate capabilities, *Studies in Higher Education, 30*, 155–170.

Kilminster, S.M., & Jolly, B.C. (2000). Effective supervision in clinical practice settings: A literature review. *Medical Education, 34*, 827–840.

King, P.M., & Kitchener, K.S. (2004). Reflective judgment: theory and research on the development of epistemic assumptions through adulthood, *Educational Psychologist, 39*, 5–18.

Knowles, M.S. (1984). *The adult learner: A neglected species.* Houston, TX: Gulf.

Ladany, N., Ellis, M.V., & Friedlander, M.L. (1999). The supervisory working alliance, trainee self-efficacy and satisfaction. *Journal of Counseling and Development, 77*, 447–455.

Lambert, M.J., & Arnold, R.C. (1987). Research and the supervisory process. *Professional Psychology: Research and Practice, 18*(3), 217–224.

Larson, L.M., & Daniels, J.A. (1998). Review of the counseling self-efficacy literature. *The Counseling Psychologist, 26*, 179–218.

Liddel, H.A. (1988). Systemic supervision: Conceptual overlays and pragmatic guidelines. In H.A. Liddel, D.C. Breunlin & R.C. Schwartz (Eds.), *Handbook of family therapy training and supervision* (pp. 153–171). New York: Guilford.

Lind, E.A., & Tyler, T.R. (1988). *The social psychology of procedural justice.* New York: Plenum Press.

Lizzio, A.J., Stokes, L., & Wilson, K.L. (2005). Approaches to learning in professional supervision: Supervisee perceptions of process and outcome. *Studies in Continuing Education, 27*, 239–257.

Lizzio, A., & Wilson, K.L. (2004). Action learning in higher education: An investigation of its potential to develop capability. *Studies in Higher Education, 29*, 469–488.

Lizzio, A., & Wilson, K.L. (2002). Outcomes in professional supervision. In M. McMahon & W. Patton (Eds.), *Supervision in the helping professions: A practical guide* (pp. 27–42). Sydney, Australia: Pearson Education.

Lizzio, A.J., Wilson, K.L., & Gallois, C.G. (1993). Training assertive communication in its social context. In K.L. Wilson & C.G. Gallois (Eds.), *Assertion and its social context* (pp. 155–169). London: Pergamon.

Lizzio, A., Wilson, K., & McKay, L. (2008). Managers and subordinates' evaluations of feedback message components. *Journal of Applied Social Psychology, 38*, 919–946.

Lizzio, A., Wilson, K., & Que, J. (in press). Relationship dimensions of professional supervision: Supervisees' perceptions of processes and outcomes. *Studies in Continuing Education.*

Magnuson, S., Norem, K., & Wilcoxon, S.A. (2000). Clinical supervision of prelicensed counselors: Recommendations for consideration and practice. *Journal of Mental Health Counseling, 22*(2), 176–188.

Marsick, V. J., & Watkins, K. (1996). *Informal and incidental learning in the workplace.* London: Routledge.

McMahon, M., & Simons, R. (2004). Supervision training for professional counselors: An exploratory study. *Counselor Education and Supervision, 43*(4), 301–309.

Milne, D., & James, I. (2000). A systematic review of effective cognitive–behavioural supervision. *British Journal of Clinical Psychology, 39*, 111–127.

Milne, D.L., Pilkington, J., Gracie, J., & James, I. (2003). Transferring skills from supervision to therapy: A qualitative and quantitative $N = 1$ analysis. *Behavioural and Cognitive Psychotherapy, 31*, 193–202.

Milne, D., & Westerman, C. (2001). Evidence-based clinical supervision: rationale and illustration. *Clinical Psychology and Psychotherapy, 8*, 444–457.

Moskowitz, S.A., & Rupert, P.A. (1983). Conflict resolution within the supervisory relationship. *Professional Psychology: Research and Practice, 14*, 632–641.

Nelson, M.L., Barnes, K.L., Evans, A.L., & Triggiano, P.J. (2008). Working with conflict in clinical supervision: Wise supervisors' perspectives. *Journal of Counselling Psychology, 55*(2), 172–184.

Nelson, M.L., & Friedlander, M.L. (2001). A close look at conflictual supervisory relationships: The trainee's perspective. *Journal of Counseling Psychology, 48*, 384–395.

Nolan, J., Hawkes, B., & Francis, P. (1993). Case studies: Windows into clinical supervision. *Educational Leadership, 51*(2), 32–36.

O'Toole, W.M. (1979). Effects of practice and some methodological considerations in training in counseling, interviewing skills. *Journal of Counseling Psychology, 26*, 419–426.

Paterson, B. (1994). The view form within: Perspectives of clinical teaching. *International Journal of Nursing Studies, 31*(4), 349–360.

Rabinowitz, F.E. (1997). Teaching counselling through a semester-long role play. *Counselor Education and Supervision, 36*, 216–223.

Schon, D.A. (1992). The crisis of professional knowledge and the pursuit of an epistemology of practice. *Journal of Interprofessional Care, 6*(1), 49–62.

Schon, D. (1983). *The reflective practitioner: How professional think in action.* New York: Basic Books.

Schwartz, R. (1981). The conceptual development of family therapy trainees. *American Journal of Family Therapy, 2*, 89–90.

Senge, P. (1990). The *fifth discipline: The art and practice of the learning organisation.* Sydney, Australia: Random House.

Skarlicki, D.P., & Folger, R. (1997). Retaliation in the workplace: The roles of distributive, procedural and interactional justice. *Journal of Applied Psychology, 82*, 434–443.

Sheikh, A.I., Milne, D.L., & MacGregor, B.V. (2007). A model of personal professional development in the systematic training of clinical psychologists. *Clinical Psychology and Psychotherapy, 14*, 278–287.

Smerdon, B.A., Burkam, D.T., & Lee, V.E. (1999). Access to constructivist and didactic teaching: Who gets it? Where is it practiced? *Teachers College Record, 101*, 5–34.

Stephenson, J. (1998). The concept of capability and its importance in higher education. In J. Stephenson & M. Yorke (Eds.), *Capability and quality in higher education*. London: Kogan Page.

Stephenson, J., & Weil, S. (1992). *Quality in learning: A capability approach to higher education*. London: Kogan Page.

Sternberg, R.J., & Horvath, J.A. (1999). *Tacit knowledge in professional practice*. Mahwah, NJ: Lawrence Erlbaum.

Teevan, K.G., & Gabel, H. (1978). Evaluation of modeling, role playing, and lecture-discussion techniques for college student mental health professionals. *Journal of Counseling Psychology, 25,* 169–171.

Vaill, P.B. (1996). *Learning as a way of being*. San Francisco: Jossey Bass.

Vygotsky, L.S. (1978). *Mind in society: The development of higher psychological processes* (M. Cole, V. John-Steiner, S. Scribner, & E. Souberman, Eds and Trans.). Cambridge, MA: Harvard University.

Watkins, C.E. Jr. (Ed.). (1997). *Handbook of psychotherapy supervision*. New York: John Wiley.

Wilson, K.L., & Gallois, C.G. (1993). *Assertion and its social context*. London: Pergamon.

Worthen, V., & McNeil, B.W. (1996). A phenomenological investigation of 'good' supervision events, *Journal of Counseling Psychology, 43,* 25–34.

Wulf, J., & Nelson, M.L. (2000). Experienced psychologists' reflections or predoctoral internship supervision and its contributions to their development. *Clinical Supervisor, 19*(2), 123–145.

—⊦⊦⊦⊦⊦—

chapter nine

Addressing Supervisee Fears in Supervision

Nadine Pelling

Tell Me Your Fears

I begin almost all my counselling and clinical skills classes in the same manner. Specifically, I ask participants to take some time and list their worst imagined client case scenarios, anonymously, on poster paper during class. In other words, I ask participants to share their fears regarding their impending work with clients. After I gain a listing of participants' worst client case scenarios I take them home and organise them into groupings that are clearly related and typed for dissemination to the entire class.

Over the next few meetings participants' concerns are directly addressed through discussion of the issues raised, exercises and related role-plays. In this manner some of the content of our supervisory work is determined by those in training. This focus honours supervisee needs. Moreover, participants can experience the fact that others also have fears when it comes to their in-the-near-future work with clients, which has a normalising and anxiety-reducing effect.

I am often amazed by the level of detail some have woven into their most concerning imagined client interactions. However, the general content presented by participants tends to be somewhat stable. What follows are the five main areas into which the worst client case scenarios of many therapists in training can be placed. This presentation includes brief suggestions relating to the therapist knowledge, self–other awareness and skills that need addressing relating to each scenario category presented. This chapter ends with a short overview of some general activities that aid in therapist knowledge, self–other awareness and skill development.

Worst Client Case Scenario Categories

I have come across five general worst client case scenario categories: harm to client/client in great pain, difficult clients, danger to therapist, ethical responsibilities and therapist competence. Of course, these categories can overlap and specific examples in each category can vary, but I have included for illustrative purposes some general examples of each that I have come across in my supervision work.

Harm to Client/Client in Great Pain

It should be no surprise that having a client demonstrate any level of suicidality or overwhelming emotional pain can be anxiety provoking for beginning-level therapists. In my classes, the most common fear listed about this category has been having a client overtly state an intention to kill him or herself. Such an issue needs to be addressed for therapist knowledge, self–other awareness and skill. Specifically, therapists need to know ethically what the limits to confidentiality entail, as well as the basic risk factors relating to self-harm and suicide. Regarding self–other awareness, therapists need to know the content areas that trigger their own emotions, and the difference between empathy and identification. Finally, all therapists need to be taught the basic skills needed to assess lethality, and follow-through actions needed to protect client wellbeing. Extensive role-play activities can be very helpful in reducing supervisee anxiety and increasing confidence when working with clients in great pain. Entire supervision sessions can be spent exploring harm to client/client in great pain factors.

Difficult Clients

What is a difficult client? According to many of my past students difficult clients include those that confront the therapist verbally, have difficulty expressing themselves verbally, those who are resistant and mandated to treatment, anyone who is sarcastic and, my personal favourite, malevolent clients who simply enjoy being difficult. Once again, the issue of difficult clients needs to be addressed for therapist knowledge, self–other awareness, and skill. Specifically, therapists need to know the roots of resistance and understand that therapy is a joint venture; not one in which a therapist can metaphorically drag a client along to experience. Through experience and support therapists can learn that basic counselling skills, such as listening and reflecting feeling, can help address the issues that difficult clients might raise. Regarding self–other awareness, I encourage therapists to remember that salt only hurts when it is rubbed in an open wound and thus, once again, therapists need to know the content areas that trigger their own emotions and the difference between empathy and identification. The supervisor can demonstrate through empathetic listening that the best way to address difficult clients is to work with, not against, client resistance. Understanding that ambivalence and self-protection are common in humans can help one to not overact to such occurrences. This type of work turns theory into practice in a manner that can be directly beneficial for clients.

Danger to Therapist

I must have been somewhat naive as a therapist in training as I do not personally remember fearing for my safety when beginning work with clients. Nevertheless, many students have indicated that they fear clients being physically confronting to, or specifically threatening the therapist if they do/do not do something that the client is against and/or requests. For instance, many students have indicated a concern over a client threatening them if they rightly engage in their mandatory reporting obligations for child abuse. Once again, therapists need to know ethically what the limits to confidentiality entail and follow through with mandatory reporting requirements. Basic safety and security measures also need to be in place when and where clients are to be seen. Regarding self–other awareness, therapists need to understand that clients may become upset in session and that we might be able to help them express their concerns in a socially appropriate manner. Therapists need to be skilled in remaining calm when working with clients, know how to excuse themselves from a dangerous situation or how to make an appropriate referral to another professional if needed. Numerous role-play scenarios, self-exploration exercises and literature searches regarding such topic areas could be conducted as part of one's supervision.

Ethical Responsibilities

Ethics are taught differently in different training programs. Some integrate ethical training across all their classes, while others have a specific class regarding professional and ethical behaviour. Each method of ethical training has its benefits and drawbacks, and experienced professionals know that ethics are not static but ever-evolving to fit our current culture and knowledge base. The most common fears about one's ethical responsibilities I have encountered as an instructor involve mandatory reporting requirements and romantic or personal (i.e., not professional) connections with clients. A lack of therapist knowledge of ethics is fairly easy to address by reading the relevant ethical codes and ethical case books, which include not just a list of 'dos' and 'don'ts', but also principles that highlight the 'why' behind such ethical codes. Also, knowing oneself and one's own vulnerabilities, as well as the need to respect clients, can be key to ethical behaviour. Role-playing scenarios in which a therapist must clearly define the professional nature of their relationship with a client or in which a mandatory reporting situation has occurred can help build one's skill in these areas. Similarly, keeping in regular collegial contact with other therapists, possibly in a supervision group, can help therapists determine what is considered standard practice and thus generally on safe ethical footing in their own geographical/specialty area. Of course, when in doubt, in practice one can contact the relevant professional organisation for advice or referral to a supervisor or colleague for discussion (please see Chapter 3 for a listing of relevant organisations).

Questioning Therapist Competence

When I first started my psychological practice a very mature female client I had just finished seeing told my supervisor that she did not want to 'see that little blonde chickie again'. In retrospect, I understand her concern since I might not like to see a psychologist in her 20s if I was in my 70s either. At the time I was at a loss for words and was not certain what to do. One needs to know referral sources in their area so that, if needed, an appropriate referral can be made. Regarding self–other awareness my supervisor challenged me to acknowledge that not every therapist can see every client and that the only way to move forward when someone questions your competence is to empathically listen to them, discuss the matter and, if needed, make an appropriate referral. This tends to be the case if you are considerably younger or older than a client, or you are or are not a parent and thus may have difficulty understanding where a client is coming from regarding parenting, or if you have just been told that therapy with you, or in general, is useless as an activity. Being skilled in listening and exploring expectations and views is a way forward. Therapist defensiveness needs to be explored personally by the therapist and supervisor, but therapy needs to remain focused on the client. Therapists need to be aware that client ambivalence and resistance can occur and that such things need to be worked with, not against. By discussing such things in supervision the supervisor can model how to be supportive, understanding and encouraging.

General Activities for Increasing Knowledge, Self–Other Awareness and Skill

Models, methods, and modes used in supervision abound. Indeed, much of this book outlines various interventions used in supervision. What follows here are simply an outlining of a few of my more favoured activities for expanding therapist knowledge, self/other awareness, and skill.

Knowledge

Reading, researching and collegial discussion are my favourite methods for increasing knowledge. Specific topic areas such as mania or addiction can be researched, one's local ethical code can be obtained and read, one can attend regular research or journal meetings at which topics are discussed.

Self–Other Awareness
Generally, one can increase self–other awareness though many of the techniques used with clients, but with a focus on how such an increase in awareness is likely to impact one's therapeutic work. For instance, timelines, genograms, an examination of personal views, counselling, keeping a journal, attending to self-care and examining multicultural issues can all be beneficial. Specifically, if working with a client with an addiction problem a therapist could examine via a time line how their views/experiences with substances commonly the focus of addiction have shaped their thinking and emotional reactions to addiction and then how this can impact their client work.

Skill
Knowledge and awareness are wonderful, but eventually one needs to develop client skill if one is to have a successful client practice. How can one build skill? Role-play activities, self-examination of one's work via video review and requesting specific feedback from colleagues, supervisors and clients can be helpful. There is also volunteer work, training placements, practice and supervised practice. Specifically, in order to increase therapeutic skill one needs to work in a reflective manner. This takes targeted time and effort as well as personal fortitude.

Concluding Statement
Therapists in training have some common fears regarding their impending work with clients. As supervisors, we can address these and thus show an acceptance of our supervisees and encourage their growth as therapists though aiding an increase in their knowledge, self–other awareness and clinical skill. Addressing common client fears can be accomplished in numerous ways but often requires therapist courage and the support of a knowledgable, understanding and supportive supervisor. What do your trainees fear and how are their fears being addressed?

Educational Questions and Activities
1. What are the five general worst client case scenario categories outlined by Dr Pelling?
   - harm to client/client in great pain
   - difficult clients
   - danger to therapist
   - ethical responsibilities
   - therapist competence.

2. Create a possible client scenario to go with each category and do either a literature search on the topic (knowledge), write your thoughts and feelings down about the topic (self–other awareness), or engage in an extended role-play as client and then counsellor regarding the topic.

3. What is your favourite way of enhancing your knowledge on a topic?
   • reading
   • discussion with colleague
   • attending a conference
   • training or other activity.

4. What is your favourite way of developing your self–other awareness?
   • journal writing
   • discussion with others
   • drawing
   • another activity.

5. What is your favourite ways of developing your counselling skills?
   • role-play
   • video playback
   • other activity.

Selected References for Further Reading

Pelling, N. J., & Renard, D.E. (1999). The use of videotaping in developmentally based supervision. *Journal of Technology in Counseling* [online serial], *1*(1). Available at http://jtc.colstate.edu/home.htm

Pelling, N., & Kocarek, C. (2003). Beyond knowledge and awareness: Enhancing counsellor skills for work with gay, lesbian, and bisexual clients. *Journal of Multicultural Counselling and Development, 31*(2), 99–112.

—++++—

People

'The People' section comprises four chapters that are generally oriented toward the more personal dimensions of clinical supervision such as relationships, modes of supervision practice, and supervisor development and training. Chapter 10 is a succinct review of the basic areas relating to the supervisory relationship and is offered in a way the reader will be encouraged to explore at greater length issues for which they have specific interest. Chapter 11 challenges the notion that individual supervision is the most appropriate mode for exploring counselling practice and offers rich descriptions of the various others modes that could be considered, each with strengths and shortcomings enumerated. A discussion is included to help supervisees gain what they need from the supervision with which they are engaged. Chapter 12 explores the development of supervisors and how supporting them in their work has become more recognised. Supervisors, of supervisors and of therapists, need to address their own personal and relational development, be experienced as therapists, engage in professional training relative to supervision, and also be in supervision themselves. Such reflective practice with clients and supervisees requires lifelong learning. Chapter 13 provides a baseline description of counsellors in Australia, information which has the potential to be used in moves to advance the professionalisation of the group.

Chapter Overview
CHAPTER 10

'The Supervisory Relationship' by Jason Dixon reviews the nature of the working relationship that is developed between supervisor and supervisee, without which useful outcomes are unlikely. This chapter examines, albeit in a cursory fashion, the very important concepts of the parallel process and transference, with a useful table that explores the developmental nature of a clinicians' increasing awareness of such issues. An inventory in the form of a list of stimulating questions that supervisors and supervisees could consider will ensure the supervisory relationship and the process of supervision are heading in the right direction.

Chapter Themes
In this chapter you will explore the following themes:
- importance and nature of the supervisory relationship
- factors affecting the supervisory relationship
- attitudes toward acculturation in the supervisory relationship
- parallel process, transference and countertransference
- a guide to parallel process and transference in supervision
- taking inventory of the supervisory relationship.

CHAPTER 11

'Modes of Supervision' by Sally Hunter and J. Randolph Bowers is a chapter with two main themes. First, the authors each present their own personal experiences in supervision in a reflective manner. Second, the authors present various modes in which supervision can occur including individual, group, and peer supervision. The positives and possible drawbacks of each mode are discussed and hints regarding getting the most out of one's own supervision are presented. This in an informative yet personally presented chapter in the true vein of the therapist as a person.

Chapter Themes

In this chapter you will explore the following themes:

• introduction
• personal experiences of counselling supervision
• Dr Sally Hunter
• Dr Randolph Bowers
• underlying assumptions about supervision
• modes of supervision
• individual supervision
• group supervision
• peer supervision
• self-supervision
• getting the most from supervision.

CHAPTER 12

How does one become a supervisor and what factors relate to supervisory identity development? In the chapter 'Supervisor Development', Nadine Pelling and Elisa Agostinelli explore the factors that relate to supervisory identity development. The Supervisor Complexity Model of Watkins is reviewed, as are the personal and relational factors related to supervision. Counselling experience, supervision training, and supervisory experience are then reviewed and presented as having an impact on one's development as a supervisor. If you are a new supervisor you will want to read this chapter, as it illustrates common supervisory development factors and the stages of development many new supervisors will encounter as they become more proficient at supervision.

Chapter Themes

In this chapter you will explore the following themes:

• introduction
• supervisor development

- SCM
- Stage 1
- Stage 2
- Stage 3
- Stage 4
- possible influences on supervisory development
- personal/relational variables
- counselling experience
- supervisory training
- supervision experience.

CHAPTER 13

'Who are Australian Counsellors and How Do They Attend to Their Professional Development?' by Nadine Pelling and Caleb Lack provides a state of the (counselling) union glimpse based on three recently published comprehensive studies. The chapter ultimately provides the reader with a baseline description of counsellors in Australia, information which has the potential to be used in moves to advance the professionalisation of counsellors as a group worthy of, and in need of, some form of statutory recognition.

Chapter Themes

In this chapter you will explore the following themes:

- Australian counselling
- method
- comparisons
- methodology
- results
- discussion.

chapter ten

The Supervisory Relationship

Jason Dixon

The nature of the relationship that is negotiated, developed and maintained between a clinical supervisor and supervisee is central to effectively engage in clinical work, to promote professional and personal development, and to ensure consistent ethical practice. In this chapter, attention is given to the challenges, importance and benefits of the supervisory relationship. The ability to form and sustain relationships in supervision and in clinical practice is more crucial than specific knowledge and therapeutic skills (Dye, 1994). Attention to parallel process, the working alliance, multiple roles, expectations and acculturative issues are addressed. This is an introduction to some of the most salient issues concerning the supervisory relationship and is a review of concepts and processes discussed in greater depth throughout this textbook. The reader is encouraged to utilise the references and suggested readings to deepen their understanding of the supervisory relationship.

Importance and Nature of the Supervisory Relationship

The significance of the supervisory relationship in therapist training and clinical practice is evident by the extensive attention given to it in the scholarly literature (e.g., Bambling, King, & Raue, Schweitzer & Lambert, 2006; Barletta, 2007; Borders, Bernard, Dye, Fong, Henderson et al., 1991; Lampropoulos, 2002; McMahon, 2002; Ronnestad & Skovholt, 1993). The impact on the supervisee's professional identity, clinical skill, self-confidence and relational style are cultivated through the quality of the supervisory relationship. Recent literature suggests there is evidence that through the supervisory relationship the attachment styles of insecure trainee therapists can be transformed in their clinical work to an identity of self-confidence and a secure relational style (Bernard & Goodyear,

2004; Renfro-Michel, 2007). New models have been proposed supporting the notion that using attachment theory is useful to enrich the supervisory working alliance and to enhance other approaches to supervisory tasks (Bennett, 2008).

The supervisory relationship has been described in different ways each emphasising certain aspects of the relationship. In general terms, supervision involves maintaining relationships while attending to the matters of supervision (McMahon, 2002). It is a relationship of utmost importance, with successful supervision experienced as being reciprocal, mutual and trusting (Safran & Muran, 2000). This relationship provides a container that holds the helping relationship within a therapeutic triad (Hawkins & Shohet, 2000). Within the supervisory relationship, specific elements should exist such as empathy, acceptance, openness with confrontation, a sense of humour and appropriate self-disclosure. Supervision is a relationship that constitutes the right balance between support and challenge (Carroll & Gilbert, 2006). This support and challenge is maintained in such a way that supervisees can freely discuss successes and failures, strengths and weaknesses. Open discussion in supervision and the flow of ideas is attained through collaboration, awareness and sensitivity, and is always respectful and nonjudgmental (Chiaferi & Griffin, 1997).

Although the purpose, style and tasks of supervision will vary, the abovementioned issues and preconditions are those that ensure quality, depth and breadth of this important professional relationship.

Factors Affecting the Supervisory Relationship

A factor that is easily attended to, and should be addressed from the outset and readdressed when necessary, is a clear understanding of the roles and expectations of both the supervisor and supervisee. Providing sufficient information on the roles of colleague, counsellor, consultant, teacher and evaluator set the way clear for expectations of all parties to be negotiated. Role ambiguity, uncertainty about expectations of performance and evaluation give rise to conflicts, work-related anxiety and dissatisfaction (Olk & Friedlander, 1992). The responsibility to resolve any ambiguity lies with the supervisor to clearly state, or restate the aspects of multiple roles and to be a ready resource to contribute to the induction of the supervisee into the profession.

When both the work of the supervisor and supervisee are challenging, the factors that affect the supervisory relationship can be sources for personal and professional development. Immediacy in attending to ambiguity and clear communication is paramount to a productive supervision experience. Helping supervisees articulate the matters that are affecting the working alliance is sometimes all that is needed to maintain and strengthen the collaborative bond. Attending to the mechanics of clinical work and to the supervisee's experience of clinical cases can reveal factors that might be affecting the supervisory relationship. For example, a supervisor does well to be concerned if a supervisee only ever presents to supervision with issues related to the experience of clinical work. Exploring and attending to the matters of the supervisee's client casework can reveal any impasse in disclosing these issues and restore balance to the working alliance.

Therapy and supervision is serious work with significant implications. While mention of the usefulness and place of humour is uncommon in the literature, there is a lighter side of clinical work. Being able to talk shop and allowing one's sense of humour to emerge (Pearson, 2004), and using humour to facilitate discussion of emotional reactions to clients (Nezu, Saad, & Nezu, 2000) diffuses a stressful environment, is an indication of trust and is an expression of a collaborative spirit. As further research emerges on humour in supervision, a more comprehensive understanding of the benefits to supervision will become evident.

Attitudes Toward Acculturation in the Supervisory Relationship

Acculturation results when groups of individuals having different cultures come into first-hand contact and, over time, there are subsequent changes in the original cultural patterns of either or both groups (Redfield, Linton, & Herskovits, 1936). Generally, culturally diverse minority groups appear to engage in four types of acculturative behaviour. *Assimilation* is an abandonment of culture of origin values and norms and an adoption of host cultural values, *integration* is an adoption of host culture values and norms and a preservation of culture of origin values and norms, *separation* is a rejection of host cultural values and norms, and *marginalisation* is an abandonment of the cultural values and norms of both the host culture and the culture of origin (Berry, 1983, 1980, 1976, 1974; Berry, Kim, Young, & Bujaki, 1989).

Although the construct validity of *marginalisation* is questionable, Dixon (2008) demonstrated that attitudes of host culture trainee therapists toward the acculturative strategies of culturally different minority groups can be validly measured. All acculturative strategies are valid, yet supervisees may be biased in that they may expect clients who are culturally different to acculturate to the host culture in a certain way. Exploring this bias and establishing an understanding that all acculturative strategies are valid promotes multicultural competence and sensitivity in the therapeutic triad. Furthermore, cultural differences are an opportunity for learning. Exploring transcultural issues with a supervisor who is culturally different from the supervisee or client conveys respect and value for ethnic identity and is an opportunity to learn the cultural aspects of social norms, protocols, cultural symbolism, morals, customs, traditions and worldview.

Parallel Process, Transference and Countertransference

Parallel process is a replication of the therapeutic relationship in the supervisory context where supervisees present themselves in a similar way as do their clients in therapy (Bernard & Goodyear, 2004; Morrissey & Tribe, 2001). Parallel process allows the process of transference and countertransference to be evident in supervision. These concepts are extremely useful, regardless of the theoretical orientation adopted. The concept of transference is rooted in the psychoanalytic literature and refers to the projections of the client onto the therapist, while countertransference refers to the needs, feelings and wishes of the therapist that are projected onto the client. Bernard and Goodyear (2004) describe transference in simple terms as a phenomenon in which a person transfers to someone in the present, the feelings and responses that have been experienced with someone in the past. Transference reactions are often triggered by something that is familiar in persons in the present to people in the past, and can be evident in the supervisory relationship. Transference is especially important in supervision when the person in the past is a client and, just as the client has sort some fulfilment of an emotional need in the supervisee, so too the supervisee seeks some fulfilment of these needs from the supervisor. A supervisee who reacts with frustration toward a client who is perceived as uncooperative may also react in a similar manner toward a supervisor who is attempting to encourage autonomy in the supervisee concerning the work with this client. In other words, the supervisor is perceived as being uncooperative and thus transference issues will become evident if they are adequately explored. A useful point of departure in ascertaining if transference is at work in supervision is for the supervisor to think along the lines of where this frustration is 'coming from' (i.e., interactions with the client or perhaps a relationship from the supervisee's personal world).

An example of parallel process is where clients and supervisees experience a halting of the therapeutic process. Supervisees do well when they are aware that both their client and themselves are stuck and then they seek guidance from their supervisor. Facilitating exploration and awareness of parallel process is dependent on supervisor skill, sensitivity and approach. Ineffective supervision or conflict can be attributed to unconscious and unrecognised dynamics in the supervisory triad (Pearson, 2000). Encouragement to work with, and not against, exploration and awareness of parallel processes (Gilbert & Evans, 2000) sometimes requires a renegotiation and mending of the supervisory alliance to enable therapist and client to re-engage and move with the therapeutic process.

McNeill and Worthen (1989), along with many others, emphasise and regard the value of the parallel process as a form of communication and a useful focus for supervision that is beneficial to both supervisee and client. The goals of working through parallel process and transference issues are to reduce the empathic impairment of the therapist, and to maintain and strengthen the working alliance between all parties in the therapeutic triad (Southern, 2007). This is achieved through a safe and emotionally contained environment where the supervisee can work through conflicts and emotions that impair empathy. There is a sense of catharsis resulting from genuine disclosure that spans both the depth and breadth of the supervisee's experience of clinical work. Supervisees are allowed to be vulnerable during these sessions. Southern points out that inexperienced therapists may be afraid of being vulnerable where an experienced therapist presents as being overconfident, technically proficient, yet lacking self-awareness. Both situations impair empathic interactions and insight. The task rests with the supervisor to be sensitive and aware of such states and respond appropriately to achieve the goals mentioned above.

Figure 10.1 is a guide I developed for exploring therapist development, parallel process and transference issues. It can be used when considering the supervisor's approach in dealing with these critical issues.

An Inventory of the Supervisory Relationship

The following is a list of questions that clinical supervisors and supervisees should consider to ensure the supervisory relationship and the process of supervision is on track. It is designed to bring attention to both the strengths of the supervisory relationship and the areas for growth that are potentially areas of conflict or threaten the supervisory working alliance.

Questions for the Supervisor

- How attentive are you to the dynamics of the relationship with your supervisee? (i.e., not just focused on the mechanics of the supervisee's practice).

- How do you know the extent to which your supervisee is freely able to disclose the experiential and emotional aspects of their work and professional development?

- To what degree is the supervisee disclosing both the depth and breadth of their clinical work?

- How does the supervisee challenge you with questions about their work? In what ways do you challenge the supervisee?

- What are the conflicts you have around the goals and processes of supervision? How are they actively dealt with in a timely manner?

Therapist Developmental Stage	Therapist Clinical Focus	Status of Parallel Process, and Transference	Supervisory Environment
Therapy student	Skills and techniques	Unaware	Reassurance, encouragement, facilitate awareness
Emerging professional	Self-awareness	Conscious and active awareness of feelings	Stimulate and differentiate awareness of client related issues
Professional therapist	Other-awareness	Conscious awareness of feelings related to self and client	Patience, orientation, exploration of self and others' feelings
Senior professional therapist	Comprehensive aspects of therapeutic relationship	Unconscious awareness and immediacy in attending to transferences and feelings	Challenge to stretch therapist's understanding of relationship and client context

FIGURE 10.1
A guide to parallel process and transference in clinical supervision.

- How are you regularly attending to the supervisee's casework, professional development and personal issues that impact their work?
- Describe the lighter moments in supervision (i.e., humour).
- In what ways is there a sense of being collegial with your supervisee?
- How are you sensitive to transcultural and acculturative factors with the supervisee and their clients?

Questions for the Supervisee
- To what extent do you feel at ease to freely disclose all aspects of your work? What holds you back?
- When do you feel empowered to discuss the success and failures of professional practice?
- To what degree do you feel respected? When do you particularly respect your supervisor?
- How is supervision challenging and edifying?
- How do you know that the supervisor understands the content and context of your clinical work, your personal experience of professional practice?
- How and when do you present ethical dilemmas to your supervisor?

- When are your needs for clinical practice and professional development being met?
- Describe the immediacy you experience in dealing with conflicts that arise with your supervisor?
- How have you identified and informed your supervisor of any transcultural aspects between you and your supervisor/clients? This includes the cultural aspects of social norms, protocols, cultural symbols, morals, customs and worldview.

Concluding Statement

This chapter has been written as a concise review of areas pertaining to the supervisory relationship as related to the field of clinical supervision. It is offered in such a way that the reader will be encouraged to explore, at great length, issues related to the supervisory relationship that specifically interests them. The references and selected further reading are an invaluable starting point for this in-depth exploration.

One important final comment. Supervisors are like 'blind seers' who usually do not have direct observation of those the therapist is engaged to help. They try to 'see' features of those who are being helped as well as facets of the therapist, try to understand aspects of gender and culture, and provide useful responses and behaviours to benefit the therapist, clinical work and client wellbeing. Both the supervisor and supervisee who value and attend to a quality relationship will ensure this insight is clear, strengthen supervisor–supervisee bond, and set the scene for a rewarding clinical practice with personal and professional development as the hallmarks.

Educational Questions and Activities

1. Classroom discussion

   Discuss the implications of supervision of clinical supervision. When and how should supervisors seek supervision for casework related to supervisees? What would be the areas of consideration that would differ from the supervisor-supervisee relationship?

2. Role play

   Using the questions from the section 'An Inventory of the Supervisory Relationship', identify and role-play scenarios where the selected questions can be answered in such a way that would strengthen the supervisory relationship.

Selected Internet Resources

- Association for Counselor Education and Supervision (ACES): http://www.acesonline.net

- The New Social Worker Online:
  http://www.socialworker.com

References and Selected Further Reading

Bambling, M., King, R., Raue, P., Schweitzer, R., & Lambert, W. (2006). Clinical supervision: Its influence on client-rated working alliance and client symptom reduction in the brief treatment of major depression. *Psychotherapy Research, 16,* 317–331.

Barletta, J. (2007). Clinical supervision. In N. Pelling, R. Bowers & P. Armstrong (Eds.), *The practice of counselling* (pp. 118–135). Melbourne, Australia: Thomson.

Bennett, C.S. (2008) Attachment-informed supervision for social work field. *Clinical Social Work, 36*(1), 97–107.

Bernard, J.M., & Goodyear, R.K. (2004). *Fundamentals of clinical supervision* (3rd ed.). Boston: Pearson.

Berry, J.W. (1974). Psychological aspects of cultural pluralism: Unity and identity reconsidered. *Topics in Cultural Learning, 2,* 17–22.

Berry, J.W. (1976). *Human ecology and cognitive style.* New York: John Wiley.

Berry, J.W. (1980). Acculturation as varieties of adaptation. In A.M. Padilla (Ed.), *Acculturation: Theory, models and some new findings* (pp. 9–25). Boulder, CO: Westview Press.

Berry, J.W. (1983). Acculturation: A comparative analysis of alternative forms. In R.J. Samuda & S.L. Woods (Eds.), *Perspectives in immigrant and minority education* (pp. 65–78). New York: University Press of America.

Berry, J.W., Kim, U., Young, M., & Bujaki, M. (1989). Acculturation attitudes in plural societies. *Applied Psychology: An International Review, 38,* 185–206.

Borders, L.D., Bernard, J.M., Dye, H.A., Fong, M.L., Henderson, P., Nance, D.W., et al. (1991). Curriculum guide for training counseling supervisors: Rationale, development, and implementation. *Counselor Education and Supervision, 31,* 58–80.

Carroll, M., & Gilbert, M.C. (2006). *On being a supervisee: Creating learning partnerships.* Kew, Australia: PsychOz.

Chiaferi, R., & Griffin, M. (1997). *Developing fieldwork skills: A guide for human services, counseling, and social work students.* Pacific Grove, CA: Brooks Cole.

Dixon, J.M. (2008). *Attitudes toward Acculturative Behaviour Scale: Development, reliability and validity* Unpublished doctoral dissertation, The Ohio University.

Dye, A. (1994). In *The Supervisory Relationship. ERIC Digest.* Retrieved December 12, 2008, from ERIC Clearinghouse on Counselling and Student Services Web Site: http://www.ericdigests.org/1995-1/relationship.htm

Hawkins, P., & Shohet, R. (2000). *Supervision in the helping professions* (2nd ed.). Philadelphia: Open University Press.

Lampropoulos, G.K. (2002). A common factors view of counseling supervision process. *The Clinical Supervisor, 21*(1), 77–92.

McMahon, M. (2002). Some supervision practicalities. In M. McMahon & W. Patton (Eds.), *Supervision in the helping professions: A practical approach* (pp. 17–26). Frenchs Forest, Australia: Pearson Education.

McNeill, B.W., & Worthen, V. (1989). The parallel process in supervision. *Professional Psychology Research and Practice, 20*(5), 329–333.

Morrissey, J., & Tribe, R. (2001). Parallel process in supervision. *Counselling Psychology Quarterly, 14,* 103–110.

Nezu, A.M., Saad, R., & Nezu, C.M. (2000). Clinical decision making in behavioral supervision. *Cognitive and Behavioral Practice, 7,* 338–342.

Olk, M.E., & Friedlander, M.L. (1992). Trainees' experiences of role conflict and role ambiguity in supervisory relationships. *Journal of Counseling Psychology, 39,* 389–397.

Pearson, Q. (2004). Getting the most out of clinical supervision: Strategies for mental health. *Journal of Mental Health Counseling, 26*(4), 361–373.

Pearson, Q. (2000). Opportunities and challenges in the supervisory relationship: Implications for counselor supervision. *Journal of Mental Health Counseling, 24,* 283–294.

Redfield, R., Linton, R., & Herskovits, M.J. (1936). Memorandum on the study of acculturation. *American Anthropologist, 56,* 973–1002.

Renfro-Michel, E.L. (2006). A relationship between counselling supervisee attachment and supervision working alliance rapport. (Doctoral dissertation, Mississippi State University). *Dissertation Abstracts International, AAT3238940.*

Ronnestad, M.H., & Skovholt, T.M. (1993). Supervision of beginning and advanced graduate students of counseling and psychotherapy. *Journal of Counseling and Development, 71,* 396–405.

Safran, J.D., & Muran, J.C. (2000). *Negotiating the therapeutic alliance: A relational treatment guide.* New York: Guilford.

Southern, S. (2007). Countertransference and intersubjectivity: Golden opportunities in clinical supervision. *Sexual Addiction and Compulsivity, 14,* 279–302.

chapter eleven

Modes of Supervision

Sally V. Hunter and J. Randolph Bowers

In Australia and the United Kingdom, lifelong supervision has become a requirement for counsellors and psychotherapists and has been built in to the professional codes of conduct as a mandatory requirement (Neufeldt, 1999, cited in Feltham, 2000). The most commonly adopted mode of supervision in Australia is the individual mode, where a less-experienced therapist consults with a more experienced therapist about their caseload face-to-face. This form of supervision, often heavily based on case discussion, is normally conducted at least once a month and is seen as vital to the ethical practice and ongoing professional development of counsellors and psychotherapists.

In this chapter we begin by describing our own personal experiences of supervision — both exceptional and ordinary. We then describe four different modes of supervision including individual, group, peer and self-supervision and the different techniques that can be used within each mode. We explore the strengths and weaknesses of each of these modes of supervision. We discuss ways of empowering supervisees to seek out the supervision that they need. In the process, we challenge the assumption that the individual mode of supervision is the most appropriate mode for counselling supervision in all cases.

Personal Experiences of Counselling Supervision
Sally Hunter

My personal experience of counselling supervision has varied enormously over the course of my career. I have received some excellent supervision, particularly when I worked in private practice and was able to choose my own supervisor. I chose a practitioner that I respected and that practiced using a theoretical approach that I wanted to learn more about. At that time, my practice was based mainly on working with couples and families and my supervisor had a lot of experience in that field. I respected her and she also respected me as a practitioner.

I experienced both the best and the worst of supervision when working in nongovernment counselling organisations. Some of my supervisors were good practitioners in their own right but did not have particular skills as supervisors. They maintained a nonthreatening supervisory environment in which I felt comfortable and unchallenged. I was able to feel confident about my level of expertise, my case management skills and the service that I offered my clients. However, I was not challenged to enhance my skills or to examine my own practice critically.

My best experience of supervision was a live supervision group that I attended for a year during the 1990s. Each member of the group brought in their ongoing clients and ran therapy sessions with them, in front of a one-way mirror. The sessions began with a case discussion before the clients arrived. On arrival, the clients were introduced to the team behind the mirror. During the counselling session, the supervisor phoned through comments and questions to direct the session. Towards the end of the allocated time, the couple or family took a short break while the therapist consulted with the team. The therapist then delivered a Milan-style opinion or summary to the couple or family on behalf of the team. This would probably now be conducted using a reflecting team approach, with the family behind the one-way mirror and the team discussing their observations of the session in front of the family.

This was a fantastic learning experience for all concerned. We had to learn to manage our anxiety about demonstrating our work in front of our peers. We had to learn to accept constructive criticism and feedback. The case discussions that we had were enormously enriched by the experience of the live sessions — and the clients universally found the experience useful and rewarding for them. They appreciated the fact that a group of therapists were interested in helping them and they often found the comments made insightful and profound.

My most difficult experiences of supervision have been in the form of group or peer supervision. When I worked in private practice, I tried to set up several peer supervision groups for myself involving local practitioners. These groups never worked particularly well or lasted for very long. Perhaps we were too democratic and unwilling for anyone to take charge of the sessions and to act as the 'supervisor'. Another complication arose because many of us came from different theoretical perspectives and practised using different modalities. While this should have enhanced the learning opportunities for all, it made any case discussion that we embarked on extremely disjointed and confusing, as each therapist tried to understand the case from their own perspective.

These experiences of supervision have taught me that the best supervision is not always to be found in a safe, one-on-one situation. The best supervision challenges the supervisee to look critically at her/his own practice. This usually involves the supervisee being willing to be open and to take the risk of exposing to others her/his work, warts and all, and to be open to receiving their feedback regardless the form that feedback may take.

Randolph Bowers

My experience of counselling supervision is on a continuum with other forms of workplace supervision. Overall, I believe that supervision is based in a human relationship of trust, learning and guidance. The supervisor often provides guidance. However, in many circumstances, and especially where supervisors take a humble and more interactive approach, guidance can sometimes be exchanged through a two-way conversation that allows the supervisee to demonstrate their strengths and their unique contributions to issues and to the supervision relationship.

The best experiences that I remember in receiving counselling supervision relate to group or peer supervision that was facilitated by a senior professor in counselling psychology. This group was conducted during my Master of Education Counselling degree in Canada. We were able to bring audiotapes of sessions and to play sections of our sessions to the group as a whole. The parts we chose were normally parts we had the most difficulty understanding. The group would give their feedback and the senior member of the group would offer advice when appropriate. Often the peer feedback was far more useful, perhaps because as peers we shared a common experience of learning about therapy and being on our learning edges together. We were able to support each other, offer critique and debate various issues that arose. The senior member of the group would often take a back seat and allow us to explore our issues and interests, giving direct advice only when he saw that we might be getting into muddy waters. The most valuable part of this experience was to not only undertake learning as a counsellor, but also to engage in providing valued feedback to other counsellors on their journey of growth and learning. This dual relationship was both healthy and proactive, empowering and energising.

Another experience of supervision was one-on-one over several years with a senior clinical social worker and professor named Redge Craig. We met on Friday afternoon each week over a 2-year period, then later in less frequent timeslots, sometimes once per month. The early years together were incredibly valuable for me. He was a fascinating man who had studied with some of the best people in the fields of Rogerian Psychotherapy, Humanistic and Existential approaches, and in strategic approaches like Neuro-Linguistic Programming and Clinical Hypnosis. He had also taught over a long career, and my time with him was toward the end of his life. He was counselling the week before he died at the age of 72. His life will always be a great inspiration to me.

The most valuable part of this relationship was my supervisor's keen skills of observation, and his ability to pick up on my weaknesses, games and ways of avoiding uncomfortable issues. He often allowed me to experience moments of intensive psychotherapy with him in order to facilitate an in-depth learning experience. My personal and professional growth was one reality for him. He believed that we bring our personal capacity into the counselling relationship with our clients, and our personal disposition, beliefs, values and perceptions impact our work, even if we deny this fact. His work assumed that we cannot bracket our personal values or beliefs and that we bring our whole selves to the work.

This framework and the presuppositions that Redge brought to supervision were grounded in humanistic, existentialist and strategic approaches to counselling and psychotherapy. He believed that through the use of strategic experiential approaches counsellors and clients could really experience moments of life-transformation. This belief made our work together dynamic and exciting. I never knew what would happen in his presence. He was like visiting a great sage or hermit in the older religious traditions. Someone who you admire and who never wastes any time, gets right to the heart of the matter and has a way of working with the 'great mystery' of life that is larger than any of us. This sense of his respect for time and space enabled him to open up a way of supervision and counselling work that facilitated and encouraged the healing potential within me, and within his clients. This kind of experience may seem rare, but it seems to me one of Redge's core beliefs was that anyone can take up the path of creating miracles in people's lives. He fundamentally believed that we could learn how to facilitate 'miracles' through modelling and demonstrating skills, and by providing opportunities to others to experience change processes that have worked in the past for others.

On the other hand, poor experiences of supervision also came my way in various contexts, including counselling supervision and supervision in the context of counsellor education. These experiences were 'poor' because they did not come from supervisors who took a humble and human empathic approach. Rather, they appeared to use their status to meet their own needs. Everyone can likely meet their own needs in many relationships. The difference that makes for a poor supervision experience comes when supervisors engage in manipulative behaviour and can not separate their personal ego needs from their roles in the workplace. One of the chief differences that I have noticed is that supervisors need to have an attitude of giving or service, combined with a personal discipline of humility and caring for their supervisees. This disposition seems important. Supervisors that expect to open up personal gain through their role as supervisors are on the wrong path in life. For this reason I have chosen to limit my practice of supervision to only a strict few relationships, acknowledging that my high personal standards for supervision demand that I am able to give much more than I receive from this type of relationship. As such, I have to acknowledge my personal limitations. I need to take my own humble approach and to understand that for me supervision is a sacred trust that I cannot enter into lightly.

My experiences of supervision lead me to conclude that really good supervision may be a relatively rare occurrence. I take a sceptical view that we can teach this form of human and spiritual relatedness in existing programs of study. It seems that most supervision in today's world is a form of line management, and that in-depth and qualitative counselling supervision raises the bar extensively. For this reason I come from a tradition where supervision is not a paid activity, but is part of our duty of care as counselling professionals. By making supervision a place of human honour, respect, humility and care we promote a very different and non-materialistic approach to the practice of helping each other maintain sustainable therapeutic practices. Most people do not know how to attain this level of quality, in part because they have never experienced or witnessed quality supervision before. In fact, there have traditionally been no schools of supervision precisely because the profound nature of quality supervision relies heavily on the personal disposition, long-term training, life experience and the spiritual awareness and capacity of the supervisor to bring their whole lives into this work.

It seems to me that to expect the counselling field to sustain quality supervision en masse is an enormous and almost impossible task. For this reason, how we define everyday (mundane) supervision needs careful consideration. In the process of building an Australian counselling field that is supported by the expectation that practitioners receive regular supervision, we need to carefully consider the impacts of the frameworks that we use. It seems to me that Australian approaches to supervision rely too heavily on payment for service, with underlying dynamics that suggest a philosophy of materialism, a practice based more in economics than in caring, and an approach that is based in fear of legal liabilities verses improving the human condition. I would hope that the field would also promote time-honoured traditions of quality, while making proactive steps to prevent economic rationalist values from dominating the field.

Underlying Assumptions About Supervision

The models that we have explored represent western approaches to supervision. We acknowledge that more work needs to be done in future to explore other cultural expressions of supervision, including indigenous and aboriginal forms of supervision. One of the underlying assumptions of western supervision is that it can be used to monitor whether or not clients are receiving appropriate treatment in therapy (Webb, 2000). It is hoped that the therapist will disclose to their supervisor any difficulties that they are having with their clients, including any transference or countertransference issues or ethical dilemmas that they are facing. In this way, the supervisor can help the supervisee to work through these dilemmas and provide a better service for their client. This process has been described as 'healing through meeting' in which the supervisor and supervisee work together to improve the outcomes for the clients (Gilbert & Evans, 2000; p. 61).

There is an underlying assumption that the supervisory relationship is effective and that the supervisee feels safe to divulge such information to their supervisor. The research evidence suggests that this underlying assumption may be questionable, given the frequency with which counsellors and psychotherapists cross ethical boundaries presumably without discussing these issues with their supervisors. For example, in a survey of 284 United States of America (US) licensed psychologists lawsuits were most common for sexual misconduct with a client, failure to warn resulting in injury, child custody decisions and client suicide. There were also a significant number of complaints filed against psychologists relating to their supervision of others (Montgomery, Cupit, & Wimberley, 1999).

There is also an assumption that the supervisor is willing to challenge their supervisees if she/he feels concerned about their practice. Research conducted with 90 US counselling supervisors demonstrated that they often did not disclose to their supervisees their negative reactions to the supervisee's counselling or to their professional performance (Ladany & Melincoff, 1999). Supervisors have also been found to make the supervisory process comfortable and unchallenging by failing to raise their concerns with their supervisees, including important professional performance issues (Ladany & Melincoff, 1999).

We know from research that 'master therapists' are able to embrace complex ambiguity and avoid premature closure. We also know that they possess strong relational skills and are, among other things, emotionally receptive in that they are self-aware, reflective, nondefensive and open to feedback (Skovholt & Jennings, 2004). Obviously, these are some of the important characteristics that the supervisor would hope to encourage and develop in the supervisee. But is this a case of the chicken and the egg?

Does the therapist need to be self-aware, reflective, nondefensive and open to feedback in the first place, in order to develop these skills further? Of course, at its best, the supervisory relationship can be transformational. The supervisor makes use of her/his instrumental self, authentic self and transpersonal self and the supervision session becomes a sacred space in which healing can occur. According to Rowan and Jacobs (2002), the instrumental self leads to healing through ego-building, the authentic self leads to development through ego-extending and the transpersonal use of self leads to opening and ego-reduction.

Modes of Supervision

There are several modes of supervision commonly practised in Australia, including individual, group, peer and self-supervision. Each of these four modes of supervision will be discussed in this chapter and analysed in terms of their strengths and weaknesses. Different supervision techniques, such as live supervision and reflecting teams, fit more easily with particular supervision modes and will also be touched on. Other techniques used in supervision such as the use of technology, 'Interpersonal Recall Process,' and online or cyber-supervision will be discussed in other chapters.

Individual Supervision

Individual supervision is the most frequently used mode of counselling supervision. It was developed out of the psychoanalytic tradition of therapy and was a natural progression from the days when analysts were expected to be in psychoanalysis themselves (Edwards, 2000). During the 1930s, psychodynamic supervision was called control analysis and was believed to be a continuation of the supervisee's personal analysis (Bernard & Goodyear, 1998). Other early models of supervision tended to see it as part of a developmental process (Bernard & Goodyear, 2004). The aim was to help the supervisee to move from dependence on the supervisor to mastery in their own right, and from competence to integration, individuation and integrity. More recently, the emphasis has been placed on the many roles of the supervisor including: setting up a 'learning relationship', teaching, evaluating the supervisee's work, monitoring professional ethical issues, counselling, consulting and monitoring administrative aspects of the work (Carroll, 1996).

In their first supervision session, the supervisor and the supervisee will normally discuss their expectations of each other and how they would like to work together. They will agree the frequency, format and venue of supervision and the ways in which both parties will prepare for the sessions. There may be some organisational requirements that need to be discussed, such as making a 6-monthly report on the supervision process, or submitting a recording of a client session for the supervisor to watch on an annual basis. The supervisor will brief the supervisee specifically in terms of how they expect them to present cases for discussion in supervision and what preparation they need to conduct before each meeting (Bernard & Goodyear, 2004). They will also ask the supervisee for their ideas about how they would like the process to work and be evaluated. Of course, there is room for a lot of flexibility within the supervision process and it can be as creative as any counselling session and involve the use of creative arts such as story-telling, use of film, letter writing, imaginary dialogue, use of metaphor, guided fantasy and so on (Lahad, 2000).

When it works well, supervision is invaluable for the supervisee and the clients involved. In these circumstances, it is also beneficial to the supervisor, although this is not the primary focus. Of course, the process relies upon the supervisee having sufficient self-awareness and honesty to disclose any issues or concerns that they have relating to their clients. However, it is also known that such disclosures produce feelings of anxiety within supervisees who do not want to be seen as 'vulnerable, ineffectual, or unlikable' (Webb, 2000, p. 69), particularly when they are training. A survey of 96 UK psychodynamic counsellors demonstrated that there was a correlation between the supervisee's perception of the strength of rapport with their supervisor and the likelihood that they would feel able to disclose sensitive issues in supervision (Webb, 2000). It was also easier for them to make such disclosures in individual rather than in group supervision and to an independent supervisor, particularly one that they had been able to choose themselves. In this study, the supervisees expressed doubt about their ability to disclose: any sexual feelings they might have towards their clients, difficulties within the supervisory process and personal feelings towards their supervisor.

Some supervisees will be able to bring their ethical dilemmas to supervision and be able to be open about their concerns. Alternatively, as supervisees discusses their caseloads, the supervisor may hear warning bells alerting her/him to possible ethical or professional practice concerns. In this situation, the supervisor needs to bring the issue into the awareness of the supervisee in order to help her/him to behave in a professional manner consistent with the ethical code for the profession (Storm & Haug, 1997). The types of minor mistakes that supervisees find relatively easy to discuss and resolve in supervision include confidentiality issues, time boundary issues, issues relating to touch and confusion or forgetting what a client had said (Daniels, 2000). Major mistakes that would be more difficult to raise in supervision include: taking sides in couple therapy, sexually exploiting a client, abusing clients emotionally, creating hugely dependent relationships or extorting money from clients (Daniels, 2000).

The way in which the supervisee chooses her/his supervisor is very important. A qualitative study conducted with eight UK counsellors showed that therapists based their selection on factors such as: convenience, gender, theoretical orientation and expertise, and the desire for safety and familiarity (Lawton, 2000). These supervisees had high expectations of having an intimate, perhaps even idealised, relationship with their chosen supervisors and demonstrated 'a tendency to view the supervisory space as a haven where the counsellor's frustration, anxieties and shortcomings would be accepted, soothed or resolved' (Lawton, 2000, p. 32–33). Even though they knew that it was not necessarily wise, they tended to want to preserve their attachment to their supervisors. The researcher concluded that 'dependency and the fear of loss may lead a counsellor to cling on to a supervisory process' (Lawton, 2000, p. 40). Unpacking the developmental needs that supervisees bring to the supervision relationship may also need to acknowledge that the supervision relationship is highly valued. As such, acknowledging the exchange of needs and desires within this relationship requires a fair degree of maturity on the part of the supervisor, who may assist their supervisees to gain greater autonomy over time. Of course, gaining such autonomy is highly prized within the western model of counselling supervision.

The main advantage of individual supervision is that it enables the creation of a safe and confidential environment in which the supervisee can appraise their own work with clients honestly and critically and thereby improve the services they offer to these clients. The supervisee–supervisor relationship mirrors the client–therapist relationship and can be used to examine transference and countertransference issues, as well as parallel processes between counselling and supervision. It provides the supervisee with a focused way of assessing their professional conduct and expert guidance from a more experienced clinician, when necessary. The supervisor has an important teaching and mentoring role that positions supervision as the cornerstone of the professional development of the therapist (Bernard & Goodyear, 2004). Attending to the human quality of the relationship may also assist supervisors and supervisees to appreciate the extent of the importance of their relationship in a holistic sense, enabling them to move beyond material and behavioural views of transference and countertransference, to explore other meanings related to their interaction.

Group Supervision

Group supervision has been defined as:

> … the regular meeting of a group of supervisees, with a designated supervisor or supervisors, to monitor the quality of their work and to further their understanding of themselves as clinicians, of the clients with whom they work, and of service delivery in general. (Bernard & Goodyear, 2004, p. 235)

These goals are achieved by the giving and receiving of feedback, mainly from interactions between the supervisees. In these days of managed care and economic rationalism, group supervision has become increasingly popular within organisations. When it successfully harnesses the power of the group process, it can be a highly effective way of conducting supervision. However, it also has the potential to be damaging to group members or to fail to meet the needs of individual therapists if the process is not well managed.

There are many advantages to group supervision, over and above the economic argument. In the right environment, supervisees can do a wonderful job of critiquing each other's work. This affords everyone in the group the opportunity for vicarious learning, by being exposed to a wide range of clients and by seeing the achievements and the mistakes that other therapists have made. Often it affords the supervisor a wider perspective on the supervisees, by seeing them interacting with their colleagues and discussing each other's cases. It can also give each supervisee a wider range of opinions about their particular case, rather than receiving feedback from one person only in the form of the supervisor. Group supervision can lead to greater accountability and improved outcomes for the client, since supervisees have the opportunity to learn from both their supervisor and their peers (Corey & Corey, 2007). Supervisees also find comfort in the fact that they are not alone in their anxieties.

One of the other great strengths of group supervision is that it enables the use of additional techniques, over and above those used in individual supervision, such as live counselling demonstrations, role-playing, role reversal, modelling, coaching, psychodrama, experiential exercises and so on (Haynes, Corey, & Moulton, 2003). Some of these methods are described in more detail in other chapters. It would be possible to use a modified form of Interpersonal Process Recall by analysing videorecordings of sessions in group supervision. The tape would be stopped and the supervisee would be invited to recall what he/she was thinking and what decisions were made about what to say and what not to say (Clarke, 1999). Obviously, it would be important for the supervisor/group leader to be trained in group processes as well as in supervision itself (Hawkins & Shohet, 2000).

In a few years time, it is likely that many therapists will be receiving group supervision via the internet using terms and techniques that have not yet been invented. A recent description of e-therapy already looks old-fashioned since it describes email and internet relay chat instead of blogs and wikis (Goss & Anthony, 2003). Online group supervision will offer new benefits, the most obvious being accessibility. Given that clients will increasingly use the internet for information, therapists will also need to embrace this technology as it develops (Walz, 2000).

Peer Supervision

The main difference between group supervision and peer supervision is that a peer supervision group is normally run by its members, who are peers, in the absence of an appointed leader or authority figure (Gomersall, 2000). As a result, there is no evaluatory process involved in peer supervision and it is closer to consultation than supervision (Bernard & Goodyear, 2004). The success of a peer group is dependent on its members being committed to the purpose of the group as demonstrated by regular attendance, and on the quality of the interactions between the members of the group. In its best form peer supervision is 'relatively free, both of collusive friendship, and dependency on expert guidance' (Gomersall, 2000, p. 110). There is a sense of freedom to describe your experiences honestly that comes with the lack of formal evaluation and the democratic structure of most peer groups.

The main strength of this type of supervision is that it affords therapists the opportunity to become more reflexive about their practice and to receive feedback from peers about their work. It provides an opportunity for ongoing education and professional development, and for the transfer of important information about the field of counselling. Often peer supervision develops when a small group of therapists who know and respect each other decide to meet regularly in order to support one another. This can be particularly useful for therapists who feel isolated in their working environments. Therapists normally meet in order to discuss complex cases, ethical dilemmas, transference and countertransference issues and in order to counteract feelings of isolation (Bernard & Goodyear, 2004). The main advantages of peer supervision are that the only cost is the therapist's time, the environment created is both convenient and supportive and there is an opportunity to learn vicariously through other people's difficulties and dilemmas. The disadvantages are that the presence of peers may disinhibit people from sharing openly about what actually happens in therapy, there is less time for each individual to get their supervisory needs met and that the dynamics of the group may impede the learning for some group members (Barletta, 2006).

Research into the therapeutic relationship (Hunter, 2002) led to an analysis of the ways in which therapists use personal, professional and organisational strategies to cope with challenging situations (Hunter & Schofield, 2006). Eight therapists who worked in nongovernment organisations were interviewed and described the value of *peer debriefing* over and above formal supervision. By this they meant talking to a carefully chosen colleague, in a confidential context, about the difficulties or challenges that they were facing with a particular client. This enabled them to defuse their anxiety, without being told how to manage the case and without being evaluated in a critical manner.

Self-Supervision

Self-supervision is another mode of supervision that can be invaluable in certain circumstances. Therapists with many years of experience who supervise less-experienced therapists and are often working in highly complex or specialised fields themselves, find it difficult to find experienced supervisors (Feltham, 2000). Geographically isolated therapists may also find it difficult to find a supervisor, although this difficulty is gradually being overcome by technological advances and e-supervision. Sometimes the supervision that is being provided by an employer does not meet the needs of the supervisee and this could be a situation where self-supervision would be useful.

Self-supervision has been used as a method for several decades (Casement, 1985). Many experienced practitioners, such as Gerald Egan, have admitted to having little or no formal supervision and choosing to consult other therapists only when necessary (Feltham, 2000). One of the goals of all modes of supervision is that the supervisee eventually learns to trust her/his own clinical judgment and becomes able to put the welfare of the client first, over and above her/his own needs. In order to achieve this goal, the supervisee needs to develop an ability to self-monitor, self-assess and self-evaluate (Haynes, Corey, & Moulton, 2003). Indeed, some therapists have argued that having a reliable internal supervisor is fundamental to good practice in the field (Gilbert & Evans, 2000).

There is an implicit link between the concept of reflexivity and the idea of self-supervision (Bernard & Goodyear, 2004). Through supervision, supervisees learn to become more reflexive and to identify areas of their own practice in which they feel a level of distress, confusion or uncertainty. In this way, they gradually become able to monitor and evaluate their own professional conduct, ethical conduct, cultural competence, responsiveness to their clients, ability to resolve conflict and so on (Haynes et al., 2003).

There are many different methods of self-supervision and, once again, it is an opportunity for the therapist to be as creative as they are with their clients. Several methods for self-supervision have been proposed — including looking at the case from three different perspectives, that of the client, the therapist and the supervisor (Lahad, 2000, p. 115–117). The use of recording can be very useful in self-supervision, since it enables an in-depth examination of the session, whereby key moments can be replayed and analysed thoroughly. The presence of the camera is less likely to place a strain on the therapist when used in self-supervision (Aveline, 1999).

A series of questions for self-supervision and self-reflection have been developed (Neufeldt 1999, cited in Bernard & Goodyear, 2004, p. 225). These are useful both for preparation for individual, group or peer supervision and for self-supervision:

1. Describe the therapy events that precipitated your puzzlement.

2. State your question about these events as clearly as you can.

3. What were you thinking during this portion of the session?

4. What were you feeling? How do you understand these feelings now?

5. Consider your own actions during this portion of the session. What did you intend?

6. Now look at the interaction between you and the client. What were the results of your interventions?

7. What was the feel, the emotional flavour, of the interaction between you? Was it similar or different from your usual experience with this client?

8. To what degree do you understand this interaction as similar to the client's interactions in other relationships? How does this inform your experience of the interaction in the session?

9. What theories do you use to understand what is going on in the session?

10. What past professional or personal experiences affect your understanding?

11. How else might you interpret the event and interaction in the session?

12. How might you test out the various alternatives in your next counselling session?

13. How will the client's responses inform what you do next?

Getting the Most From Supervision

'Supervision is traditionally a process, over time, which in turn, mirrors and directs another process, such as counselling or psychotherapy' (Goss, 2000, p. 75). In that sense, supervision is an indirect process that requires openness and honesty on the part of the supervisee and a willingness to ask difficult questions on the part of the supervisor, for it to work effectively. In order to get the most from supervision, the supervisee needs to be open to learning, be able to admit when she/he does not know the answer or is operating beyond her/his level of competence and be assertive in getting her/his supervision needs met (Corey & Corey, 2007).

The issue of power is evident in supervision, just as much as it is alive and well in therapy (Gilbert & Evans, 2000). A minority of therapists continue to try to change the sexual orientation of gay and lesbian clients or to engage in sexual activity with their clients, 'and if the client protests, the therapist has a number of finely honed tools for putting them back in their place' (Totton, 2006, p. 86). Supervision literally means overseeing and, like all human activities, it has its shadow side. Supervision that is developmentally inappropriate for the supervisee will not work well. In addition, if the supervisor is intolerant of differences, fails to model good professional and/or personal attitudes, does not manage boundary issues or difficult interpersonal exchanges well in supervision, or appears to be professionally apathetic then supervision will fail (Magnuson, Wilcoxen, & Norem 200, cited in Nelson-Jones, 2005).

Lifelong supervision is not mandatory in the US (Feltham, 2000) and in the UK the supervisory role has been described as moving towards more of a policing role and some therapists have been obliged to attend mandatory supervision as a penalty for misconduct (Daniels, 2000). As a result, the necessity for counsellors to receive career-long supervision has recently been challenged (Wosket, 2006) for the following reasons:

- a lack of evidence of the efficacy of supervision
- the unintended message that counsellors need surveillance and cannot be trusted to work independently
- infantilising senior members of the profession
- the lack of motivation when mandated to attend supervision
- the second-hand nature of the reports of client issues in supervision that may enable unethical practitioners to censor what they bring to supervision.

Conclusion

In this chapter we have described the modes of supervision that are currently used in Australia. Individual supervision remains the most popular mode of supervision and has many advantages, given that the supervisee receives the individual attention of the supervisor and an opportunity to disclose sensitive issues within a confidential context. Group and peer supervision are becoming increasing popular, mainly for financial reasons. These modes also offer different, creative opportunities for mutual learning and for enriching each other's clinical practice. The ability to use self-supervision as a method of monitoring one's own professional development is also a vital tool for therapists to develop. Supervision, at its best, can be an invaluable support to therapists and enhance their clinical practice, as well as their sense of wellbeing as a result of their work.

Individual supervision is not necessarily the best method of supervision for all supervisees, depending on their level of expertise. Often different modes of supervision will complement each other.

Educational Questions and Activities

1. What has been your personal experience of different modes of supervision, both as a supervisee and as a supervisor?
   - Which modes have you found most useful?
   - Which have you found least useful?
   - What made it more/less useful?

2. What mode of supervision did you find most useful during your training or as an early career therapist?
   - What did you need from supervision most at that time?
   - What helped/stopped you from getting your needs met?

3. What mode of supervision would suit you best now?
   - What do you need most from supervision now?
   - What do you envisage your needs being over the next 5 years?

4. How can you get the most out of your supervision over the next 5 years?
   - Do you need to change supervisor?
   - If so, what qualities or attributes would you want in your new supervisor?
   - If not, how can you change your behaviour in supervision in order to receive better supervision?

5. Does self-supervision really work?
   - What would you need to put in place to ensure that self supervision was really working?
   - How would you know when it was working?
   - How would you know when it was not working?

Selected References for Further Reading

Bernard, J.M., & Goodyear, R.K. (2004). *Fundamentals of clinical supervision* (3rd ed.). Boston: Pearson Education.

Lahad, M. (2000). *Creative supervision: The use of expressive arts methods in supervision and self-supervision.* London: Jessica Kingsley.

Haynes, R., Corey, G., & Moulton, P. (2003). *Clinical supervision in the helping professions: A practical guide.* Pacific Grove, CA: Brooks/Cole.

References

Aveline, M. (1999). The use of audiotapes in supervision of psychotherapy. In G. Shipton (Ed.), *Supervision of psychotherapy and counseling: Making a place to think* (pp. 80–92). Buckingham, England: Open University Press.

Barletta, J. (2006). Clinical supervision. In N. Pelling, R. Bowers & P. Armstrong (Eds.), *The practice of counselling* (pp. 118–135). Melbourne, Australia: Thomson.

Bernard, J.M., & Goodyear, R.K. (1998). *Fundamentals of clinical supervision.* Boston: Allyn and Bacon.

Bernard, J.M., & Goodyear, R.K. (2004). *Fundamentals of clinical supervision* (3rd ed.). Boston: Pearson Education.

Carroll, M. (1996). *Counselling supervision: Theory, skills and practice.* London: Cassell.

Casement, P. (1985). *On learning from the patient.* London: Tavistock/Routledge.

Clarke, P. (1999). Interpersonal process recall in supervision. In G. Shipton (Ed.), *Supervision of psychotherapy and counselling: Making a place to think* (pp. 93–104). Buckingham, England: Open University Press.

Corey, M.S., & Corey, G. (2007). *Becoming a helper* (5th ed.). Belmont, CA: Thomson Brooks/Cole.

Daniels, J. (2000). Whispers in the corridor and kangaroo courts: The supervisory role in mistakes and complaints. In B. Lawton & C. Feltham (Eds.), *Taking supervision forward* (pp. 74–91). London: Sage.

Edwards, D. (2000). Supervision today: The psychoanalytic legacy. In G. Shipton (Ed.), *Supervision of psychotherapy and counselling: Making a place to think* (pp. 11–23). Buckingham, England: Open University Press.

Feltham, C. (2000). Counselling supervision: Baselines, problems and possibilities. In B. Lawton & C. Feltham (Eds.), *Taking supervision forward: Enquiries and trends in counselling and psychotherapy* (pp. 5–24). London: Sage.

Gilbert, M., & Evans, K. (2000). *Psychotherapy supervision.* Buckingham, England: Open University Press.

Gomersall, J. (2000). Peer group supervision. In G. Shipton (Ed.), *Supervision of psychotherapy and counselling: Making a place to think* (pp. 107–118). Buckingham, England: Open University Press.

Goss, S. (2000). A supervisory revolution? The impact of new technology. In B. Lawton & C. Feltham (Eds.), *Taking supervision forward* (pp. 175–189). London: Sage.

Goss, S., & Anthony, K. (Eds.). (2003). *Technology in counselling and psychotherapy.* Basingstoke, England: Palgrave Macmillan.

Hawkins, P., & Shohet, R. (2000). *Supervision in the helping professions* (2nd ed.). Buckingham, England: Open University Press.

Haynes, R., Corey, G., & Moulton, P. (2003). *Clinical supervision in the helping professions: A practical guide.* Pacific Grove, CA: Brooks/Cole.

Hunter, S.V. (2002). *Walking in sacred spaces: The experiences of the counsellor in the client-counsellor relationship.* Armidale, Australia: University of New England.

Hunter, S.V., & Schofield, M.J. (2006). How therapists cope with challenge: Personal, professional and organisational strategies. *International Journal for the Advancement of Counselling,* 28(2), 121–138.

Ladany, N., & Melincoff, D.S. (1999). The nature of counselor supervisor nondisclosure. *Counselor Education and Supervision, 38,* 161–176.

Lahad, M. (2000). *Creative supervision: The use of expressive arts methods in supervision and self-supervision.* London: Jessica Kingsley.

Lawton, B. (2000). 'A very exposing affair' : Exploration in counsellors' supervisory relationships. In B. Lawton & C. Feltham (Eds.), *Taking supervision forward* (pp. 25–41). London: Sage.

Montgomery, L.M., Cupit, B.E., & Wimberley, T.K. (1999). Complaints, malpractice, and risk management: Professional issues and personal experiences. *Professional Psychology: Research and Practice, 30*(4), 402–410.

Nelson-Jones, R. (2005). *Practical counselling and helping skills* (5th ed.). London: Sage.

Rowan, J., & Jacobs, M. (2002). *The therapist's use of self.* Buckingham, England: Open University Press.

Skovholt, T.M., & Jennings, L. (2004). *Master therapists: Exploring expertise in therapy and counseling.* Boston: Pearson Education.

Storm, C.L., & Haug, I.E. (1997). Ethical issues: Where do you draw the line? In T.C. Todd & C.L. Storm (Eds.), *The complete systemic supervisor* (pp. 26–40). Boston: Allyn and Bacon.

Totton, N. (2006). Power in the therapeutic relationship. In N. Toton (Ed.), *The politics of psychotherapy: New perspectives* (pp. 83–93). Maidenhead, England: Open University Press.

Walz, G.R. (2000). Summing up. In J.W. Bloom & G.R. Walz (Eds.), *Cybercounselling and cyberlearning: Strategies and resources for the Millennium* (pp. 405–413). Alexandria, VA: American Counseling Association.

Webb, A. (2000). What makes it difficult for the supervisee to speak? In B. Lawton & C. Feltham (Eds.), *Taking supervision forward* (pp. 60–73). London: Sage.

Wosket, V. (2006). Clinical supervision. In C. Feltham & I. Horton (Eds.), *The Sage handbook of counselling and psychotherapy* (pp. 165–173). London: Sage.

—┼┼┼┼┼—

chapter twelve

Supervisor Development

Nadine Pelling and Elisa Agostinelli

The practice of clinical supervision has a well-established history (Bernard & Goodyear, 1992). It was the first educational method in which more experienced colleagues would supervise new and less-experienced colleagues to increase their knowledge and competence as practitioners. It was also a way for colleagues to meet and discuss particularly difficult client cases and monitor their own responses to particular issues.

Today the practice of supervision has become more structured and complex. Dealing with a supervisee's personal, professional and ethical issues is not an easy task. It can be difficult to meet supervisee expectations. Supervision can also be exhausting as, 'during the process of supervision, Supervisors make their personality, acquired clinical and theoretical knowledge, and emotional and mental resources available to the learning process' (Yerushalmi, 1999, p. 427).

Recently, the idea of supervising supervisors and aiding in their development has emerged in our profession as a possible support for supervisors, but also as a way to control the quality of supervision offered (Ellis, 2006; Emilsson & Johnsson, 1997). It is now widely recognised that supervisors of counsellors can benefit from supervision (BAC, 1996; BACP, 2007; Emilsson & Johnsson, 2007). This recognition fulfils Styczynski's (1980) assertion years ago that as the field of supervision developed, more attention would have to be paid to the training and credentials of supervisors. In other words, if an informed perspective on clinical supervision is to be obtained then an understanding of supervisory development must also be acquired (Watkins, 1997a). This chapter outlines a popular model of supervisor development and then reviews four main influences on supervisory development.

Supervisor Development

In most supervisory developmental models, supervisors progress from being vulnerable and anxious about supervising to becoming more autonomous supervisors wherein a supervisory identity takes form (Watkins, 1995b, 1995c, 1995d). At earlier stages of their own development supervisors require more structure and a more secure holding environment, whereas at later stages the developing supervisor requires more of a collaborative relationship with their supervisor of supervision (Watkins, 1995b, 1995c, 1995d). Both of these statements are true for the supervisory complexity model as outlined as follows.

Supervisor Complexity Model

The most written about and elaborate model of supervisor development is the supervisor complexity model (SCM). This model was based on the counsellor development models by Hogan (1964) and Stoltenberg (1981), later further developed into the IDM of Stoltenberg, McNeill, and Delworth (1998). According to the SCM (Hillman, McPherson, Swank, & Watkins, 1998; Watkins, 1990a, 1990b, 1993, 1994, 1995a, 1995b, 1995c, 1995d), supervisors progress through four different stages of development in their progression from novice to more competent and expert supervisors. During each of these stages supervisors have specific tasks to accomplish and responsibilities (Watkins, Schneider, Haynes, & Nieberding, 1995). At each stage the supervisor develops greater professional identity, increased acceptance of the supervisee, a less dogmatic approach regarding theory and an increasing confidence in supervisory skills. Development is viewed as both qualitative and quantitative in nature. Development occurs in the form of an increased sense of professional identity.

Stage 1: Role shock. This stage is encountered by a new supervisor when first entering the supervisor role and is characterised by questions of role boundaries and definitions. Counsellors may feel like imposter supervisors and wonder if they are professionals or students. Supervisors at this stage are also likely to be concrete in their provision of supervision and thus interventions may appear superficial in nature. Supervisors of supervision trainees at this stage of development are best advised to provide a clear and strong holding environment and thus provide a stabilising and soothing function for supervision trainees. Supervision trainees need to be helped to define the supervision relationship at this stage of development.

Stage 2: Role recovery and transition. This stage is characterised by a more realistic perception of one's weaknesses and strengths as a supervisor. Some confidence in one's abilities as a supervisor develops. However, process and transference/countertransference issues are still not well addressed by supervisors at this stage of development. Supervisors of supervision trainees are urged to loosen the hold of their relationship with the supervision trainee at this stage of development and encourage the trainee's development of autonomy.

Stage 3: Role consolidation. At this stage supervisors have reached a level of increasing consistency in their supervision provision. Supervisors at this level are more realistic about their strengths and weaknesses and can function as a resource for counselling trainees. Supervisors of supervision trainees at this level are more likely to adequately address transference, process and countertransference issues with their counselling trainees.

Stage 4: Role mastery. A supervisor at this stage has a sense of mastery about their supervisory competence. Various issues can be addressed competently by supervisors at this level. If supervision is provided for supervisors at this level it is likely to be collaborative, challenging in nature and on an as-needed basis.

Possible Influences on Supervisory Development

There are four main influences on supervisory competence: personal variables, counselling experience, supervisory training, and supervisory experience.

Personal and Relational Factors

Looking at fitness to practice, the personal characteristics of the counsellor trainee 'invariably affect the supervisory and treatment process' (Haber, 1996, p. 21). According to Bernard and Goodyear (1992), personal growth is part of supervision. It is important to encourage counsellor trainees' personal growth as they learn to encourage parallel growth in their clients (Emerson, 1996). Edwards and Bess (1998) stated, 'the development of a therapist's self-awareness must carry at least as much weight in his or her professional education and training as the accumulation of knowledge about theories and methodologies established by the leaders of the profession' (p. 98). R.N. Wendt (personal communication November 17, 1997) stated that if the therapist measures her self-growth based on her perceived competence as professional, personal development may be impeded. Consequently, counsellor trainees need a training process that integrates personal and technical competencies (Aponte & Winter, 2000).

Personal issues are seen as potential 'handicaps' and resources at the same time. They are considered 'handicaps' when they prevent the counsellor trainee in establishing a therapeutic relationship with the client and seeing the underlying dynamics between the members of the client's family. They are considered resources when they facilitate the counsellor trainee in making a shift in the affective relationship between members of the client-family (Andolfi, 1985). Wendt (1999) suggested that to be able to achieve greater self-awareness and open the boundaries to personal transformation, counsellors and supervisors need to experience vulnerability and failure in their professional life. Through the discussion of personal issues during counselling training, the supervisor may identify counsellor trainees that are hampered in their performance as counsellors because their personal issues are too great to be overcome (Bernard & Goodyear, 1992). This can be a delicate and difficult decision for a supervisor to make and the possibility to discuss the issue with another colleague during the supervision of supervisors could make the process more objective. In addition, to be able to look at the supervisees' personal issues, the supervisors need to constantly look at his or her personal issues and how they affect work as a supervisor.

Supervisors need to 'develop their own capacities for self-observation and to learn more about their own strength and weaknesses' (Whitman & Jacobs, 1998, p.172). As counsellors, we have to be aware of our limits. We need to be able to recognise that we cannot work with certain kind of clients because of our personal experience or because of specific issues we are going through in a specific time of our life. According to Aponte and Winter (2000), counsellors' effectiveness is not only related to what the counsellor has been able to resolve in his or her life, but also to what the counsellor has learned to recognise and work with in his or her self. 'By resolving individual issues, or by learning to work with unchangeable or unresolved issues, a clinician attains greater freedom and ability in the use of self with clients' (Aponte & Winter, 2000, p. 148).

If we think about a therapy session, 'ultimately, our single most important instrument is the person we are' (Corey, 2001, p. 38).Competent counsellors are those are able to recognise their own limitations and refer the client to someone else. As a supervisor we have to do the same. Professionally and personally we cannot be fit to interact with every supervisee. We have to be able to recognise that some of our personal issues in specific times of our life can interfere with our supervisory work with specific supervisees. In this case we need to be able to recognise the problem and refer the supervisee to another supervisor. 'Supervisors should be aware that they are participants in the supervisory process, and that their style, inner conflicts, or enactments may directly affect the supervisory relationship and patient treatment' (Whitman & Jacobs, 1998, p. 172). However, at times supervisors may not be able to recognise the effect of their personal issues on the supervisory relationship. Therefore, it is essential for supervisor to have supervision so they can be helped to recognise the reasons for possible impasse in the supervisory relationship and to assure quality services to the counsellor and a safe and effective treatment to the client.

Discussion of personal issues during counselling training reduces the prospect of burnout and increases successful therapeutic outcome (Aponte & Winter, 2000). Similarly, the discussion of personal issues can help the burnout of supervisors. Fear and Woolfe (1999) found that counsellors need to 'integrate the epistemological beliefs of their chosen orientation with personal philosophy' (p. 254). If this does not occur it may lead to 'a loss of optimal functioning, or in the individual suffering a level of intrapsychic conflict which in turn may result in burnout or abandonment of career' (Fear & Woolfe, 1999, p. 256).

According to Gee (1996), part of the supervisory process is the interpretation of the counsellor trainee's countertransference in relation to the client's transference. In doing so, the supervisor has to focus on aspects of counsellor trainees' personal development related to the relationship between the counsellor trainee and the client, and not on other aspects of their personal development. In the psychoanalytic orientation, countertransference refers to the counsellor's personal issues and 'knowing that a counselor reaction emanates from an area of unresolved conflict requires the counselor to examine his or her own personal issues' (Rosenberger & Hayes, 2002, p. 269). The supervisor should help the counsellor trainee examine personal issues, but only if these issues relate to problems occurring in the therapeutic relationship between counsellor trainee and client. The focus of recent psychodynamic supervision is to examine and explore during the supervisory experience the intrapersonal and interpersonal dynamics that occur between counsellor trainee and client. 'Intrapersonal dynamics consist of covert behaviors and sensory processes such as feelings, thoughts, and perceptions' (Bradley, 1989, p. 68). The supervisor has to focus on counsellor trainees' reactions to clients' transference/countertransference issues. He or she has to be aware of transference and countertransference dynamics between and client that could cause an impasse in the therapeutic process (Borders & Leddick, 1987).

Because of the nature of the relationship, it is likely that counsellor trainees' resistance emerges during the supervisory session and the interpretation of this dynamic by the supervisor is a therapeutic necessity (Bradley, 1989). The processes that occur in the relationship between patient and therapist are often reflected in the relationship between therapist and supervisors (please see the chapter on Alliance Supervision to Enhance Client Outcomes for further discussion of this topic). This is called parallel process and it is the most unique dynamic in supervision. The same dynamic could occur during supervision of supervisors: A beginner supervisor can experience parallel issues from her own supervision session with a beginner counsellor when she has her own supervision of supervision (Stoltenberg & Delworth, 1987). In this case it is essential that a third parson (the supervisor of supervisors) will analyse and interpret the dynamic between supervisee and supervisor.

Where is the line between therapy and supervision relating to personal and relational variables? Aponte (1992) tried to define the line between supervision and therapy, stating that 'because the trainers ... consistently redirect the focus of personal exploration to clinical practice, they do not become personal therapists' (p. 275). The supervisor points out to the student the problem he or she had during the session and connects the problem with the student's personal issues and family issues (Aponte, 1992). This should be translated into the supervision of supervisor relationship.

Counselling Experience

Many believe that to be a competent supervisor one must be a competent counsellor. Styczynski (1980) reports that therapist skills are important as they can be imparted to the trainee and also because many of the skills successful in therapeutic interventions are also relevant to the supervisory relationship to 'optimize change and development of the student' (p. 31). Watkins (1997a, 1997b) echoes this sentiment.

Whereas being a competent counsellor may be a necessary component of being a competent supervisor, counselling skills do not sufficiently enable one to work as an effective supervisor (Farrell, 1996; Watkins, 1991). Indeed, Stoltenberg, McNeill, and Delworth (1998) indicate that being a counsellor does not sufficiently enable one to supervise others' work. Thus, training and experience as a supervisor are also viewed as important aspects of developing supervisory competence in conjunction with counsellor development (Pelling, 2008; Stoltenberg & Delworth, 1987). Research supports the idea that counsellors develop as they gain experience, namely supervised experience. Similarly, supervisors are expected to develop a more balanced view of themselves and their supervisees as they develop (Watkins, 1993).

Supervisory Training

Many authors indicate that training in supervision is needed for therapists to develop their supervisory skills (Bernard & Goodyear, 1992; Farrell, 1996; Stoltenberg & Delworth, 1987; Watkins, 1997a, 1997b). Research also supports the need for training by indicating that systematic training is more likely to facilitate counsellor growth than less systematic training (Lambert & Ogles, 1997). Some authors also advocate that continuing education should be sought by those who perform supervision (Davies, 1997). As indicated by Stoltenberg and Delworth (1987, p. 154), 'It seems reasonable at this point to believe that higher functioning supervisors are more effective and that, as with counseling skills, training may improve supervisor functioning'. However, as Watkins (1991) states there is a paradox in psychotherapy supervision training, namely, while the supervisory role is considered important, training in how to be a supervisor is very limited.

The SCM specifically identifies training as an agent capable of advancing supervisory identity and skill development, as it can aid the acquisition of competencies in interventions and appropriate supervisory tasks and roles. Supervisory training could be especially helpful for supervisors in the first stage of supervisory development, role shock. Such training can serve as a buffer for supervisors by indicating what the transition from counsellor to supervisor might entail.

Supervisory Experience

Experience as a supervisor has long been believed to have a positive influence on one's development as a supervisor (Stoltenberg & Delworth, 1987). Research supports the idea that supervisory experience can aid supervisory development. Stone (1980) as well as Marikis, Russell, and Dell (1985) indicate that more experienced supervisors made more planning statements. However, Watkins (1993) points out that research indicates that supervisors may not develop and become more competent simply because they conduct supervision. Nevertheless, the more supervisory experience a supervisor accumulates the greater opportunity they will have to confront more developmental challenges and issues and thus prompt supervisory identity development.

It is possible that supervised supervision experience aids one's development as a supervisor more than independent experience due to the greater amount of reflection, support and feedback provided by the additional supervisory relationship. Supervision of supervision can provide attachment components that allow for safety and exploration of supervisory behaviours.

Conclusion

Supervision has a long history in the therapeutic professions. Recently, the importance of developing supervisors and supporting them in their work has been recognised. Supervisors of supervisors and supervisors of clinicians need to address personal and relational variables, be experienced clinicians, engage in professional developmental training in relation to supervision and can also benefit from supervision of their own supervision. Reflective practice with clients and/or supervisees means continuous and lifelong learning, as well as development.

Educational Questions and Activities

1. What does the Supervisor Complexity Model have to say about supervisor development?
   - that growth progresses through four different states and that during each stage supervisors have specific tasks to accomplish and responsibilities.
2. What are the SCM stages?
   - role shock
   - role recovery and transition
   - role consolidation
   - role mastery.
3. List four influences on supervisory competence.
   - personal/relational variables
   - counselling experience
   - supervisory training
   - supervisory experience.
4. Which of the four variables above do you see as most influential and why?

Selected References for Further Reading

Watkins, C. (1995b). Psychotherapy supervisor and supervisee: Developmental models and research nine years later. *Clinical Psychology Review, 17*(7), 647–680.

Watkins, C. (1995c). Psychotherapy supervisor development: On musings, models, and metaphor. *The Journal of Psychotherapy Practice and Research, 4*, 150–158.

Schofield, M., & Pelling, N. (2002). Supervision of counsellors. In M. McMahon & W. Patton (Eds.), *Supervision in the helping professions: a practical approach* (pp. 211–222). Sydney, Australia: Prentice Hall.

Pelling, N. (2008). The relationship of supervisory experience, counseling experience, and training in supervision to supervisory identity development. *International Journal for the Advancement of Counselling, 30*(4), 235–248.

References

Andolfi, M. (1985). L'hadicap dello studente come strumento di formazione. In M. Andolfi & D. Piccone (Eds.), *La formazione relazionale: Individuo e gruppo nel processo di apprendimento* (pp. 218–238). Roma: Terapia Familiare.

Aponte, H.J. (1992). Training the person of the therapist in structural family therapy. *Journal of Marital and Family Therapy, 19*(3), 269–281.

Aponte, H.J., & Winter, J.E. (2000). The person and the practice of the therapist: Treatment and training. In M. Baldwin (Ed.), *The use of self in therapy* (pp. 127–165). New York: The Haworth Press.

Bernard, J.M., & Goodyear, R.K. (1992). *Fundamentals of clinical supervision* (2nd ed.). Boston: Allyn & Bacon.

Borders, L., & Leddick, G.R. (1987). *Handbook of counseling supervision.* Alexandria, VA: Association for Counselor Education and Supervision.

Bradley, L.J. (1989). *Counselor supervision: Principles, process, and practice* (2nd ed.). Muncie, IN: Accelerated Development Inc.

British Association for Counselling (BAC). (1996). *Code of Ethics and Practice for Supervisors of Counsellors.* Rugby, England: Author.

British Association for Counselling and Psychotherapy (BACP). (2007). *Ethical framework for good practice in counselling and psychotherapy.* Leicestershire, England: Author.

Corey, G. (2001). *Theory and practice of counseling and psychotherapy* (6th ed.). Pacific Grove, CA: Brooks/Cole

Davies, D. (1997). *Counselling in psychological services.* Buckingham, UK: Open University Press.

Edwards, J.K., & Bess, J.M. (1998). Developing effectiveness in the therapeutic use of self. *Clinical Social Work Journal, 26,* 89–105.

Ellis M.V. (2006). Critical incidents in clinical supervision and in supervisor supervision: Assessing supervisory issues. *Training and Education in Professional Psychology, 8*(2),122–132.

Emerson, S. (1996). Creating a safe place for growth in supervision. *Contemporary Family Therapy,* 18, 393–403.

Emilsson, U.M. & Johnsson, E. (2007). Supervision of supervisors: on developing supervision in postgraduate education. *Higher Education Research & Development, 26,* 163–179.

Farrell, W. (1996). Training and professional development in the context of counselling psychology. In R. Wolfe & W. Dryden (Eds.), *Handbook of counselling psychology* (pp. 581–604). London: Sage.

Fear, R., & Woolfe, R. (1999). The personal and professional development of counselors: The relationship between personal philosophy and theoretical orientation. *Counselling Psychology Quarterly, 12,* 253–262.

Gee, H. (1996). Developing insight through supervision: Relating, than defining. *Journal of Analytical Psychology, 41,* 529–552.

Haber, R. (1996). *Dimensions of psychotherapy supervision: Maps and means.* New York: W.W. Norton.

Hillman, S.L., McPherson, R.H., Swank, P.R., & Watkins, C.E.J. (1998). Further validation of the Psychotherapy Supervisor Development Scale. *The Clinical Supervisor, 17*(1), 17–32.

Hogan, R.A. (1964). Issues and approach in supervision. *Psychotherapy, theory, research, and practice, 1,* 139–141.

Lambert, M., & Ogles, B. (1997). The effectiveness of psychotherapy supervision. In C.E. Watkins (Ed.), *Handbook of psychotherapy supervision* (pp. 421–446). New York: John Wiley & Sons.

Marikis, D.A., Russell, R.K., & Dell, D.M. (1985). Effects of supervisory experience level on planning and in session verbal behavior. *Journal of Counseling Psychology, 30,* 403–412.

Pelling, N. (2008). The relationship of supervisory experience, counseling experience, and training in supervision to supervisory identity development. *International Journal for the Advancement of Counselling, 30*(4), 235–248.

Rosenberger, E.W., & Hayes, J.A. (2002). Therapists as subject: A review of the empirical countertransference literature. *Journal of Counselling and Development, 80,* 264–270.

Schofield, M., & Pelling, N. (2002). Supervision of counsellors. In M. McMahon & W. Patton (Eds.), *Supervision in the helping professions: A practical approach* (pp. 211–222). Sydney, Australia: Prentice Hall.

Stoltenberg, C.D. (1981). Approaching supervision from a developmental perspective: The counselor complexity model. *Journal of Counseling Psychology, 28,* 59–65.

Stoltenberg, C., & Delworth, U. (1987). *Supervising counselors and therapists: A developmental approach.* San Francisco: Jossey-Bass.

Stoltenberg, C., McNeill, B., & Delworth, U. (1998). *IDM Supervision: An integrated developmental model for supervising counselors and therapists.* San Francisco: Jossey-Bass.

Stone, G.L. (1980). Effects of experience on supervision planning. *Journal of Counseling Psychology, 27,* 84–88.

Styczynski, L. (1980). The transition from supervisee to supervisor. In A. Hell (Ed.), *Psychotherapy supervision: Theory, research & practice* (pp. 29–40). New York: John Wiley & Sons.

Watkins, C. (1990a). Development of the psychotherapy supervisor. *Psychotherapy, 27*(4), 553–560.

Watkins, C. (1990b). The separation-individuation process in psychotherapy supervision. *Psychotherapy, 27*(2), 202–209.

Watkins, C. (1991). Reflections on the preparation of psychotherapy supervision. *Journal of Clinical Psychology, 47*(6), 145–147.

Watkins, C. (1993). Development of the psychotherapy supervisor: Concepts, assumptions, and hypotheses of the supervisor complexity model. *American Journal of Psychotherapy, 47*(1), 58–74.

Watkins, C. (1994). The supervision of psychotherapy supervisor trainees. *American Journal of Psychotherapy, 48*(3), 417–431.

Watkins, C. (1995a). Psychotherapy supervision in the 1990s: Some observations and reflections. *American Journal of Psychotherapy, 49*(4), 568–581.

Watkins, C. (1995b). Psychotherapy supervisor and supervisee: Developmental models and research nine years later. *Clinical Psychology Review, 17*(7), 647–680.

Watkins, C. (1995c). Psychotherapy supervisor development: On musings, models, and metaphor. *The Journal of Psychotherapy Practice and Research, 4,* 150–158.

Watkins, C. (1995d). Researching psychotherapy supervisor development: Four key considerations. *The Clinical Supervisor, 13*(2), 139.

Watkins, C. (1997a). *Handbook of psychotherapy supervision.* New York: John Wiley & Sons.

Watkins, C. (1997b). The ineffective psychotherapy supervisor: Some reflections about bad behaviors, poor process, and offensive outcomes. *The Clinical Supervisor, 16*(1), 163–180.

Watkins, C., Schneider, L., Haynes, J., & Nieberding, R. (1995). Measuring psychotherapy supervisor development: An initial effort at scale development and validation. *The Clinical Supervisor, 13*(1), 77–90.

Wendt, R.N. (1997, March). *Failure, loss, and marginalization: Toward therapist transformation and therapeutic honesty.* Unpublished paper presented at the IX International Family therapy Association World Conference, Jerusalem.

Whitman, S.M., & Jacobs, E.G. (1998).Responsibilities of the psychotherapy supervisor. *American Journal of Psychoterapy, 52*(2), 166–175

Yerushalmi, H. (1999). The roles of group supervision of supervision. *Psychoanalytic Psychology, 16*, 426–447.

—++++—

Who are Australian Counsellors and How Do They Attend to Their Professional Development?

Caleb Lack and Nadine Pelling

Australian counselling is still a developing profession and, as of 2008, three workforce surveys have been conducted in an effort to identify the characteristics of Australian counsellors and describe their activities. Two published workforce surveys used as their foci members of two different counselling organisations, the Australian Counselling Association (ACA) and the Psychotherapy and Counselling Federation of Australia (PACFA) (Pelling, 2005; Schofield, 2008). The third published workforce survey examined individuals advertising themselves as counsellors in the *Australian Yellow Pages* (Pelling, Brear, & Lau, 2006). All three studies illustrate methodological strengths and limitations and purport to describe counsellors in Australia. In this chapter we compare and contrast the methods used and the results obtained in these published workforce surveys to date. Results show many similarities among the findings, possibly illustrating a fairly homogeneous group despite the different organisational affiliations/ populations used to sample counsellors. It is suggested that a baseline description of Australian counsellors has thus been obtained and it is therefore recommended that counselling organisations in Australia, most notably the ACA and PACFA, work together to advance the profession as they appear to be representing similar groups of people. Recommendations for future counselling workforce surveys are provided and include a strong suggestion to survey larger samples of the counselling workforce in Australia. Accurate workforce descriptions can aid supervisors in providing targeted and appropriate supervision to specific groups of supervisees. Results regarding counsellor participation in supervision and professional development activities are also presented.

Australian Counselling

Counselling is a developing profession without statutory regulation in Australia. Despite this, or maybe because of it, a number of organisations exist that purport to represent counselling and counsellors in Australia, each with differing educational and general membership requirements (Pelling, 2006; Pelling & Sullivan, 2006; Pelling & Whetham, 2006). For counsellors who do not affiliate with the psychological or social work professions there exist a number of specialty, state and national counselling organisations. This includes two primary national general counselling organisations: the Australian Counselling Association (ACA) and the Psychotherapy and Counselling Federation of Australia (PACFA) (Armstrong, 2006; Pelling, 2006; Schofield, Grant, Holmes, & Barletta, 2006). The ACA represents approximately 3,000 individual counsellors (personal communication, P. Armstrong, April 28, 2008) and PACFA is an umbrella organisation that represents various member organisations (Schofield, 2008).

Historically, some have viewed the ACA and PACFA as competitors, despite one organisation being an individual membership association and the other a federation of medium- and smaller sized associations, respectively. However, currently the ACA and PACFA are working collaboratively to develop a joint register for counsellors to aid in their common goal of having counselling recognised as a profession by the Australian government for the purposes of government health (Medicare) service rebates (personal communication, P. Armstrong, April 28, 2008). This is a welcome development, one that was called for by Pelling and Sullivan (2006) in a special issue of the *International Journal of Psychology* on counselling in Australia.

With surveys available, and the two largest counselling organisations in Australia collaborating, it both became possible and was deemed timely to compare and contrast the methods and findings of the three published workforce surveys on Australian Counselling.

Method

Two clean copies of the three published workforce surveys were obtained. One set was provided to Dr Lack for methodological review and the other to Dr Pelling for a results comparison. As Dr Pelling is the lead author of two of the published workforce surveys under examination, it was deemed inappropriate for her to lead the methodological critique. Both of the individuals involved in this methodological and results comparison are employed as clinical psychologists in a university setting, with one having published on the topic of Australian counselling previously. The methodological review examined general methodology/procedure, sample population and return rates. The results were compared regarding demographics, education and professional activities, and work settings.

Comparisons

All three recently published studies (Pelling, 2005; Pelling et al., 2006; Schofield, 2008) have attempted to identify who is providing service to the public using the term 'counsellor'. While all have relied on survey data to reach their conclusions, each has differed in terms of their methodology, sample population and other factors. The aim of this section is to provide a critique of the methods used, describe the differences and similarities of these studies, and provide information to assist in improving such research in the future. Following this methodological comparison, the results of the three workforce studies are compared. The chapter ends with a general description of Australian counsellors and some recommendations for counselling representation and future workforce studies.

Methodology

Studies will be discussed chronologically, with comparisons following. Pelling's (2005) article focused on self-identified members of the ACA. Using a similar survey to Pelling, Brear and Lau (2006), this article focused on gathering information from those ACA members who received the journal *Counselling Australia*, although those who received electronic communication from the ACA were also sent the survey. The survey asked about multiple demographic characteristics (e.g., gender, age, racial/ethnic group, religious affiliation and marital status), training and professional development, provision of services, involvement in professional organisations and comfort with six topics likely to be encountered by counsellors (i.e., use of electronic means to provide services, sexual orientation issues, service provision to Indigenous populations, and comfort treating depression, anxiety and substance use). The data were collected over a 1-month period in April 2004, with no reported follow-ups or reminders to increase the return rate. A total of 241 (out of 1,000) responses were received from those who were given the survey through the mail, with only 48 (out of 2,000) responses from those who received the electronic communication. These 48 were excluded from all analyses.

Pelling, Brear, and Lau's (2006) article used a highly similar survey, but did not report questions concerning comfort level with likely encountered issues. For their sample, the respondents were drawn from those persons who advertised themselves as counsellors in the *Australian Yellow Pages*, with a total of 587 surveys sent to a randomly selected portion of all advertised counsellors across the country. These data were collected between March and April 2004 and used a specified reminder procedure to increase return rate (see below). A total of 317 (out of 510 deliverable surveys) were returned to the authors. Schofield (2008) focused on members of PACFA member associations for her research. All 41 PACFA member associations, approximately 3,000 persons in total, were involved in this survey. The survey itself had 48 questions that covered multiple areas: limited demographic information (i.e., gender and age), priorities for the future of PACFA, work setting, experience and training background, involvement in professional organisations, professional development activities, work setting and practices, and information about private practice. In Schofield's (2008) study, data were also collected during 2004, with the first mailings occurring in January and stretching over the next 6 months, during which 'several e-mail reminders' (Schofield, 2008, p. 6) were sent to the PACFA member associations. A total of 316 surveys were returned out of over 3,000 sent; only 122 identified themselves as counsellors or psychotherapists, corresponding to a return rate of 10.5%.

As can be seen, all studies focused on self-reported survey data. In addition, all three studies, despite their varied publication dates, collected their survey data in the first half of 2004. Of the three, two (Pelling, 2005; Schofield, 2008) focused on members of a particular organisation and only one attempted a random sample of counsellors (Pelling et al., 2006), although this was drawn from those advertised as providing counselling services in a telephone directory. As such, each of these studies has threats to the ability to generalise to the total population of self-identified counsellors. The low rates of returned surveys for the two studies focusing on members of the ACA and PACFA could indicate high rates of self-selection, particularly given the high rates of advanced degrees (masters or doctoral, see below) in both samples. Given that counselling is a nonregulated profession, the random sampling method used (Pelling et al., 2006) likely represents a more accurate assessment of the population in question.

Also concerning in terms of applicability to wider samples and populations is the fact that two of the studies had very low return rates (10% or less of total sample for Pelling, 2005; Schofield, 2008), even though the information was requested under the auspices of an organisation to which the persons belonged. The third used multiple mailings to gather information and remind people to return the survey, resulting in a much higher return rate (62.2%; Pelling et al., 2006). Again, this contributes to this study being more likely representative of the counsellor population as a whole. It is also important to note that, as the total estimated number of counsellors in Australia is over 16,000 (Australian Bureau of Statistics,

2003), each study has sampled only a tiny percentage of the total counsellors in the nation — from 0.008% (Schofield, 2008) to 0.015% (Pelling, 2005) to 0.019% (Pelling et al., 2006). Thus, although all three publications represent workforce surveys, none could be said to profile the actual profession of counselling in Australia. Instead, the surveys appear to simply describe, to varying degrees of accuracy, specific sections of the profession.

A last fact concerning the accuracy of these three studies on reflecting the counselling population as a whole concerns the types of persons sampled. Each study had widely varying rates of other types of mental health professionals who responded to the survey as a counsellor. For example, Pelling (2005) had 4.1% of her sample comprising psychologists, while psychologists made up 41.9% and 6.5% of the other studies (Pelling et al., 2006 and Schofield, 2008, respectively). Also, the Schofield (2008) study included social workers (5.7%), nurses (9.8%) and medical practitioners (0.8%) in the sample. In addition, the Pelling (2005) and Schofield (2008) studies included students in their sample, at quite different rates (16.6% and 1.7%, respectively). This, combined with the differences in rates of regulated professions described above, undoubtedly impacted the findings on educational level, possibly resulting in under- (Pelling, 2005) and overestimation (Schofield, 2008) of the average educational qualifications held by counsellors.

In future research, using a randomised sample, similar to that used by Pelling et al. (2006), is highly recommended. Going beyond only sampling those who are advertised in the *Yellow Pages* should be undertaken, as anyone is able to call themselves a counsellor due to the nonregulated status of the term. Such work could involve focusing on one particular city or state/territory, starting with those who advertise their services in the phone directories, but also asking those who are advertised if they are aware of any counsellors who do not advertise in the directory. Also, obtaining lists from the city government of all persons listed as having permits to operate within the city in a counselling capacity, if possible, might allow for a wider sampling of people providing counselling services. Surveys of the major counselling organisations (such as ACA or PACFA) should also be repeated, with a focus on getting much higher rates of returned information to gain a better understanding of the members. Alternatively, these organisations could require all members, either joining for the first time or renewing their membership, to complete a survey as part of their application packet. Lastly, a survey that attempts to gather information from a larger percentage of the total counsellor population should be undertaken, as the current surveys have all surveyed much less than 1% of the total populace.

Results

Demographics

In spite of the differences in sampling techniques and populations, much information can be gained by comparing the results of these three studies. Perhaps the most glaring similarity across the studies was the demographic results. For all, a vast majority of the respondents were female (between 70.3% and 78%) and middle-aged (mean ages between 49 and 53 years old). Those studies that reported on other demographics (Pelling, 2005; Pelling et al., 2006) found a majority of the sample to be married or partnered (66.8% and 75.7%), heterosexual (90.5% and 93.4%), and living in urban environments (69.3% and 73.8%) in New South Wales (28.2% and 30.6%) or Victoria (24.1% and 28.4%). In terms of racial characteristics, both studies reported a majority of Caucasians, although Pelling (2005) reported only 14.9% of her sample identifying as such, while the other study reported 86.1% of respondents identifying as Caucasian (Pelling et al., 2006). Similarly, both reported a preponderance of religious affiliations being Christian, at rates of 7.5% (Pelling, 2005) and 55.8% (Pelling et al., 2006). As noted in the methodology section above, the Pelling (2005) and Pelling et al. (2006) studies provided greater detail regarding the demographic characteristics of the samples than the Schofield (2008) study.

Education and Professional Activities

Training and education results across the three studies differed significantly. For baccalaureate, master's, and doctorate degrees, Pelling (2005) found rates of 34.4%, 18.3%, and 4.6% respectively; Pelling et al. (2006) found rates of 36.9%, 31.2%, and 8.8%; and Schofield (2008) found rates of 34.1% and 43.9% (master's/doctorate combined). The lower rates of higher education in the Pelling (2005) study may reflect that fact that over 16% of the sample comprised students and, thus, may be in the process of completing a degree. The Pelling (2005) and Pelling et al. (2006) studies reported similar rates of engaging in supervision, between 70% and 72%. Additionally, the Pelling (2005) and Pelling et al. (2006) studies report that conference attendance and reading books/journals are popular professional development activities, reported by 65–86% and 89–96% respectively. The top three journals in both the Pelling (2005) and Pelling et al. (2006) studies remained the same, although their order differed according to study: *Australian Psychologist, Counselling Australia* and *Psychotherapy in Australia.*

The average number of years working as a counsellor ranged from a low of 8.6 to a high of 14.8 in the Pelling (2005) and Pelling et al. (2006) studies respectively. The Schofield (2008) study indicated an average of 13 years. Given that there was a fairly significant number of students included in the Pelling (2005) study, once again there appears to be a great deal of similarity among the samples in terms of counselling experience. The Pelling (2005) and Pelling et al. (2006) studies report individual (81–95% of the respondents engaged in individual counselling as a professional activity) and couple/family counselling was popular in all three surveys (51–70% engaged in this professional activity). Between 23–35% of respondents in all three surveys reportedly engaged in specialised practice.

One glaring difference in the results of the three studies was on theoretical orientation. For the Pelling (2005) and Pelling et al. (2006) studies the main theoretical influence was eclectic, with cognitive–behaviour or narrative influences. However, the Schofield (2008) study reported a preponderance of psychoanalytic theorists. It is not possible to know why this difference specifically exists but this may identify a point of real divergence between the samples and thus populations examined.

Work Setting

Solo private practice was a popular activity with 43% to 63% of the respondents in the three studies working in this setting. Income information was not reported in the Schofield (2008) study, however the respondent in the sample reported, on average, holding 1.7 employment positions. The Pelling (2005) and Pelling et al. (2006) studies reported samples that indicated an average salary of $40,000 or less per year, with an average fee between $58 and $80 an hour, respectively.

Discussion

As of 2008, three counselling workforce surveys have been conducted and published in Australia. The current examination shows that all of these studies sampled only a very small proportion of the ABS-reported number of counsellors in Australia. The studies themselves vary regarding the sampling procedures used, participants used as the foci for their data collection and return rate obtained. Nevertheless, great similarities are reported in the results of all three studies.

Who are Australian counsellors? Generally speaking, Australian counsellors are women of middle-age. They tend to be married or in a partnered relationship, heterosexual and living in urban environments. In terms of education, most counsellors tend to hold some type of baccalaureate degree. Differences in reported postgraduate (master's/doctorate) degrees existed and are likely to be a result of studies including/excluding students, in addition to the inclusion of members of regulated professions thus seemingly lowering/artificially raising the educational levels reported. A fuller examination of educational level obtained in terms of specific counselling (vs. psychological) training and examination of degrees in progress versus obtained degrees could be illuminative in regards to the educational levels held by Australian counsellors, especially those counsellors who do not identify with a different, regulated profession (e.g., psychologists). Similarities were also demonstrated between studies in terms of supervisory activities, professional development activities and experience level. Indeed, counsellors in Australia appear to have a fairly high level of experience in terms of years of practice, with about a decade being fairly standard. Once again, similarities existed in professional activities including the popularity of individual as well as couple/family counselling. Differences were reported in terms of theoretical orientation with eclectic/cognitive–behavioural and psychoanalytic theories being reported by the Pelling (2005) as well as Pelling et al. (2006) studies and the Schofield (2008) research, respectively.

Conclusion

Due to the similarities in the findings obtained by the three published Australian counselling workforce surveys, we propose that a baseline description of Australian counsellors has been obtained. As a result, it might be in the best interest of the Australian counselling industry to have the ACA and PACFA work together, as they are reported to be doing currently, as what will benefit one group is likely to benefit the other (personal communication, P. Armstrong, April 14, 2008; Pelling & Sullivan, 2006).

Future counselling workforce surveys are encouraged to focus on increasing, first, the return rate obtained possibly by using a multimailing technique, such as that engaged by Pelling et al. (2006). Second, a wider sampling of the existing number of counsellors in Australia needs to be obtained in any future survey. As a result, surveys may best avoid focusing on one specific association's membership or one limited listing of counsellors but employ a snowballing technique to sample a large number of counsellors who could be contacted by various methods.

Regardless, Australian counselling can be said to be developing smoothly with a number of published workforce surveys and the two main representative counselling bodies in Australia now working in collaboration.

Educational Questions and Activities

1. True or False: The three published workplace surveys of Australian counsellors show more similarities than differences.
   A. true.

2. List one main difference found among the three discussed workplace surveys.
   • theoretical orientation.
3. Is your favourite journal listed among the most popular for Australian counsellors?
4. Describe the general Australian counsellor in terms of demographic characteristics.
   • Generally speaking, Australian counsellors are women of middle-age. They tend to be married or in a partnered relationship, heterosexual and living in urban environments. In terms of education, most counsellors tend to hold some type of baccalaureate degree.

Selected Internet Resources
• Australian Counselling Association
  http://www.theaca.net.au
• Psychotherapy and Counselling Federation of Australasia
  http://www.pacfa.org.au

Selected References for Further Reading
Pelling, N. (2005). Counsellors in Australia: Profiling the membership of the Australian Counselling Association. *Counselling, Psychotherapy, and Health* [Online serial], *1*(1), 1–18. Available via http://www.cphjournal.com
Pelling, N., Brear, P., & Lau, M. (2006). A survey of advertised Australian counsellors. *International Journal of Psychology, Special Issue Counselling in Australia, 41*(3), 204–215.
Schofield, M. (2008). Australian counsellors and psychotherapists: A profile of the profession. Counselling & Psychotherapy Research, Special Issue *Australian Counselling and Psychotherapy Research, 8*(1), 4–11.

References
Armstrong, P. (2006). The Australian Counselling Association: Meeting the needs of Australian Counsellors. *International Journal of Psychology* [Special Issue 'Counselling in Australia'], *41*(3), 153–155.
Australian Bureau of Statistics. (2003). 2001 *Census basic community profile and snapshot, Australia.* Retrieved September 14, 2004, from http://www.Australian Bureau of Statistics.gov.au/Ausstats/Australian Bureau of Statistics@census.nsf/Lookup2001Census/7DD97C937216E32FCA256BBE00837
Pelling, N. (2005). Counsellors in Australia: Profiling the membership of the Australian Counselling Association. *Counselling, Psychotherapy, and Health* [Online serial], *1*(1), 1–18. Available at http://www.cphjournal.com

Pelling, N. (2006). Professional counselling organisations. In N. Pelling, R. Bowers, & P. Armstrong (Eds.), *The practice of counselling* (pp. 442–453). Melbourne, Australia: Thomson Publishers.

Pelling, N., & Sullivan, B. (2006). The credentialing of counselling in Australia. *International Journal of Psychology* [Special Issue 'Counselling in Australia'], *41*(3), 194–203.

Pelling, N., & Whetham, P. (2006). The professional preparation of Australian counsellors. *International Journal of Psychology* [Special Issue 'Counselling in Australia'], *41*(3), 189–193.

Pelling, N., Brear, P., & Lau, M. (2006). A survey of advertised Australian counsellors. *International Journal of Psychology* [Special Issue 'Counselling in Australia'], *41*(3), 204–215.

Schofield, M. (2008). Australian counsellors and psychotherapists: A profile of the profession. *Australian Counselling and Psychotherapy Research* [Special Issue 'Counselling & Psychotherapy Research'], *8*(1), 4–11.

Schofield, M., Grant, J., Holmes, S., & Barletta, J. (2006). The Psychotherapy and Counselling Federation of Australia: How the federation model contributes to the field. *International Journal of Psychology* [Special Issue 'Counselling in Australia'], *41*(3), 194–203.

—++++—

Evaluation

Section 5 — 'Evaluation' is a word often dreaded by supervisees and supervisors alike. It can be unnerving to be evaluated and also to complete evaluations. This section provides both general and specific information about evaluation. For instance, Chapter 16 provides a general overview of the topic of competence and assessment while Chapter 15 specifically discusses managing student competence problems. Chapter 14 is also a targeted chapter which argues that assessment must be purposeful and linked to the purposes in place for the current supervisory contacts. The chapters included in this section provide scaffolding upon which supervisors and supervisees can build their understanding of evaluation and its complexity while also providing some specific details for supervisors regarding the 'how to' of evaluation and managing competency problems.

Chapter Overview

CHAPTER 14

'Purposeful Assessment: An Integral Aspect of Supervision' by Piet Crosby asserts that evaluation in supervision needs to be tied to the purpose of supervision. He reviews how one should assess and decide on supervisory goals and how this relates to the selection of a supervisor and initial, as well as ongoing, assessment of the supervisee. Piet Crosby also outlines the desirability of providing assessment of and feedback to the supervisor.

Chapter Themes

In this chapter you will explore the following themes:
- what is supervision and what are its purposes?
- what should assessment comprise during supervision programs?
- assessing and deciding the goals and requirements of the supervision program
- assessing and selecting the supervisor
- initial assessment of the supervisee
- assessment of developing competencies
- assessment of and feedback to the supervisor
- assessment of outcomes for clients
- summary.

CHAPTER 15

'Supervision as Gatekeeping: Managing Professional Competency Problems in Student Supervisees' by Brian Sullivan discusses the often feared aspect of evaluation relating to student professional competency problems. In a gentle manner he reviews the three main domains of counselling competence; affective, relational, and performance and argues for the use of clear and shared terminology regarding competency problems. The use of supervision in decisions to remediate or dismiss students is reviewed.

Chapter Themes

In this chapter you will explore the following themes:

- introduction
- professional training standards
- beginning with the end in sight
- the 'self' of the counsellor
- the three dimensions of counselling mastery
- affective domain
- relational domain
- student performance concerns
- clear, shared, and consistent terminology
- our role as gatekeepers
- remediation
- dismissal
- recommendations.

CHAPTER 16

'Assessment of Competence' by Nadine Pelling is a literature analysis regarding how the counselling and psychology professions struggle to define what makes therapists competent in their applied work. Additionally, the controversy over whom and for what purpose competency is defined and how it is measured is presented. This is a broad introduction to the issues of assessment and therapist competence.

Chapter Themes

In this chapter you will explore the following themes:

- introduction
- defining competence
- assessment of competence
- purpose of assessment
- who will assess competence?
- training/supervisor assessment
- manager assessment
- external judge assessment
- self-assessment

- peer assessment
- client assessment
- how do we measure competence?
- questionnaires/rating scales
- journals
- exams
- identifying a minimum level of counsellor competence
- enforcing minimum levels of counsellor competence
- can/does licensure and certification ensure counsellor competence?

chapter fourteen

Purposeful Assessment: An Integral Aspect of Supervision

Piet Crosby

What is Supervision and What are its Purposes?

Supervision programs can be designed to meet a multiplicity of purposes. Licensing or credentialing authorities and professional organisations (e.g., the Psychologists Registration Board of Victoria [PRBV, 2005], the Psychotherapy and Counselling Federation of Australia [2006], and the New Zealand Association of Counsellors [2007]), variously state supervision programs are designed to develop and support supervisees in their clinical roles, reflect on and develop ethical practice, ensure delivery of competent services to clients, inform decisions about whether a trainee is ready for independent practice, maintain the standards of the profession and ensure services are culturally appropriate. Additionally, codes of ethics and supervision guidelines reflect the interests of several parties involved, typically the supervisee, the supervisor, clients working with the supervisee and the community and professional bodies who are reliant on the quality of supervision programs to ensure maintenance of standards and service delivery. This diversity is reflected in Bernard and Goodyear's (2004) definition of supervision as:

> an intervention provided by a more senior member of a profession to a more junior member or junior members of that same profession. This relationship is evaluative, extends over time, and has the simultaneous purposes of enhancing the professional functioning of the more junior person(s), monitoring the quality of professional services afforded to the client, she, he or they see, and serving as a gatekeeper of those who are to enter the particular profession. (p. 8)

This definition extends adequately to peer supervision, especially when defined as bringing (the in total greater) expertise of the peer group to '*formal review* [my emphasis] of the work of a member that is requested by that member' (Australian Psychological Society [APS], 2007, p. 2) rather than as a less hierarchical peer collaboration (which the APS entitles 'peer consultation'). Accordingly, this chapter does not consider peer supervision separately.

What Should Assessment Comprise During Supervision Programs?

The purposes of any particular supervision program and the included stakeholders imply several aspects of appropriate assessment. For instance, role development and supporting functions require repeated assessment of skill levels and knowledge shown by supervisees and ongoing feedback. This is so that supervisee and supervisor can consider implications of observations, and develop suggestions for improvement, regardless of whether the competence level is moving towards or beyond 'satisfactory' level. Developing ethical practice awareness can be served by involving the supervisee in self-assessment and reflection. Gatekeeping (e.g., licensing and accreditation) and maintaining standards functions require assessment of competence against an understanding of what is satisfactory for an independent practitioner or association member. Protection of the client requires knowing what is being done with clients and consideration of client outcomes. Given this range of purposes it is unsurprising that Magnusson, Norem and Wilcoxon (2000) state that despite the existence of 'a variety of assessment protocols ... available to augment appraisal procedures ... supervisors and supervisees must rely on individually defined criteria and procedures for formally and finally assessing progress' (p. 183). This chapter provides only limited reference to psychometric instruments that may be used in particular programs, in accord with absence of such requirements by supervision guidelines of licensing, credentialing, or professional associations. Baird (2002) cites Kadushin's (1985) recommendations that assessment should be continuous, agreed on in advance, occur in a positive and supportive environment, recognise strengths and weaknesses, viewed as progress reports rather than final scores and be a shared responsibility between supervisor and supervisee. He recommends that supervisees adopt a commitment to learning and acceptance of assessment, and that both supervisees and supervisors adopt a commitment to facilitating mutual exploration, learning and development.

Assessing and Deciding the Goals and Requirements of the Supervision Program

Supervision programs may be established to meet requirements of (licensing) registration boards, meet membership requirements of (credentialing) professional associations, or meet tertiary course requirements. They may contribute to ongoing (postlicensing) professional development (Page, Dale, & Sutton, 2001), which is required by some professional associations, such as the British Association for Counselling and Psychotherapy (BACP; 1996). Supervision may be required in competence programs following competence reviews by a licensing authority (e.g., New Zealand Psychologists Board, 2006). Supervision programs may also be designed to suit specific and relatively limited purposes, such as to assist a supervisee develop a specific skill or group of skills. Accordingly, the first step in developing a supervision program and the assessment processes it will incorporate, is considering the goals of the supervision program, simultaneously noting assessment requirements required by any relevant authorities. Particular care should be taken to note documentation requirements for later applications to licensing and credentialing bodies. Botti (2002) provides an eloquent account of the need to consider these requirements fully from the outset, and of the consequences of not doing so.

Psychologists require registration or licensing by statutory (government) boards in order to practice legally in Australia, New Zealand, the United States of America, and Canada. A total of 49 American states require licensing for Counselors (American Counselling Association, 2006). These authorities require evidence of supervised experience and define requirements such as the number of hours required for internship and supervision, required competencies and breadth of practice setting requirements. They may stipulate inclusion of particular assessment processes and tasks.

As examples, The Alaskan Board of Professional Counsellors (2007) requires 3,000 hours of supervision subsequent to graduation with a master's degree. The Supervision Program Guidelines of the (Australian) Psychologists Registration Board of Victoria (PRBV, 2005) list knowledge of the discipline, psychological assessment and diagnosis, intervention strategies, communication, research and assessment, and ethics as required competencies. The guidelines define each competency and stipulate tasks and activities by which competence can be demonstrated and assessed. The South Australian Psychological Board (2006) guidelines stipulate breadth of placement experience across age ranges and presenting issues. Reporting requirements and documentation to be included in the supervisee's eventual application for accreditation are stipulated.

In all jurisdictions professional associations exist to support practice of counselling and psychology. Qualifications for membership of these bodies include generally similar, but often more specific, required evidence of supervised experience to those of the licensing authorities above. Some have component specialist colleges/divisions with additional requirements. Supervision programs may therefore also need to address requirements of professional associations to which the supervisee aspires, and which, in some jurisdictions, especially those where licensure does not exist, serve to regulate access to the profession through representing membership of professional associations (credentialling) to society, employers and clients as evidence of competence. Tertiary institutions training counsellors and psychologists include supervision requirements in placement units, which again resemble those of licensing authorities.

Assessing and Selecting the Supervisor

Licensing authorities and professional associations may require formal licensing or credentialing of approved supervisors. There are an increasing number of postgraduate courses to train supervisors (Emilsson & Johnsson, 2007), but course assessments are not discussed here. Licensing and professional association requirements may include training in supervision, supervised experience of supervision, professional licensing and credentials, areas of expertise, or length of experience (Magnuson, Norem, & Wilcoxon, 2000; Wheeler & King, 2000). Some authorities and associations require provision of such information when a supervision program is developed. Additionally, codes of ethics note the need to practice within areas of competence (supervision being an area of practice) and the need to avoid issues such as dual relationships (e.g., Australian Psychological Society, 2004). Falender, Cornish, Goodyear, Hatcher, Kaslow et al. (2004) provide an exhaustive list of knowledge, skills, values and other supervision competencies that could be used as a checklist in considering whether a potential supervisor is appropriate for a particular supervision program.

Initial Assessment of the Supervisee

Supervisees come to their supervision programs with a range of pre-existing skills, attitudes beliefs and developmental levels (Heppner & Roehlke, 1984; Stoltenberg, 2005). In order to match input and style of supervision the supervisor will need to conduct some initial assessment of the supervisee, perhaps through an initial discussion of past experiences, desires for the supervision program, beliefs about areas of strength and development needs, and particular interests. It also provides an opportunity for a supervisor to share similar information, understanding of the complexities of the various goals of supervision programs, the importance of considering the interests of parties involved, and the potential conflicts in the supervisor's roles in addressing the above. This will be the beginning of ongoing assessment of a supervisee's developing competencies and development, allowing appropriate adjustment of processes, and hopefully the beginning of a collaboration aimed at their further development towards and beyond basic competence. An instrument such as the Supervision Utilization Rating Scale (Vespia, Heckman-Stone, & Delworth, 2002) could be used, for example, to facilitate discussion of approaches to supervision and identify facilitative and inhibitory tendencies.

Assessment of Developing Competencies

Having developed agreed goals and requirements to be met in the supervision program the supervisee and supervisor can negotiate, develop and clarify appropriate assessment strategies, incorporating those stipulated by relevant licensing and accreditation bodies. The Psychotherapy and Counselling Association of Australia (2006), for example, lists written assignments, oral presentations, case studies, live supervision, recorded interviews and relevant and detailed feedback. Strategies should be adequately comprehensive to allow assessment of all required competencies and knowledge, and address the interests of those involved, including clients.

Record-keeping competence, for example, might be assessed through supervisee presentation of selected case files for examination, through randomly examining files on clients seen by the supervisee, and through incidental observations, for example when a supervisor countersigns correspondence. Assessment could be based on a checklist of record-keeping requirements. Counselling skills might be assessed through observation, participation in co-counselling sessions, or through viewing recordings of sessions, perhaps using instruments such as the Counselor Interview Rating Form (Russell-Chapin & Sherman, 2000), skills checklists or 'flow of consciousness' comments. Ethical awareness might be assessed through preparing written material, or discussion of ethical issues that arise during the supervision program, or oral presentations. Knowledge of, and ability to implement, interventions might be assessed through observation, viewing session recordings, examination of data gathered during sessions, use of instruments developed to evaluate adherence to manualised treatments (such as the Motivational Interviewing Supervision and Training Scale, Madsell et al., 2005), or from client feedback and data.

Particular assessment activities may, of course, contribute to assessment of more than one competence. Baird and Kadushin recommend that assessments of each competency should be based on several observations and data sources, as is required by some authorities. The New South Wales Psychologist Registration Board Supervision Guidelines (2006), for example, require that communication skills are assessed using at least three direct observations and at least one other method (such as review of a range of written reports, case notes and correspondence, discussion or review of workshop learning, review of interactions with colleagues and other professionals). Baird recommends that both supervisee and supervisor should be involved in development and implementation of all assessment processes, perhaps by shared discussion and review, perhaps by independent completion of assessments before discussion, perhaps by contributing to complementary processes. He stresses that ongoing supervisor feedback and supervisee–supervisor discussions throughout the program should identify and reflect on strengths and areas for improvement, providing 'specific suggestions for continued growth' (p. 80).

Grading and reporting systems that will be used in final assessments should also be discussed and clarified from the outset. Periodic reviews with reference to the standards that will be used in the final assessments and reporting should be conducted on a regular basis to ensure that remedial action, either competency building or documentation, can be taken in timely manner. Baird cites Lazar and Mosek's (1993) recommendation of pass/fail grading systems, reflecting the complexity of the supervisor's multiple roles (including mentor, coach, assessor and overseer of client welfare). Additionally, their research findings that assigned grades were affected by factors such as the relationship between supervisor and supervisee or perceived experience (Dohrenbusch & Lipska, 2006) rather than being determined solely by the quality of the supervisee's work. Many licensing and credentialing bodies require only pass/fail assessments. For example, the Psychologists Registration Board of Victoria requires a supervisor statement that each competency has been met, and on what date. Baird (2002) provides a sample assessment form for using a 5-point grading system ranging from *Far below expectations* to *Far above expectations*, as well as space for comments and suggestions for further study. Baird points out that there should be clarity about the reference points supervisors use when making such judgments (for example whether an 'acceptable' grade means acceptable for a supervisee at this stage of development, or acceptable for a professional in independent practice), and there should also be discussion of what information will be considered in assessing a particular competency. Supervisees should not, for example, believe that assessments will be based solely on specific assessed activities if observations throughout a placement, incidental feedback from colleagues or other professionals, and client outcome measures and feedback will also be considered.

Assessment of, and Feedback to, the Supervisor

Assessment of supervisor qualifications in order to meet licensing or accreditation requirements has been briefly discussed above. Falender et al. (2004) suggest that assessment of supervisors include self-assessment, direct observation of supervision via recordings or live observation, review of documentation, review of supervision outcomes and supervisee feedback. Baird (2002) recommends supervisors seek feedback from their supervisees, both of an ongoing nature raising concerns, issues and successes during supervision sessions, and through more formal instruments, such as Baird's Supervisor Assessment Form.

Assessment of Outcomes for Clients

A core purpose of supervision is preparation for, or enhancing, independent practice with real clients. It involves work with real clients. Supervisees and supervisors have responsibilities to these clients, and supervisors have legal and personal interest in ensuring the quality of work done with clients as the work done is ultimately the responsibility of the supervisor (Magnusson et al., 2000). Saptya, Riemer and Bickman (2005) reviewed the effectiveness of various forms of feedback, and the importance of including client outcomes in evaluating performance and the positive impact of having direct client health status feedback on improving service effectiveness. Assessment should therefore include consideration of outcomes for, and experiences of clients, a process that may also instil this interest as an ongoing aspect of independent practice. Examples include examination of data gathered during intervention programs and seeking feedback from clients at the end of their involvement with the supervisee, or after a delay. The University of South Australia's (2006) *Psychology Clinic Procedural Manual*, for example, includes a 'Client Satisfaction Survey' that is given or sent to each client when therapy is completed or a case closed.

Summary

To summarise, assessment is an integral aspect of supervision. Like other processes in supervision, assessment is intended to both assess and facilitate professional development. This is most likely to happen when it is a collaborative process designed and implemented by both supervisor and supervisee. At the same time, assessment must be comprehensive and rigorous, reflecting the seriousness of the supervision enterprise in its impact in present and future clients, and the many requirements and interests that must be satisfied. This chapter has supported an approach of embarking on supervision and assessment with a close eye for the eventual outcomes, in accord with the overarching purpose of developing competent and effective independent practitioners. Appendix A presents a framework for purposeful assessment in supervision along with an example application and evaluation for your review.

Educational Questions and Activities

1. List two reasons a supervision program may be established:
   * to meet licensing/registration requirements
   * to meet tertiary course requirements or ongoing professional development requirements.

2. Indicate a few ways in which counselling skills can be assessed:
   * observation
   * participation in co-counselling sessions
   * viewing recordings of sessions
   * use of a standard instrument.

References

Australian Psychological Society. (2004). *Peer consultation network guidelines.* Melbourne, Australia: Author. Retrieved May 5, 2007, from http://www.psychology.org.au/prac_resources/practice_resources/?ID=1223.

Australian Psychological Society. (2004). *Guidelines on Supervision.* Melbourne, Australia: Author. Retrieved May 5, 2007, from http://www.psychology.org.au/Assets/Files/guidelines_on_supervision.pdf

Alaskan Board of Professional Counselors. (2007). *Professional Counselor Licensure Application.* Juneau, Alaska: Author. Retrieved 13 May, 2007, from http://www.commerce.state.ak.us/occ/ppco.htm

Baird, B.N. (2002). *The internship, practicum, and field placement handbook: A guide for the helping professionals.* Upper Saddle River, NJ: Prentice Hall.

Bernard, J.M., & Goodyear, R.K. (2004). *Fundamentals of clinical supervision* (3rd ed.). Boston: Allyn and Bacon.

Brotto, L. (2002). Chronicles of a clinical psychology internship applicant — Part I: Things I wish I had known earlier. *Psynopsis, Winter*, 20–21.

British Association for Counselling and Psychotherapy. (1996). *Code of Ethics and Practice for Counsellors.* Leicestershire, England: Author. Retrieved May 14, 2007, from http://www.bacp.co.uk/ethical_framework/index.html

British Association for Counselling and Psychotherapy. (2006). BACP *Counsellor/psychotherapist accreditation scheme: Criteria for application.* London: Author. Retrieved 9 May, 2007, from http://www.bacp.co.uk/accreditation/index.html

Dohrenbusch, R., & Lipska, S. (2006). Assessing and predicting supervisors' evaluations of psychotherapists: An empirical study. *Counselling Psychology Quarterly, 19*(4), 395–414.

Emilsson, U.M., & Johnsson, E. (2007). Supervision of supervisors: on developing supervision in postgraduate education. *Higher Education Research & Development, 26*(2), 163–179.

Falender, C.A., Cornish, J.A., Goodyear, R., Hatcher, R., Kaslow, N.J., Leventhal, G., et al. (2004). Defining competencies in psychology supervision: A consensus statement. *Journal of Clinical Psychology, 60*(7), 771–785.

Heppner, P.P., & Roehlke, H.J. (1984). Differences among supervisees at different levels of training: Implications for a developmental model of supervision. *Journal of Counseling Psychology, 31,* 76–90.

Hong Kong Psychological Society. (2006). *Statutory registration.* Hong Kong: Author. Retrieved May 15, 2007, from http://www.hkps.org.hk/www/upload// 0603141516305501.pdf

Madson, M.B., Campbell, T.C., Barrett, D.E., Brondino, M.J., & Melchert, T.P. (2005). Development of the Motivational Interviewing Supervision and Training Scale. *Psychology of Addictive Behaviors, 19*(3), 303–310.

Magnusson, S., Norem, K., & Wilcoxon, A. (2000). Clinical supervision of prelicensed counsellors: Recommendations for consideration and practice. *Journal of Mental Health Counselling, 22*(2) 176–188.

New Zealand Association of Counsellors. (2007). *Code of ethics.* Hamilton, NZ: Author. Retrieved May 15, 2007, from http://www.nzac.org.nz/

New Zealand Psychologists Board. (2006). *Competence.* Wellington, NZ: Author. Retrieved May 10, 2007 from http://www.psychologistsboard.org.nz/conduct/ competence.html

Page, B.J., Dale, R.P., & Sutton, J.M. (2001). National survey of school counselor supervision. *Counselor Education and Supervision, 41,* 142–150.

Psychotherapy and Counselling Federation of Australia. (2006). *Psychotherapy and Counselling Federation of Australia training standards January 2007.* Melbourne, Australia: Author. Retrieved May 10, 2007, from http://www.pacfa.org.au/ files/PACFA%20Training%20Standards%202007%20v1.pdf

Russell-Chapin, L.A., & Sherman, N.E. (2000). The counsellor interview rating form: A teaching and evaluation tool for counsellor education. *British Journal of Guidance and Counselling, 28*(1), 115–124.

Saptya, J., Riemer, M., & Bickman, L. (2005). Feedback to clinicians: Theory, research and practice. *In Session, 61*(2), 143–153.

South Australian Psychological Board. (2006). *Guidelines on supervision for accredited training supervisors and trainee psychologists.* Adelaide, Australia: Author. Retrieved May 5, 2007, from http://www.sapb.saboards.com.au/supervisionguide.pdf

Stoltenberg, C.D. (2005). Enhancing professional competence through developmental approaches to supervision. *American Psychologist, 60*(8), 857–864.

The New South Wales Psychologist Registration Board. (2006). *Supervision Guidelines.* Sydney, Australia: Author. Retrieved 10 May, 2007, from http://www.psychreg. health.nsw.gov.au/hprb/psych_web/psy_supervisionguidelines.htm

University of South Australia. (2006). *Psychology Clinic Procedural Manual.* Unpublished manuscript, University of South Australia, Adelaide.

Vespia, K.M., Heckman-Stone, C., & Delworth, U. (2002). Describing and facilitating effective supervision behaviour in counselling trainees. *Psychotherapy: Theory, Research, Practice, Training, 39*(1), 55–65.

Wheeler, S., & King. D. (2000). Do counselling supervisors want or need to have their supervision supervised? An exploratory study. *British Journal of Guidance and Counselling, 28*(2), 279–290.

Supervision as Gatekeeping: Managing Professional Competency Problems in Student Supervisees

Brian Sullivan

Supervision is an essential component of any professional counsellor training program (Psychotherapy and Counselling Federation of Australia,
2009). The key characteristics of a profession are to: 'screen and select new
members; to educate, train, and socialize those who are selected; and to
articulate standards of ethical practice' (Forrest, Elman, Gizara, & Vacha-
Haase, 1999, p. 628). Yet while the counselling literature acknowledges
this critical role of counsellor education programs, there is little substantive
direction for faculty in directing that process (Wilkerson, 2006). This
chapter is about the broad concept of supervision in regards to counsellor
trainees, the students in our counsellor education programs. In this specific
context, supervision includes the tripartite work of counsellor educators in
facilitating training in traditional coursework (theoretical and skills-based),
personal development, and supervised practice with program-based and
on-site supervisors and trainers (Rønnestad & Skovholt, 2001). In particular, this chapter is about how we as counsellor educators, trainers and
supervisors, manage students who are manifesting problematic performance in the program — be that academic difficulties, skills deficits,
personal limitations, interpersonal problems, mental health issues, ethical
concerns or any combination of these, as they may overlap (Forrest et al.,
1999; Ladany, Friedlander, & Nelson, 2005).

The two most critical tasks of counsellor educators are the selection
screening and ongoing evaluation of student counsellors (Enochs &
Etzbach, 2004; Forrest et al., 1999). If we do not attend prudently to
these twin tasks, we run the risk of graduating students who may not be

appropriate candidates to be professional counsellors, and ultimately this is potentially harmful to the public who use counselling services. Not only is there the potential of harm to clients and future clients, but also to the reputation of the training program and faculty, the counselling profession itself and, of course, the negative consequences of career unsuitability on the individual graduate. These supervisory tasks involve not only academic and attitudinal considerations, but ethical and legal implications as well (Enochs & Etzbach, 2004; Ladany, et al., 2005).

As counsellor educators, we need to begin with the end in sight. We need to have specific key performance indicators, clearly articulated to our students, so that there are no surprises, no catches and no hidden agenda in our counselling programs (Bhat, 2005; Kaslow, Rubin, Forrest, et al., 2007). What should a graduate from our programs be able to do? What kind of person (cognitively, ethically, attitudinally and behaviourally) should our candidates and graduates be? Ensuring that students who graduate from our programs are likely to be professionally competent is a basic objective of counsellor trainers and supervisors. This is a foundational principle of ethical and accountable counsellor education programs (Kaslow et al., 2007).

Professional Training Standards

The Psychotherapy and Counselling Federation of Australia (PACFA), in its 2009 Professional Training Standards, states that 'students need to demonstrate the presence of some fundamental human capacities for beginning training as a counsellor/psychotherapist'. The capacities so important for selection of suitable candidates may be demonstrated for those who are doing the selection via live interviews, observing student's participation in experiential workshops, referees' reports among other means. Whatever means a training program chooses to select candidates, students 'need to demonstrate the capacity to relate in a facilitative way with others and to reflect on and examine the impact of these action' (PACFA, 2009). The PACFA professional standards continue to enunciate student requirements of self-awareness, maturity and ethical behaviour. The standards emphasise the importance of students 'being open to positive and challenging feedback'.

While these standards provide counsellor educators and supervisors guidelines for the selection of suitable candidates and an example of means to undertake that selection process, they do not elucidate gatekeepers on the specifics of the management of those who are accepted onto the program and then show diminished functioning in any of the relational skills, self-awareness, maturity and/or ethical behaviour aspects of student development.

Working Towards the Goal

As professional counsellors, our noble vocation (Skovholt & Jennings, 2005) is:

> to understand; to help; to speak the truth; to make a meaningful connection with our clients that fosters their sense of agency, their capacity for enjoyment and mastery, and their ability to tolerate grief and limitation, whether or not their behaviour is unconventional and inconvenient according to ordinary cultural norms. (McWilliams, 2005, p. 140)

Obviously, this work is *not* for everyone. So counsellor educators and those responsible for the supervision of trainees need to ensure that it *is* for those who have been selected and have embarked on their training to become professional counsellors. Supervisors need to work with their supervisees to ensure that those who are in training are being true to and growing in that vocation. This, of course, is for the good of our clients, both present and future. It is also for the good of our trainees; for the good of our training institutions and supervisory faculty; and ultimately, it is for the good of the counselling profession.

Good counsellors are both born and bred. However, our natural proclivities and personal qualities should be nurtured in and through the quality of our training and supervision. It is not an either/or situation. Our training and what we bring to that training are both vital for our development as counsellors (Sullivan, 2008; Wheeler, 2002). Wheeler (2002) has employed a culinary analogy that captures this synthesis of trainer, trainee and training:

> … the way the pudding is stirred and baked has much to answer for, but without handpicked, good-quality ingredients, the result may be less than satisfactory. So it is with counsellor training: the outcome depends not only on the program delivered but also on the suitability of the participants. (p. 427)

For the best end product, we need good programs of training, with highly effective trainers and supervisors, and we need good quality candidates. Good training and supervision provides structured learning experiences and professional direction for those with innate personal qualities. Good training and supervision will enhance and deepen those innate personal qualities (Sullivan, 2008; Wheeler & Richards, 2007).

The 'Self' of the Counsellor

In counselling, we typically work with those who have been 'bruised by life' to varying degrees, both with 'the walking wounded' and 'the worried well' (Aveline, 2005, p. 157). There is much at stake for our clients when they access our services. However, we must not lose sight of the fact that as human beings and as trainees, or counsellors, we too are 'wounded', albeit aspiring to be 'wounded healers' (Wheeler, 2002, p. 435). As counsellors we are not somehow outside of, immune to, or exempt from the human condition, the struggles and pain of human living and relating. We wrestle with the questions, issues and challenges that concern most people. They are concerns about the meaning of our lives, about the ways of achieving and living good and happy lives, about how to be healthy both physically and mentally and being in good and happy relationships (Sullivan, 2008). With that in mind then, let us briefly consider the qualities and characteristics of good counsellors that have been shown to be effective with clients. It is critical for us as trainers and supervisors to consider these qualities and characteristics, especially when selecting trainees for our programs, and when dealing with trainees who may be exhibiting cognitive difficulties, problematic behaviours and ethical deficiencies? There is much at stake for us when we select, accept and commit to train students to become professional counsellors. We should also remember that there is much at stake for students who embark on this journey to become professional counsellors.

The Three Dimensions of Counselling Mastery

The research of Skovholt, Jennings and colleagues (Jennings & Skovholt, 1999; Ronnestad & Skovholt, 2003; Skovholt, 2005; Sullivan, Skovholt, & Jennings, 2005; Skovholt & Jennings, 2005; Jennings, Goh, Skovholt, Hanson, & Banerjee-Stevens, 2003) has largely sought to find answers to the question of 'What are the personal characteristics of expert counsellors?'

Three dimensions or domains have been identified that belong to the highly effective counsellor (Jennings & Skovholt, 1999; Skovholt, 2005). These domains — the cognitive, emotional and relational — are integral areas of functioning for the effective counsellor. Master therapists blend these three domains and have them available to them in their work with clients. In their qualitative research with 'master therapists', Jennings and Skovholt (1999) identified that within each of these three domains there were three categories:

Cognitive domain:
- master therapists are voracious learners
- accumulated experiences have become a major resource
- master therapists value cognitive complexity and the ambiguity of the human condition

Affective domain:
- master therapists are self-aware, reflective, nondefensive and open to feedback

- master therapists are congruent, mentally healthy and mature individuals who attend to their own emotional wellbeing
- master therapists are aware of how their emotional health affects the quality to their work; they are willing to work on their own emotional health

Relational domain:

- master therapists possess strong relational skills, such as warmth, respect, caring and a genuine interest in people
- master therapists believe that the foundation for therapeutic change is a strong working alliance
- master therapists are experts at using their exceptional relationship skills in therapy. They provide safety and support for their clients and also are not afraid to challenge them. They are not afraid of strong emotion and, having the courage to deal with their own painful areas, can be present with their clients' pain

When considering the type of students we admit to our counselling programs, these characteristics and qualities of master counsellors could be a reliable guide in the selection and screening of candidates. While not expecting trainees to be instant experts or immediate master counsellors, counsellor educators and supervisors are looking for trainees and supervisees who are open to growth, receptive of feedback and capable of achieving a developmental trajectory in that direction. And for our trainees to graduate, as supervisors and educators we are saying to the public and to the profession that at this stage of their development these graduates are professionally competent, personally sound and ethically appropriate in their practice. They are 'good enough' to practise as professional counsellors.

In balancing the needs of potential counsellor trainees and other stakeholders (e.g., the profession, the public and the counsellor education program), Russell and her colleagues (2007) posed three questions that counsellor educators and supervisors might ask themselves. These questions are: (1) Would I be comfortable hiring this person? (2) Would I be willing to supervise this person as my employee? (3) Would I refer a family member to this counsellor? (cf., p. 239). If, as counsellor educators and supervisors, we honestly discussed our responses to these questions about our students with the counselling faculty, we may in fact save ourselves (and others) much grief and anxiety later in the program.

Student Performance Concerns

As educators and supervisors in graduate programs we are also aware of some students about whom we have serious professional concerns, in regards to their clinical competency, personal soundness and/or ethically appropriateness. These concerns may arise through our direct observation, observation of other faculty, practicum supervisor reports, other student feedback, or indeed from information that the trainee gives to us directly (Forrest et al., 1999). In their Code of Ethics and Standards of Practice F.3, the American Counseling Association (1995) has used the term 'personal limitations' of supervisees that are likely to negatively affect professional competence. The rates of problematic students in programs, at least from American research, run at about 5% (Forrest et al., 1999; Rapisarda & Britton, 2007). If this statistic was similar in our Australian counselling programs, it would mean that out of 40 students over a 2-year full-time equivalent program, there would be 2 students who are presenting with professional problems. At any rate, the literature suggests that most graduate programs have at least one trainee who is not meeting a satisfactory standard of professional performance (Elman & Forrest, 2007). These students demand an inordinate amount of the faculty's time, energy and resources. How we manage them, and what we in fact do with them and for them, is critical for all stakeholders.

Forrest and her colleagues (1999) summarised the ethical mandates incumbent upon trainers, educators and supervisors, in managing problematic student performance. These include: (a) attending to the possibility that their trainees' personal problems might lead to harm of others; (b) making sure that trainees are not harming clients or others under their care; (c) attending to the possibility that trainees may misuse their influence; (d) evaluate whether trainees are performing responsibly, competently and ethically; (e) articulating a clear set of professional standards and (f) evaluating trainees based on these relevant and established requirements (cf. p. 636).

Clearly, being aware of potential harm, articulating performance criteria and standards, and evaluating student performance are essential aspects of ethical counsellor education and supervision. The faculty of responsible and ethical counsellor education programs needs to respond to the following questions:

1. How do we identify and respond to the trainee who is showing serious limitations in any or all of the domains: cognitive, relational or affective?

2. How do we understand the difference and overlap between impaired, incompetent and unethical behaviours in our trainees (Forrest et al., 1999)?

3. Are these problems, with appropriate intervention, always surmountable?

4. Or do they indicate that a trainee may in fact be unsuitable for the profession and should be counselled off or even dismissed from the program?

5. What if, in our supervisory evaluation and with faculty consultation, a trainee is deemed not professionally 'good enough' and so unsuitable for the profession?

6. When is dismissal warranted and necessary for the protection of clients, the trainee and the profession?

7. What is the threshold for dismissal on our program?

8. What are our professional, ethical and legal responsibilities as trainers and supervisors to this trainee, to the public, to the profession and to our training institutes?

Certainly it has been my experience in discussing these questions with colleagues that as a profession, counsellor educators and supervisors are struggling to fully comprehend and implement their role and responsibilities as gatekeepers for professional counselling quality control (Forrest et al., 1999). As educators and supervisors, we are accountable to and for our programs, to our trainees, to the profession and ultimately to future clients. How we operationalise our accountability is crucial to our role as gatekeepers to and for the profession. There is a tension between our need to support and nurture students and facilitate their growth as professionals, and our evaluative role as gatekeepers. It may be that there is a tension between university requirements to maintain full occupancy in academic programs for economic viability (the 'innkeeper' role) and our professional roles to screen and evaluate. This means that not everyone who begins the program is necessarily fit for graduation as a competent and ethical professional counsellor. Counselling certain students out of the program or even their dismissal are real options.

Clear, Shared, and Consistent Terminology

Over the past 20 years or so, there has been much conjecture and controversy over which terminology we as counsellor educators and supervisors use when referring to students who are not 'measuring up' to program and professional expectations. When looking at the problem emotions, behaviours and attitudes that students can manifest, it is obvious that these problems are on a continuum, ranging 'from interpersonal skill deficits to major psychopathology' (Ladany et al., 2005, p. 183). These problems have been referred to as: (a) *impairment*, where students have shown prior professional competency, but are experiencing diminished functioning due to some external stressors; *incompetence*, where students have never shown a level of competent professional functioning; *unethical behaviour*, where students have shown they are not performing in accord with the counselling profession's code of ethics. Impairment, incompetence and unethical behaviour are not mutually exclusive and may of course overlap (Forrest et al., 1999). Other terminology that has been used includes: *undesirable, unsuitable, emotionally troubled, personality problems* (Elman & Forrest, 2007). The problem with these terms is that they lack specificity and precision, blur behaviour and personality, and mix up cause and consequences. These terms can be seen as labels that are detrimental to the career future of the student, not only in the counselling profession (cf. Elman & Forrest 2007 for a complete discussion on this). Elman and Forrest have proposed and argued for a more behaviourally precise term, *professional competence problems*. This term may cover the breadth and depth of the problems and concerns that counsellor educators and supervisors encounter in students who are not, for whatever reason, meeting professional standards of practice. Because it is behaviourally focused, the term may lead to more attentive monitoring and evaluation of students, which will in turn lead to 'improved identification, remediation, and effective outcomes' (Elman & Forrest, 2007, p. 508).

Our Role as Gatekeepers

Let us now discuss our gatekeeper role, which may be fraught with difficulties for many of us. Within the metaphor of the 'gatekeeping' role are three contributing components worth noting. Firstly, there is the 'gate' or the expectations, obligations and standards of professional and ethical practice that are evaluated via a set of criteria within the structured program of counsellor education and professional bodies. Secondly, there is the one trying to access and progress through the gate, that is the student who is being evaluated and assessed, and is attempting to meet professional competency and ethical standards. Thirdly, there is the 'gatekeeper' who is the evaluator, the trainer or supervisor who is responsible for professional quality control in the form of evaluation. Ultimately, the purpose of the process of gatekeeping is twofold: to protect the profession for which training is being provided and to protect the public who will access the profession.

Brear, Dorrian, and Luscri (2008) have identified the twofold challenge for gatekeepers: 'to develop a set of relevant and explicit criteria against which students can be measured, and to develop a fair and valid framework within which the gatekeeping mechanism can operate' (p. 94). They go on to summarise the seven functions of effective gatekeeping for the counselling profession as:

- promoting student equity
- fulfilling the educational and ethical responsibilities of the educator
- guarding the integrity of training programs
- ensuring the quality of graduates

- enhancing the quality of the profession
- maintaining societal sanction
- protecting the interests of the community, particularly consumers of counselling services (i.e., our clients and future clients).

Bemak, Epps and Keys (1999) designed a five-step model of gatekeeping, with the goal being ongoing evaluation of students. The five steps are:

1. Before the application process begins, potential applicants have the program's expectations clearly clarified and communicated to them, where unacceptable or inappropriate behaviours, attitudes and outlooks that could lead to dismissal are explicitly stated.

2. A contractual agreement, signed by the student, indicating comprehension of and agreement to the above.

3. Early identification of problematic concerns, where prompt review with the student and faculty staff is undertaken.

4. Remediation recommendations in the form of a plan are designed with the student and counsellor educators and supervisors.

5. Ongoing monitoring and evaluation of progress and outcomes, where this student is informed of this. At this stage is satisfactory progress is not made, then dismissal becomes a real possibility.

Christine Suniti Bhat's (2005) idea of designing performance appraisals for student counsellors has much merit. They are used for evaluating employees and could in fact be a useful tool for us as gatekeepers of the profession, as they are defined in terms of behavioural and measurable objectives. A performance appraisal process encapsulates much of the Bemak, Epps, and Keys' five-step model.

Remediation

Counsellor educators and supervisors need to know when to initiate remediation assistance for students who are manifesting professional competence problems — the earlier the better (Bhat, 2005). While there is some literature that refers to remediation in terms of 'sanctioned' or 'mandated' supervision (Cobia & Pipes, 2002; Rapisarda & Britton, 2007), it may be better to use the term *required performance* or *clinical monitoring*, which in reality is an increased and focused level of supervision (cf., Rapisarda & Britton, 2007). 'Sanctioned' and 'mandated' suggest a sense of being involuntary, punitive and coercive. And, as such, may indicate the student lacks motivation and commitment to the process. While this may be the case for some students presenting with performance problems, it is not necessarily the case for all. If the student's performance and functioning has diminished, he or she may welcome remediation steps to regain or achieve satisfactory performance standards, and so be able to continue successfully to graduation.

In summarising the remediation literature, Forrest and her colleagues (1999) suggested that remediation plans should:

1. identify and describe deficiencies that are directly tied to the program's evaluation criteria

2. identify specific goals or changes that need to be made by the trainee

3. identify possible methods for meeting those goals

4. establish criteria for judging whether remediation has been successful

5. determine a timeline for re-evaluation.

The remediation plans generally include increased mentoring and advising, intensified and focused supervision, additional field experience, remedial or repeating coursework or practicum and personal counselling is often encouraged. Forrest and her team believe that while remediation plans are discussed in the literature, there has not been the data gathering or research to support how we should design, implement and monitor remediation plans designed to manage and address students' performance problems (Forrest et al., 1999).

Dismissal

When remediation plans do not achieve positive outcomes for students, we need to face the fact that these students need to be counselled off the program, or even dismissed from the program as being unsuitable for the profession, in that they never had or have not been able to achieve an adequate level of professional competence. If such students are known to the faculty and to other students, and are permitted to continue to graduation, then the training institute, university and program faculty may be held legally liable (as well as the graduate) for malpractice, for any harm done to clients in the future (Enochs & Etzbach, 2004). Due process obviously needs to be followed according to the policies of the university or training institute, where students have been duly informed of professional competencies, standards and expectations, remedial plans that have not achieved sufficient change in the student's professional competency levels are recorded, extensive and detailed documentation is completed and placed in the student's file (Wilkerson, 2006).

Some of the reasons for dismissal include continued poor academic performance, poor clinical performance, failed competency tests, ethical violations, psychopathology, emotional instability, personality disorder, unprofessional demeanour, poor interpersonal skills, sexual misconduct and substance abuse (Forrest et al., 1999). Obviously, these are serious issues and are going to affect a student's ability to successfully meet professional competency standards, and could lead to potential harm done to clients, the profession and the program itself. Ultimately, we do no favour to a student who is professionally incompetent to permit him or her to graduate.

Recommendations

The following recommendations are a compilation of recommendations from some of the relevant literature. If implemented, these could contribute positively to the selection, review, remediation and retention policies and practices in our programs (Bhat, 2005; Bemak, Epp, & Keys, 1999; Enochs & Etzbach, 2004; Russell et al., 2007). They include:

- Screening and selection procedures are clearly outlined and defined, including required professional and personal characteristics, students' openness to feedback and willingness to undertake personal counselling.

- Screening and selection should not be an isolated process at the program's beginning, but the evaluation and review process needs to be ongoing. Just because a student wins initial selection into the program should not ensure certain graduation. He or she may exhibit such behaviour on the program that indicates the individual is not appropriate to continue in the program.

- Counsellor educators and supervisors should establish clear performance-based contracts with students early in training, where learning objectives and professional competencies are unequivocally articulated, performance reviews and competency interviews regularly undertaken. Students are informed of the gatekeeping role of the faculty and onsite supervisors. Students are also alerted to the expectations of professional codes of conduct and standards of practice.

- Counsellor educators and supervisors require regular and ongoing opportunities to consult together about students' dispositions and progress.

- The gatekeeping role of counsellor educators and supervisors is an ethical obligation so as to take appropriate action to protect clients and future clients from harm. Therefore, the faculty need to be professionally developed and trained in the gatekeeping role. The role needs to be defined in a systematic and structured way, with clear policies and procedures.

- Universities need to have 'clear and precise procedures for dismissing students who are inappropriate for the program' (Enochs & Etzbach, 2004, p. 399) because of continued professional competency problems.

These recommendations are intended to strengthen our role as gate-keepers and lessen the stressful effects of not dealing early enough or adequately with students' professional competency problems.

Conclusions

The review of supervision literature (mainly examining studies undertaken with trainees) by Wheeler and Richards indicated that supervision has positive effects on the supervisee where their growth and development is enhanced. Supervisees' self-efficacy and skills are improved via supervision. 'Supervision does seem to offer opportunities for supervisees to improve practice and gain in confidence' (Wheeler & Richards, 2007, p. 63). This is evidence that: as supervisors of trainees we need to take this role seriously; we need to consider the recommendations from the literature for our programs; we need to professionally develop ourselves as gatekeepers; we need to articulate professional performance standards, requirements and program expectation; and finally, we need to communicate clearly, strongly and early to our students that this is one of our key roles in the program. In this way, we are likely to manage problematic performance better in our programs and protect the public, the program and the profession from incompetent professionals in the future.

Educational Questions and Activities

1. If the three domains of counselling mastery are the cognitive, the affective, and the relational (Jennings & Skovholt, 1999), how can we best evaluate if our program applicants are likely to be effective in these areas? In what ways can counsellor educators and supervisors assist potential students fairly in demonstrating their capacities to be worthy candidates for a postgraduate counselling program?

    A. A combination of the following: Live panel interviews? Experiential group exercises? Referee reports? Academic transcripts? Other ways? This should not be a quick process but we should take time over this entry point, and faculty wide consultation should be part of the process. Well-considered and comprehensive selection processes will save us time and resources later on in the program in dealing with students who lack competency.

2. Forrest and her colleagues (1999) summarised the ethical mandates incumbent upon trainers, educators and supervisors, in managing problematic student performance. These include:

    • attending to the possibility that their trainees' personal problems might lead to harm of others

- making sure that trainees are not harming clients or others under their care
- attending to the possibility that trainees may misuse their influence
- evaluating whether trainees are performing responsibly, competently, and ethically
- articulating a clear set of professional standards
- evaluating trainees based on these relevant and established requirements (cf. p. 636).

Discuss how your program attends to these mandates effectively.

3. Discuss the significance of the language we use in defining and labelling certain behaviours and/or individuals who are problematic. What are the benefits and dangers in using the following terminology in regards to students? (a) 'incompetence', (b) 'impairment', (c) 'personal limitations', (d) 'inappropriateness', (e) 'unsuitability', (f) 'unfit to practice', (g) 'professional competence problems'?

   - (a)–(f): The problem with these terms is that they: lack specificity and precision, blur behaviour and personality, mix-up cause and consequences. These terms can be seen as labels that are detrimental to the career future of the student, not only in the counselling profession.
   - (g): This term may cover the breadth and depth of the problems and concerns that counsellor educators and supervisors encounter in students who are not, for whatever reason, meeting professional standards of practice. Because it is behaviourally focused, the term may lead to more attentive monitoring and evaluation of students, which will in turn lead 'improved identification, remediation, and effective outcomes' (Elman & Forrest, 2007, p. 508).

4. Discuss how you can design, implement and monitor remediation plans shaped to manage and address individual student's performance problems. Who should take responsibility for these plans on your program? Should the three tasks of design, implementation and monitoring be undertaken by different individuals on the faculty?

   A. Forrest and her colleagues (1999) suggested that remediation plans should:
      - identify and describe deficiencies that are directly tied to the program's evaluation criteria
      - identify specific goals or changes that need to be made by the trainee
      - identify possible methods for meeting those goals

- establish criteria for judging whether remediation has been successful
- determine a timeline for re-evaluation.

5. Discuss with your colleagues what behaviours, attitudes and contexts demand the dismissal of a student from your program. What are our professional, ethical and legal responsibilities as trainers and supervisors to this trainee, to the public, to the profession and to our training institutes?

A. This is a demanding and difficult decision to come to for most counsellor educators. When remediation plans do not achieve positive outcomes for students, we need to face the fact that these students may need to be counselled off the program, or even dismissed from the program as being unsuitable for the profession, in that they never had or have not been able to achieve an adequate level of professional competence during the required time period. Some of the reasons for dismissal include continued poor academic performance, poor clinical performance, failed competency tests, ethical violations, psychopathology, emotional instability, personality disorder, unprofessional demeanour, poor interpersonal skills, sexual misconduct and substance abuse (Forrest et al., 1999).

Due process obviously needs to be followed according to the policies of the university or training institute, where students have been duly informed of professional competencies, standards and expectations, remedial plans that have not achieved sufficient change in the student's professional competency levels are recorded, extensive and detailed documentation is completed and placed in the student's file (Wilkerson, 2006).

References

American Counseling Association. (1995). *Code of Ethics and Standards of Practice F.3.* Alexandria, VA: Author.

Aveline, M. (2005). The person of the therapist. *Psychotherapy Research, 15*(3), 155–164.

Bemak, F., Epp, L.R., & Keys, S.G. (1999). Impaired graduate students: A process model of graduate program monitoring and intervention. *International Journal for the Advancement of Counseling, 21,* 19–30.

Bhat, C.S. (2005). Enhancing counseling gatekeeping with performance appraisal protocols. *International Journal for the Advancement of Counselling, 27*(3), 399–411.

Brear, P., Dorrian, J., & Luscri, G. (2008). Preparing our future counselling professionals: Gatekeeping and the implications for research. *Counselling and Psychotherapy Research, 8*(2), 93–101.

Cobia, D.C., & Pipes, R.B. (2002)/ Mandated supervision: An intervention for disciplined professionals. *Journal of Counseling & Development, 80*(2), 140–144.

Elman, N.S., & Forrest, L. (2007). From trainee impairment to professional competence problems: Seeking new terminology that facilitates effective action. *Professional Psychology: Research and Practice, 38*(5), 501–509.

Enochs, W.K., & Etzbach, C.A. (2004). Impaired student counselors: Ethical and legal considerations for the family. *The Family Journal: Counseling and Therapy for Couples and Families, 12*(4), 396–400

Forrest, L., Elman, N., Gizara, S., & Vacha-Haase, T. (1999). Trainee Impairment: A review of identification, remediation, dismissal, and legal issues. *The Counseling Psychologist,* 27, 627–686

Jennings, L., & Skovholt, T.M. 1999. The cognitive, emotional, and relational characteristics of master therapists. *Journal of Counseling Psychology, 46*(1), 3–11.

Jennings, L., Goh, M., Skovholt, T.M., Hanson, M., & Banerjee-Stevens, D. (2003). Multiple factors in the development of the expert counselor and therapist. *Journal of Career Development, 30*(1), 59–72.

Kaslow, N.J., Rubin, N.J., Forrest, L., et al. (2007). Recognizing, assessing, and intervening with problems of professional competence. *Professional Psychology: Research and Practice, 38*(5), 479–492.

Ladany, N., Friedlander, M.L., & Nelson, M.L. (2005). *Critical events in psychotherapy supervision: An interpersonal approach.* Washington, DC: APA

McWilliams, N. (2005). Preserving our humanity as therapists. *Psychotherapy: Theory, Research, Practice, Training, 42*(2), 139–151.

Psychotherapy and Counselling Federation of Australia, (2009). *PACFA training standards.* Available at http://www.pacfa.org.au/

Rapisarda, C.A., & Britton, P.J. (2007). Sanctioned supervision: Voices from the experts. *Journal of Mental Health Counseling, 29*(1), 81–92.

Rønnestad, M.H., & Skovholt, T.M. (2001). Learning arenas for professional development: Retrospective accounts of senior therapists. *Professional Psychology: Research and Practice, 32,* 181–187.

Rønnestad, M.H., & Skovholt, T.M. (2003). The journey of the counselor and therapist: Research findings and perspectives on professional development. *Journal of Career Development, 30*(1), 5–44.

Russell, C.S., Beggs, M.A., Peterson, C.M., & Anderson, M.P. (2007). Responding to remediation and gatekeeping challenges in supervision. *Journal of Marital and Family Therapy, 33*(2), 227–244.

Sullivan, B.F. (2008). *Counsellors and counselling: A new conversation.* Sydney, Australia: Pearson Education.

Skovholt, T.M. (2005). The cycle of caring: A model of expertise in the helping professions. *Journal of Mental Health Counseling, 27*(1), 82–93.

Skovholt, T., & Jennings, L. (2005). Mastery and expertise in counseling. *Journal of Mental Health Counseling, 27*(1), 13–18.

Wheeler, S. (2002). Nature or nurture: Are therapists born or trained? *Psychodynamic Practice, 8*(4), 427–441.

Wheeler, S., & Richards, K. (2007). The impact of clinical supervision on counsellors and therapists, their practice and their clients. A systematic review of the literature. *Counselling and Psychotherapy Research, 7*(1), 54–65.

Wilkerson, K. (2006). Impaired students: Applying the therapeutic process model to graduate training programs. *Counselor Education and Supervsion, 45*(3), 207–217.

chapter sixteen

Counsellor Competence

Nadine Pelling

The topic of counselling competence has increased in importance in recent years along with a growing demand for quality counselling, an increase in credentialing efforts and a focus on the professionalisation of counselling. There are many ways of defining and assessing counsellor competence. This chapter describes some of the main issues relating to the definition and assessment of counsellor competence, including who is assessing competence and for what purpose.

The Importance and Complexity of Counsellor Competence

The topic of counsellor competence became very important in the 1990s in the United States (McLeod, 1992). In fact, a plethora of professional ethical codes regarding counsellor competence developed — a synopsis of which can be found in Corey, Corey, and Callanan (1992). Anderson (1992, p. 22) states that this was due to five discernible forces influencing the counselling profession in the United States, namely:

- a growing demand for quality mental health counseling
- an increasing public awareness of specific issues in mental health care and general health care consumerism
- increasing demands for quality assurance, accountability, and containment of mental health care cost
- a progressive state-by-state wave of credentialism and licensure
- increasing national emphasis on counselor professionalism.

As a result, counsellor licensure and certification have long been viewed as a validation of qualifications needed for effective and competent counselling in the United States (McLeod, 1992). Counsellor licensure and certification have become expected in the United States. The goal of counsellor licensure and certification is to increase counsellor professionalism and protect consumers from incompetent practitioners.

A similar focus on counselling competency is currently developing in Australia. This is evident in the two main generalist counselling associations' recent focus on educational standards and credentialing efforts. These two associations are often seen as competitors due to their overlapping and similar functions as well as, at times, different philosophies regarding the credentialing of counselling. It is sufficient to say that different counselling associations in Australia are defining competence or readiness for counselling differently. This is not surprising given that counsellor competence is so difficult to define and measure. Add this to indecisiveness regarding who will measure counsellor competence and the complexity of assessing competent counselling services in Australia becomes clear (Armstrong, 2006; Pelling, 2003, 2006; Pelling & Sullivan, 2006; Pelling & Whetham, 2006; Pelling, Brear, & Lau, 2006; Schofield, Grant, Holmes, & Barletta, 2006; Sullivan, 2003).

Defining Competence

How does one define counsellor competence? The literature on counsellor competence centres on the idea of skill (Egan, 1990; Ivey & Authier, 1978) — thus, a competent counsellor would be one who has mastered a set of counselling skills. The National Counsellor Examination's testing of professional knowledge on basic counselling information and skills in eight basic areas of counselling practice seems to subscribe to this view of competence as skill (Corey, Corey, & Callanan, 1992).

However, there are those who believe that competence cannot be reduced to the level of skill and that counselling is not simply the accumulation of a set of skills. As stated by McLeod (1992, p. 360) 'the person of the counselor, including her values and philosophy, is a key factor in the counseling relationship, and that this factor is not readily observable within discrete, "micro" interactions'.

Thus, although the literature on competence focuses on the idea of skill it also seems agreed upon that competence subsumes skill and refers (McLeod, 1992, p. 360) 'to any qualities or abilities of the person which contribute to effective performance of a role or task'. As stated by McLeod (p. 359) 'Counselling is an activity in which, almost uniquely, the quality of work and the outcome of effort is largely hidden from external scrutiny and affirmation'. This sentiment is echoed by Gross and Robinson (1985) who view counsellor competence as containing five basic aspects (the fourth issue being most closely associated with competence as skill) which are an:

(1) accurate representation of professional qualifications; (2) professional growth through involvement in continuing education; (3) provision of only those services for which one is qualified; (4) maintenance of accurate knowledge and expertise in specialized areas; and (5) assistance in solving personal issues which impede effectiveness.

As stated by McLeod (1992, p. 367)

> Within the thousands of counseling and psychotherapy trainers, tutors and supervisors there certainly must exist a deep well of experience and knowledge about how best to assess the competence of counselors. Very little of this knowledge is written down, however, and even less of it has been subject to systematic research.

Thus, obviously, defining counsellor competence is difficult and one's definition clearly depends on many factors, including the purpose of one's definition. Capturing the essence of, and what is meant by competence is elusive (Goh, 2005). Nevertheless, this difficulty has not prevented many efforts at measuring counsellor competence.

The Assessment of Competence

The measurement of counsellor competence is complicated by its very nature. First, there is no precise definition of competence. Second, the purpose of competence measurement will affect the definition of competence and thus the assessment technique used. Third, the measurement of competence will also be influenced by who is measuring competence.

Purpose of Assessment

The measurement of counsellor competence takes two forms, formative and summative, depending on what function the assessment is to serve. Summative assessment's purpose is to evaluate the competence of a person and formative assessment's purpose is to generate information concerning the developmental needs of the counsellor. Summative assessment would therefore most likely be used in evaluating a counsellor's competence to perform a particular job or whether the person should receive a professional certification or license. In contrast, formative assessments are designed to generate information about the developmental needs of the counsellor that could be used to define learning objectives in work settings or in continuing education programs (McLeod, 1992).

Who Will Assess Competence?

Counsellor competence can be assessed by counsellor trainers, managers, supervisors, external judges, themselves, peers and clients. These varied assessors usually differ in their purpose, their corresponding definition of competence and their measurement techniques. Some general statement concerning the advantages and disadvantages of each of the before mentioned competence evaluators are as follows (McLeod, 1992).

Trainer/supervisor assessment. Competence assessment is a necessity when one is in a training program. Unfortunately, the validity and reliability of assessment by a trainer or supervisor may be negatively impacted by many factors. For example, trainers may not have equal exposure to all their trainees and the contact they do have may be coloured by 'impression management' on the trainee's part who want to be evaluated favourably. Moreover, supervision is said to involve aspects of assessment, training, support and personal therapy which can complicate the assessment process (Corey, Corey, & Callanan, 1992; McLeod, 1992).

Manager assessment. Some managers are not members of the counselling profession and thus their assessment of counsellor competence might be resisted due to the belief that only counsellors should judge counsellor competence. Such managers might consider a counsellor effective if they work well with other staff members, engage in professional development and if clients return to see the counsellor in question.

External judge assessment. Judgments made by an external judge are less likely to be biased. However, the counselling work they are exposed to is likely to be limited and thus may not be representative of the counsellor's overall competence.

Self-assessment. The main argument against counsellor self-assessment of competence is that incompetent counsellors are not likely to know how to make accurate judgment of their own competence (McLeod, 1992). In contrast, Gross and Robinson (1987) purport that an internal frame of reference is best used to ensure competence, although the necessity for some level of external enforcement is conceded. Gross and Robinson (1987) believe that each counsellor should take full responsibility for their own conduct and their adherence to the rules and regulations of their profession. Self-assessment, of course, depends on the honesty of the assessor or counsellor. In Australia, counsellors themselves are likely the most common assessors of competence as counselling is an unregulated activity. Thus, in Australia competence assessments are not specifically required for counselling practice.

Peer assessment. This type of assessment is less impacted by the 'impression management', which can influence supervisory assessment. However, if peer assessment is to be used an appropriate culture regarding the giving and receiving must be created and maintained.

Client assessment. As stated by McLeod (1992, p. 363) 'The ultimate criterion of counselor competence must be that of client benefit'. In other words, did the client benefit from his or her counselling experience? Unfortunately, research in this area is limited and can be very expensive.

How Do We Measure Competence?

The measurement of competence is very complicated, depends on the definition of competence utilised and can be accomplished in a number of ways. Moreover, the multifarious measurement of competence is even further complicated by the general exclusion of validity and reliability data on counsellor competence measurements (McLeod, 1992). In general, the measurement of counsellor competence is best assessed in a safe and open environment, when assessment techniques are based in research, target competencies are specific and multitudes of measurement techniques are used, such as with 'Centre Data' in Bray's (1982) study. The main techniques used for the measurement of counsellor competence are as follows: questionnaires and rating scales, video/audio tapes, role-play exercises/simulations, journals and exams (McLeod, 1992).

Questionnaires/rating scales. There are two types of questionnaires/rating scales: those with an evaluative component and those designed to estimate how often a counsellor does something (i.e., reflect the client's feelings), whose results would then be interpreted in relation to the theory the counsellor is using. Both Carkhuff (1969) as well as Ivey and Authier (1978) have developed rating scales that assess various counselling skills. Similarly, specific scales have been devised and used to measure different types of counselling competence, such as multicultural competence (Holcomb-McCoy, 2005). In contrast, Sachs (1983) has developed a rating scale designed to measure the absence of competence via its focus on therapist errors. It seems that those using questionnaires and rating scales as supervising counsellors set cut-off levels between acceptable and unacceptable levels of competence. The counselling behaviour assessed can be 'live', on video/audiotape, or role-play/simulation situations.

Journals. Learning journals and diaries containing the participant's subjective record of their development and learning can also be used to assess counsellor competence. Competence is assessed by examining the amount of insight the counsellor has into his or her actions and interventions.

Exams. Formal examinations are widely accepted as able to assess dimensions of cognitive skill and knowledge, rather than interpersonal skill that is required for working with clients. This technique assumes that counsellor competence is largely due to one's ability to learn difficult theoretical material. However, empirical testing of this assumption has not been flattering and many sources believe that 'too high an emphasis on theoretical knowledge may distract the counselor from her primary task, that of establishing a therapeutic relationship with her client' (Chevron & Rounsaville, 1983; McLeod, 1992, p. 366). In fact, Chevron and Rounsaville (1983) found, in their study of psychotherapy evaluating techniques, that only supervisors' ratings were correlated with patient outcome.

Identifying a Minimum Level of Counsellor Competence

To summarise, there is a lack of information regarding the reliability and validity of assessments of counsellor competence. The research findings of Chevron and Rounsaville (1983) suggest that competence assessments and client outcome lack a relationship. Thus, developing counsellor competence and designating a minimum level of counsellor competence to be measured does not, at this time, seem realistic. It seems more logical to focus on the gradations of competence, rather than on identifying various absolute levels of competence when skill and direct work with clients is concerned. It is easier to judge whether a counsellor is grossly incompetent versus designating competence. This is the reasoning behind Sachs' (1983) study of negative factors in psychotherapy. Nevertheless, there are authors that have proposed minimum standards of competence for counsellors; one example is Anderson (1992) who has proposed eight minimum standards.

Enforcing Minimum Levels of Counsellor Competence

How does one ensure counsellor competence given the lack of consensus regarding a definition of competence and the multitude of assessors as well as assessment techniques? It seems that the most efficient and common method of ensuring counsellor competence is the counsellors' self- and peer assessment; if an open, safe and honest environment can be maintained. This is important to ensure that a 'police state' does not result in the counselling profession. Yes, we want to ensure that only competent counsellors are practicing counselling, but a professional emphasis in assessment must be on formative versus summative assessment aimed at continuously increasing counsellor competence if the counselling profession is to be an inclusive occupation and not exclusive in Australia. This is the approach taken by Nagy (1989) who has proposed nine guidelines for counsellors to avoid practicing beyond their limits of competence, including skills areas and personal problem management.

Can/Does Licensure and Certification Ensure Counsellor Competence?

Unfortunately, legal regulation and certification cannot ensure counsellor competence. They may serve to create very general minimum standards of competence but they certainly cannot confer overall competence (Corey, Corey, & Callanan, 1992). As pointed out by Nagy (1989), counsellor competence can be exceeded both on purpose as well as accidentally and steps must be taken by the counsellor him/herself to ensure that one does not work outside their boundaries of competence. Evidently, we must patrol ourselves to ensure that our peers and we learn how to stay within our boundaries of competence when working with clients. We must understand and believe that this is in our own and our clients' best interests.

Within the profession 'incompetence' is generally recognisable by both the counsellor him/herself and also his/her peers. Differing levels of competence are less definable due to the subjective nature of defining competence, differing reasons for competence measurement and the plethora of people who may be in charge of competence assessment. Given all this subjectivity it seems impossible to decisively measure competence with purely objective measures and thus designate a minimum level of competence, as well as objective gradations of competence. Counsellors subjectively know what competence and incompetence are and how to evaluate them: an objective measurement and testing of this is less likely and some would argue not desired. A starting point for competence assessment is clearly stating our definition of competence and who and for what purpose competence is to be assessed, while keeping in mind the difficulty in assessing such a concept.

Acknowledgment

The contents of the present chapter have been previously published as follows.

Pelling, N. (2006). Counsellor competence: A survey of Australian counsellor self perceived competence, *Counselling Australia, 6*(1), 3–14.

Pelling, N. (2007). Counsellor competence. In N. Pelling, R. Bowers, & P. Armstrong (Eds.), *The practice of counselling* (pp. 36–45). Melbourne, Australia: Thomson.

Educational Questions and Activities

1. Discuss how you define competence.

2. List two forms of assessment:
   * formative
   * summative.

3. Who are some stakeholders who can assess competence?
   * trainers/supervisor
   * manager
   * external judge
   * self
   * peer
   * client.

References

Anderson, D. (1992). A case for standards of counselling practice. *Journal of Counselling & Development, 71*, 22–26.

Armstrong, P. (2006). The Australian Counselling Association: Meeting the needs of Australian counsellors. *International Journal of Psychology, 4*(3), 156–162.

Bray, D.W. (1982). The Assessment Center and the study of lives. *American Psychologist, 37*(2), 180–189.

Carkhuff, R. (1969). *Helping and human relations* (2nd ed.). New York, Holdt.

Chevron, E., & Rounsaville, B. (1983). Evaluating the clinical skills of psychotherapists. *Archives of General Psychiatry, 40*, 1129–1132.

Corey, G., Corey, M., & Callanan, P. (1992). *Issues and ethics in the helping professions* (4th ed.). Belmont, CA: Brooks/Cole.

Egan, G. (1990). *The skilled helper* (4th ed.). San Francisco: Brooks/Cole.

Goh, M. (2005). Cultural competence and master therapists: An inextricable relationship. *Journal of Mental Health Counseling, 27*(1), 71–82.

Gross, D.R., & Robinson, S.E. (1985). Ethics: The neglected issue in consultation. *Journal of Counseling and Development, 64*(1), 38–41.

Holcomb-McCoy, C. (2005). Investigating school counselors' perceived multicultural competence. *Professional School Counseling, 8*(5), 414–424.

Ivey, A., & Authier, A. (1978). *Microcounselling: Innovations in interviewing, counselling, psychotherapy and psychoeducation* (2nd ed.). Springfield, IL: Thomas.

McLeod, J. (1992). What do we know about how best to assess counsellor competence? *Counselling Psychology Quarterly, 5*(4), 359–372.

Nagy, T. (1989, February). Boundaries of competence: Training and therapist impairment. Selected proceedings of the Annual Meeting of the California Sate Psychological Association, San Francisco.

Pelling, N. (2003). Counselling in Australia [Comment]. *Counselling Today, 45*(7), 4 & 30.

Pelling, N. (2006). Introduction to the special issue on counselling in Australia. *International Journal of Psychology.*

Pelling, N., & Sullivan, B. (2006). The credentialing of counselling in Australia. *International Journal of Psychology, 41*(3), 194–203.

Pelling, N., & Whetham, P. (2006). The professional preparation of Australian counsellors. *International Journal of Psychology, 41*(3), 189–193.

Pelling, N., Brear, P., & Lau, M. (2006). A survey of advertised Australian counsellors. *International Journal of Psychology, 41*(3), 204–215.

Sachs, J. (1983). Negative factors in brief psychotherapy: An empirical assessment. *Journal of Consulting and Clinical Psychology, 51*, 557–564.

Schofield, M., Grant, J., Holmes, S., & Barletta, J. (2006). The Psychotherapy and Counselling Federation of Australia: How the federation model contributes to the field. *International Journal of Psychology, 41*(3), 163–169.

Sullivan, B. (2003). Counselling in Australia [Comment]. *Counselling Today, 45*(7), 30.

—+−+−+−+−+−

Emerging and Specialist Issues

This section, 'Emerging and Specialist Issues', demonstrates the ever evolving nature of applied supervisory practice. In Chapter 17 Arthur and Collins discuss the importance of infusing culture into counselling supervision thus honouring the broadly defined multicultural nature of clients, supervisees, as well as supervisors. Chapter 18 is the largest chapter in the book. This chapter was created by 5 different authors and reviews the unique aspects of supervision in five specialisation areas: marriage and family therapy, school counselling, alcohol and drug abuse counselling, supervision in university-based training clinics, and supervision in community agencies. In reality this large chapter is five chapters in one, but the material is presented together to highlight how supervision needs to be adjusted to the context in which it takes place. Chapter 19 is truly unique in that it reviews the use of technology in supervision including videoconferencing and the internet. Finally, Chapter 20 reviews clinical placement supervision in detail and provides some tools for supervision in this context. Together, these chapters present supervision on the 'cutting edge' in terms of newness and targeted practice.

Chapter Overview

CHAPTER 17

'Culture-Infused Counselling Supervision' explores the impact of culture not just on counselling but on the supervisory relationship. With a skilful use of scenarios the importance of culture in the supervisory relationship is demonstrated. The chapter provides information on addressing cultural influences in supervision and conducting a cultural audit of counselling supervision. Thus, this is a very practical chapter regarding the application of culture in counselling supervision.

Chapter Themes

In this chapter you will explore the following themes:

- introduction
- our model of culture-infused counselling
- defining culture-infused supervision
- competence for culture-infused supervision
- enhancing culture-infused supervision through collaborative inquiry
- working with cultural expectations in supervision
- supervision scenarios
- Scenario 1
- Scenario 2
- Scenario 3

- Scenario 4
- addressing cultural influences in supervision
- tools for reflective practice
- cultural auditing of counselling supervision
- conducting a Cultural Audit of Supervision Practices.

CHAPTER 18

Clinical supervision takes place in a multitude of settings and 'Supervision of Applied Specialities' acknowledges this fact. Five leading experts in five separate applied specialities come together in this chapter to outline what is unique about supervision in their area. This chapter is truly informative to supervisors and supervisees alike in that it illustrates the diverse nature of supervision relating to context. While this is a large chapter, each speciality section can be read in isolation. Conversely, read together the entire chapter illustrates the importance of organisational context to supervision.

Chapter Themes

In this chapter you will explore the following themes:

- marriage and family therapy supervision
- MFT historical development and core values
- family systems-informed emphases in MFT supervision
- MFT-informed strategies in supervision
- current trends and future developments
- school counselling supervision
- current status and unique challenges
- models of school counsellor supervision
- supervisor competency
- supervision of alcohol and drug counselling
- alcohol and other drug abuse counsellor competencies
- alcohol and other drug abuse clinical supervision
- supervision in university training clinics
- overview of university training clinics
- overview of the Department of Counselor Education and Counseling Psychology at WMU
- an uncommon faculty appointment
- in-house supervision of master's-level practica and internships
- supervision of doctoral students

- the association of directors of psychology training clinics
- community mental health supervision
- unique challenges for the community mental health supervisor
- organisation of the supervision experience
- evaluation
- protocol for handling emergencies and crisis situations
- marriage and family therapy educational questions and activities
- alcohol and drug counseling educational questions and activities
- university training clinics educational question
- community mental health counseling educational questions and activities.

CHAPTER 19

Technology is everywhere and clinical supervision is no exception. In 'The Use of Technology in Supervision' the reader is provided with an overview of the use of technology in supervision and the new ways of delivering clinical supervision. Practical information and illustrations are provided which make the use of technology in supervision concrete and under-standable. This chapter is a must read for supervisors working in the technological age.

Chapter Themes

In this chapter you will explore the following themes:

- technology-assisted supervision
- enhancing use of video and audio through analytical and research software
- extending direct observation
- delivering clinical supervision via technology
- phone
- e-mail
- bulletin board/forum/listserv
- IM/chat
- videoconferencing/webcam
- virtual worlds
- considerations for the use of technology in supervision
- review of current standards
- contracting/informed consent
- ethical/legal concerns

- encryption/confidentiality
- verbatim material
- transference/countertransference
- suitability of the supervisor
- technical competencies
- training and education
- other suitability considerations.

CHAPTER 20

'Supervising Clinical Placement' by John Barletta and Jason Dixon brings this text to a close by exploring the crucial role of internship and practicum experiences in the development of trainees. It is in these contexts that students are happily inducted into the profession and supervisors perform the potentially burdensome role of gatekeeper. This chapter educates the novice as to the possible supervisory approaches they will be exposed to, while providing a useful template on how to provide a client history to a supervisor, group or peer. The table which highlights the development of the therapist will be an invaluable resource to normalise and validate the feelings and steps of trainees on their professional journey.

Chapter Themes
In this chapter you will explore the following themes:
- definition and purpose
- what to expect from the supervision experience
- approaches a supervisor may employ
- live supervision and supervision with pre-recorded work
- characteristics of effective supervisors
- case conceptualisation, critical thinking and note taking
- client history intake form
- therapist development
- the journey of professional therapists
- critical incidents and case studies
- case presentations
- circumstances requiring immediate action to prevent imminent harm
- sample suicide contract.

chapter seventeen

Culture-Infused Counselling Supervision

Nancy Arthur and Sandra Collins

Although there is now abundant literature on multicultural counselling, attention to multicultural competence issues has only recently surfaced in the supervision literature (Norton & Coleman, 2003). Supervision is an important learning context for examining the influence of culture in counselling relationships. In our model of Culture-Infused Counselling (Collins & Arthur, 2005b; Collins & Arthur, in press a; in press b), we have emphasised the importance of cultural influences on the working alliance between counsellors and clients. We have also argued that an examination of cultural influences on counselling relationships must go beyond counsellor–client dyads to include all roles in which counsellors are involved. This includes the roles associated with counsellor supervision. We believe that culture is an ever-present dynamic in the ways that client issues and interventions are conceptualised. Culture is also an ongoing influence in the supervisory relationship.

If we work from the premise that the central goal of supervision is to improve the welfare of clients through facilitating the responsiveness of professionals (Bernard & Goodyear, 1998), it follows that supervision must be concerned with promoting multicultural counselling competence (Ancis & Ladany, 2001; Chen, 2001, Constantine, 1997; D'Andrea & Daniels, 1997). The implication is that supervisors must also increase their level of competence for multicultural counselling supervision. Effective multicultural supervision holds the additional goals of enhancing the training experiences of supervisees and supporting more satisfying supervisory relationships (Constantine, 2003; Pope-Davis, Toporek, & Ortega-Villalobos, 2003).

The purpose of this chapter is to familiarise readers with the importance of incorporating cultural influences into the supervision process. First, we provide an overview of our model of Culture-Infused Counselling. Second, we develop a rationale for incorporating cultural auditing in counselling supervision. In doing so, we highlight the multicultural counselling competencies of both supervisors and supervisees, cultural expectations in supervision and ways for supervisors to increase competence in culture-infused counselling supervision. The chapter ends with a cultural auditing tool that is designed to promote discussion between supervisors and counsellors about the influences of culture in their work together.

Our Model of Culture-Infused Counselling

The emphasis on multicultural counselling supervision has emerged in response to the establishment of multicultural competence in counselling as a core mandate for professional practice. To understand the process and implications of multicultural supervision it is important to briefly overview the broader context of multicultural counselling generally.

A number of key authors have mapped out competencies for multicultural counselling over the past several decades. The most well-known documents were developed by members of the Division of Counseling Psychology of the American Psychological Association (APA), specifically Arredondo and colleagues (1996) and Sue and colleagues (1992, 1999). Although the competencies have continued to evolve over time and have been applied in documents like the more recent APA (2002) *Guidelines on Multicultural Education, Training, Research, Practice, and Organizational Change for Psychologists*, the basic model has remained relatively stable over time. Three core categories have been identified as essential to the development of multicultural counselling competence: (a) awareness of one's own cultural assumptions, values and biases; (b) understanding of client world-views and perspectives and (c) implementation of interventions strategies and techniques that are appropriate to the cultural context of the client (Sue, Arredondo, & McDavis,1992).

Over the years there have been many criticisms of the current paradigm, based primarily on the following issues. First, the definition of what constitutes culture has evolved over time, and most writers now accept that other dimensions of personal cultural identity must be more fully integrated into the model (Arredondo & Perez, 2006; Weinrach & Thomas, 2002). The continued primacy of race and ethnicity in the current frameworks is problematic in reserving discussions about culture for certain clients, for example, in instances when there are visible differences between the counsellor and client. This focus fails to take into account the importance of other cultural factors such as gender, ability, sexual orientation, age, socioeconomic status and so on, as well as the complexity of working with clients with multiple nondominant identities (Lowe & Mascher, 2001; Silverstein, 2006).

Second, while the most recent guidelines do incorporate other key areas of professional practice, including supervision, little effort has been made to clearly articulate how the current competencies models should be adapted to include these expanded areas of practice (Collins & Arthur, in press a). Our model maintains the self-awareness and awareness of client cultural identities as the first two core competency domains, but integrates the broader definition of culture and frames the specific competencies in a way that allows for easy expansion to other domains of practice, such as organisational consultation, counsellor education, supervision or social justice roles (Arthur & Collins, 2005a; Collins & Arthur, 2005b).

The third common criticism of the traditional models, and perhaps the most important in the context of the current discussion on supervision, is the argument that effective practice involves more than the application of appropriate intervention strategies and techniques (Collins & Arthur, in press a). We have proposed the concept of the working alliance to replace the earlier, narrower focus on interventions as the third core domain of cultural competency. The working alliance is a broader, pantheoretical construct that elevates the relationship between counsellor and client to its rightful place as one of the most significant predictors of counselling outcomes (Coleman, 2004; Roysircar, Hubbell, & Gard, 2003). It is in the context of the working alliance relationship between counsellor and client that counsellor self-awareness and awareness of the culture of the client(s) are manifest, negotiated and applied. For a more detailed rationale for our model of culture-infused counselling, see Collins and Arthur (in press a).

Developing a culturally-sensitive working alliance involves: (1) agreement on the goals to be addressed through the relationship, (2) agreement on the tasks required to reach those goals and (3) a context of mutual respect and trust in the pursuit of those goals (Collins & Arthur, 2005a). Selection of appropriate interventions is only one component of the process of establishing and implementing an effective working alliance. The collaborative nature of the counselling working alliance highlights the importance not only of acquisition of appropriate strategies and techniques, but of their application only within the context of active negotiation about their cultural relevance for a particular client, with a particular cultural world-view, in a particular context, to address particular presenting concerns (Meissner, 2006).

Culture-infused counselling is defined as the 'conscious and purposeful infusion of cultural awareness and sensitivity into all aspects of the counselling process and all other roles assumed by the counselling psychologist'

(Arthur & Collins, 2005b, p. 16). A core assumption of this model is that all humans are cultural beings whose world-views are affected by personal identity factors (e.g., family dynamics or personal experiences), cultural factors (e.g., ethnic heritage, gender, ability, sexual orientation, etc.), and contextual factors (e.g., social norms or historical context; Collins & Arthur, 2005b). Given this premise, we join other writers who argue that any encounter between counsellor and client, supervisor and supervisee, consultant and organisation, and so on is necessarily multicultural in nature.

In summary, our model of culture-infused counselling requires the development of specific competencies (attitudes, knowledge and skills) in three core domains (Collins & Arthur, 2005; in press a):

1. Counsellor self-awareness (which includes awareness of one's personal cultural identities, of the differences between one's identities and those of members of other dominant and nondominant groups, of the impact of culture on the theory and practice of counselling, of the personal and professional impact of the discrepancy between dominant and nondominant groups in society, and of one's own level of multicultural counselling competence).

2. Awareness of the cultural world-view of the client(s) (which includes awareness of their cultural identities, of the relationship of personal cultural identity to health and well-being, and of the sociopolitical influences that impinge on the lives of nondominant populations).

3. A culturally-sensitive working alliance (which includes establishing trusting and respectful relationships with clients that take into account cultural identities, collaboration with clients to establish counselling goals that are responsive to salient dimensions of cultural identities, and collaboration with clients to establish counsellor and client tasks design to facilitate attainment of those goals).

Defining Culture-Infused Supervision

There are three ways that supervision has been characterised in the multicultural counselling literature. In the first perspective, the interplay of cultural forces between the counsellor/supervisee and the client is examined. From this perspective on supervision, the dynamics between counsellors and their clients are the central focus. The supervision process emphasises the best ways to support clients who present with diverse cultural identities. This view of supervision takes into consideration more traditional views of multicultural counselling in which the counsellor–client dyad is examined to enhance an effective therapeutic alliance. Supervision might entail discussions of client issues, presenting concerns and cultural implications of counselling approaches.

In the second perspective on supervision, the focus shifts to the cultural dynamics that exist between the counsellor/supervisee and the supervisor. An underlying assumption is that culture is a central force in the interpersonal process of supervision (Chen, 2001). From this perspective, supervision takes place within a multicultural relationship. Due to their personal life experiences and affiliations with different cultural groups or cultural identities, counsellors/supervisees and their supervisors hold different world-views. Multicultural supervision from this second perspective emphasises how to address and incorporate the diversity between counsellors/supervisees and their supervisors.

A third, and more dynamic perspective, takes into account the interplay of cultural forces that shape the professional relationships in the triadic process between clients, counsellors/supervisees and their supervisors. We argue that counselling supervision has to address the ways that culture is infused through the interactions among all three parties. We maintain that the central priority in supervision is to ensure the welfare of clients, and the majority of time in supervision is focused on the counsellor/supervisee and client dyad. However, addressing cultural influences in the counsellor/supervisee–supervisor relationship can not only facilitate a stronger supervisory process but also improve the delivery of multicultural counselling to clients. From this perspective, discussions of cultural influences in the supervisory relationship can be leveraged to consider how differing world-views impact counselling processes and goals (Brown & Landrum-Brown, 1995). This helps to model to counsellors/supervisees the skill of reflective practice and opens up the scope of possible interpretations of client behaviour and appropriate interventions. Supervision from this culture-infused perspective is intended to promote collaboration and reciprocal learning between supervisors and counsellor/supervisees. It is through modelling open exploration of multiple perspectives that multicultural counselling competencies can be enhanced through supervision.

The terms multicultural supervision and crosscultural supervision tend to be used interchangeably in much of the literature on supervision. However, Brown and Landrum-Brown (1995) distinguish them as follows. The term *multicultural supervision* 'alludes to the study and practice of supervision in and for different cultures. Multicultural supervision would involve the study of different cultural patterns of supervision as pertaining to its content, process, and outcomes' (p. 264). Crosscultural supervision refers to 'supervision content, processes, and outcomes pertaining to the client–counsellor–supervisor triad in which at least one of the parties in the triadic relationship is culturally different from one or both of the other parties' (p. 264). Constantine (2003) appears to blend these approaches: 'Multicultural supervision competence is characterized by supervisors' awareness, knowledge, and skills in addressing multicultural issues both within the context of supervision relationships and with regard to supervisees' relationships with their clients' (p. 384).

We prefer the term *culture-infused counselling supervision* and focus on how the cultural characteristics of the supervisor, supervisee and client triad are all relevant for counselling and supervision. An underlying assumption in culture-infused counselling supervision is that all counselling and supervision relationships are multicultural in nature (Norton & Coleman, 2003). Culture-infused counselling supervision emphasises that culture permeates the supervisory relationship and the influences of that relationship on the multicultural counselling process. Both the supervisor and the counsellor/supervisee bring their own personal cultural identities to the relationship. This is likely to result in diverse professional views, even though they may both have similar training within the helping professions.

Based on our model, culture-infused counselling supervision can be defined as the conscious and purposeful infusion of awareness of supervisor, counsellor/supervisee and client cultural identities into all aspects of the supervision process. From the perspective of supervisors' multicultural competence, there are then three core components to the model:

1. supervisors' awareness of their own cultural identities, including potential cultural biases and assumptions
2. supervisors' awareness of the personal cultural identities of both the counsellor/supervisee(s) and the client(s) and
3. establishment of a supervisory relationship that reflects the mutuality, trust and active negotiation of goals and tasks for supervision that are core to a culturally sensitive working alliance.

In this case, the specific competencies required will build on the core competencies for culture-infused counselling but will include additional competencies required to establish and maintain an effective supervisory relationship that meets the specific needs of counsellors/supervisees from a range of cultural backgrounds. Some of those specific competencies will be explored in this chapter, along with suggestions for continued competency development.

Competence for Culture-Infused Counselling Supervision

There are several learning contexts that support the development of multicultural counselling competencies. Critical learning processes occur in courses on multicultural counselling and in the field during practicum supervision when counsellors-in-training work directly with clients. One overriding assumption in culture-infused counselling supervision is that both the counsellor/supervisee and the supervisor have received prior training about cultural influences in counselling. Through exposure to curriculum, both parties enter the supervisory relationship in a state of readiness for exploring more about cultural factors in counselling practice (Stone, 1997). However, the extent to which prior training prepares either students or supervisors for crosscultural supervision is questionable, as reflected in the variety of approaches and divergent levels of cultural infusion within counsellor education curriculum (Arthur, 1998; Parham & Whitten, 2003).

Numerous studies have suggested that the curriculum of counsellor education programs does not adequately prepare graduates to work with clients from diverse cultural backgrounds (Arthur & Januszkowski, 2001; Sue & Sue, 1999). Although strides have been made to integrate multicultural counselling curriculum, and many programs offer specialist courses, counsellor education programs tend to emphasise the self-awareness and knowledge domains of multicultural competence. Students in counsellor education programs benefit from supervision to help them translate concepts about multicultural counselling into skills for practice.

We view multicultural competence as an ongoing learning process and not an end result that is attainable through one program of study. Consequently, multicultural content should not be limited to counsellor education curriculum, and in particularly not to a single course within those programs. It needs to be integrated into continuing education and professional development programs (Parham & Whitten, 2003). To this end, we have developed a competency framework for use in professional development planning aimed at both preservice and postgraduate levels (Collins & Arthur, in press a).

Supervision practices can support cultural learning during counsellor education programs or through ongoing professional practice in the workplace. However, it is of concern that supervisors may not have received education about either multicultural counselling or supervision practices. Without deliberate attempts to improve their multicultural counselling competencies through professional development, some supervisors may lack foundation competencies essential to effective culture-infused counselling supervision (Berkel, Constantine, & Olson, 2007; Bernard, 1992; Parham & Whitten, 2003). Additional training about the supervision of multicultural counselling is crucial (Cary & Marques, 2007).

An integral part of culture-infused counselling supervision is constant assessment of the boundaries of the counsellor/supervisee's multicultural counselling competence (Chen, 2001). However, we are advocating that more attention needs to be paid to the boundaries of supervisors' capacity for multicultural counselling. A main concern is whether supervisors are held to the same standard in recognising and limiting their professional practice to areas where they have sufficient background knowledge and experience. Falender and Shafranske (2007) expressed concerns about the lack of attention to culture and the lack of cultural competence of supervisors as an important area for attention in the practice of clinical supervision.

The first core domain of culture-infused counselling supervision is counsellor self-awareness. This domain forms a foundation for cultural understanding of others and for the development of a culturally sensitive working alliance. One key factor in supervision is the level of cultural identity development of the supervisor (Norton & Coleman, 2003). As in the counselling relationship, it will be difficult for supervisors to facilitate development of student cultural identity beyond the level that they have themselves attained (Constantine, Warren, & Milville, 2005; MacDougall & Arthur, 2001). This holds true whether the emphasis of supervision is placed on the needs of clients, or whether the emphasis is placed on cultural dynamics that operate in the supervisory relationship.

Supervisor–supervisee interpersonal interaction dynamics have been explored for the potential impacts of cultural identity mismatches on the supervision relationship and outcomes for clients (Ancis & Ladany, 2001; Brown & Landrum-Brown, 1995). Ideally, the negotiation of cultural differences between counsellors/supervisees and their supervisors strengthens their working relationship. Within the supervisory relationship, discussion of issues of world-view, power and salient cultural dimensions such as gender, sexual orientation and ethnic affiliation may be leveraged to deepen the supervisory relationship and, ultimately, enhance multicultural counselling competencies. A consistent finding in the literature on supervisory relationships is that trust in supervisory working alliance is an essential prerequisite for counsellors/supervisees to engage in discussion about cultural issues (Nilsson, 2007).

Conversely, lack of attention to cultural dynamics that matter to students in supervision may lead to greater defensiveness, misunderstandings and invisible and unspoken barriers of power differences in supervisory relationships. The supervision of lesbian, gay, bisexual or transgendered counsellors/supervisees, for example, may be compromised if supervisors are uninformed about identity development, or supervisors are unwilling to encourage supervisees to integrate their personal experiences into their professional identity (Messinger, 2007). Religion and spirituality is another area often overlooked in preparing students for multicultural counselling, and supervisors require related competencies (Berkel et al., 2007). Failing to attend directly to these and other cultural factors in supervision may also perpetuate the marginalisation of cultural factors in the counsellor/supervisee's work with clients (Estrada, Frame, & Williams, 2004).

Barriers to Infusing Culture into Supervision Practices

In additional to the level of supervisor and supervisee competence, there are other barriers to effectively infusing culture into supervision practices. To a large degree, these barriers reflect cultural biases and assumptions on the part of either supervisors or supervisees that have not been adequately addressed, a reminder again about the importance of self-awareness on the part of the supervisor.

Even though counsellors/supervisees and their supervisors may have been exposed to multicultural counselling concepts in their training programs, it should not be assumed that either member of the supervision dyad necessarily embraces multiculturalism as a positive or desirable direction in their professional practice (Steward, Morales, Bartell, Miller, & Weeks, 1998). Opponents to the multicultural counselling movement have challenged the need for such an approach in counselling (Pedersen, 1991). It is conceivable that some counsellors/supervisees have higher levels of interest and expertise in examining cultural influences in supervision than their supervisors, or vice versa (Constantine, 1997; D'Andrea & Daniels, 1997; Priest, 1994).

As instructors, we have experienced this issue with some students who resist the expectation to examine their personal level of competency for professional practice, as well as with the instructors and field supervisors with whom they work. This situation has prompted discussions with our colleagues about pedagogical issues related to instructing multicultural counselling and how far we should go with infusing culture into supervisory practices. For example, in the role of practicum seminar supervisor there are responsibilities for overseeing the experiences of students at their practicum sites, where they are also supervised by an on-site practitioner. Considerable independence is offered to site supervisors regarding the content of supervision and the nature of the supervisory relationship. The extent to which examination of culture enters into supervisory practices may differ at the practicum site or in the context of a course-related practicum seminar. We would advocate for a more proactive approach to working with site supervisors to extend the focus on culture in practicum site supervision. In turn, the extent to which practicum instructors examine culture in their course seminars appears to be entirely based on interests and varying levels of expertise with multicultural counselling.

Even if there is a willingness on behalf of supervisors to explore cultural influences through supervision, disparate levels of competency can be problematic for counsellors/supervisees. There is a risk of exploitation when supervisors depend upon their supervisees, often students, as the main source of education about culture or about the multicultural counselling process (Estrada et al., 2004). We will discuss this issue in more detail in the next section as we explore ways to share expertise in a collaborative supervisory relationship.

Many authors have pointed to the existence and impact of bias in assumptions, beliefs and attitudes of supervisors (Brinson, 2004). Several potential consequences occur when supervisors are unaware of their personal cultural biases and assumptions (Garrett et al., 2001). First, supervisees may be inappropriately judged according to the supervisor's world-view and the viewpoints of the supervisee may not be seen as valid. In this instance, supervisees may feel compelled to work as if in agreement, even though the approach does not resonate with them or the supervisors' perspective contradicts their personal and professional world-view. Second, miscommunication or cultural misunderstandings often pose barriers to effective interactions. This includes lack of understanding about the verbal or nonverbal communication patterns used by the counsellor/supervisee. Such misinterpretations may be channelled into evaluations about the competence level of the counsellor/supervisee when rigid standards for communication skills are upheld (Brown & Landrum-Brown, 1995; Hird, Cavalieri, Dulko, Felice, & Ho, 2001).

Inherent power differences in supervision roles make it difficult for counsellors/supervisees to feel comfortable and confident about challenging their supervisor's views of multicultural counselling (D'Andrea & Daniels, 1997). Power differences related to race and privilege can easily spill over into case conceptualisation and impact whose views are considered to be more expert and legitimate (Fong & Lease, 1997). These differences can also impact assessment of counsellor/supervisee competence. The imposition of power differences may be unintentional; supervisors who have not explored cultural influences may also be unaware of how they use power in the supervisory relationship and inadvertently dominate supervisees (Brown & Landrum-Brown, 1995; Hird et al., 2001). It may also be important for supervisors to learn specific skills for engaging in dialogue about cultural issues while expressly acknowledging the power differentials in the supervisor relationship (Toporek, Ortega-Villalobos, & Pope-Davis, 2004).

The extent to which counsellors/supervisees view their supervisors as culturally aware and receptive to alternate points of view can either strengthen or detract from a satisfactory supervisory relationship (Constantine, 1997). Supervisees' perceptions about the multicultural competence of their supervisors impact the supervisory working alliance and are related to perceived supervision satisfaction (Inman, 2006). A breakdown of trust between supervisor and supervisee may result in important client cultural issues or multicultural dynamics between counsellor and client also remaining unexamined.

These observations raise the question of how to leverage discussion about cultural influences to a central place on the agenda for counsellor supervision. In order to do that, we must engage in open dialogue about the interest and competency levels of supervisors for managing culture-infused supervision.

Enhancing Culture-Infused Supervision Through Collaborative Inquiry

There are a number of positive ways that the supervisors and counsellors/supervisees can work together to enhance competencies for multicultural counselling. For example, even when counsellors/supervisees are more knowledgable, supervisors can initiate and facilitate shared learning through collaborative inquiry (Chen, 2001). Negotiating a stance of co-discovery promotes greater levels of collaboration and mutuality between supervisees and supervisors in their respective roles. However, to be effective, both supervisors and their counsellors/supervisees need to carefully examine their expectations about expertise in the supervisory relationship.

There is usually an expectation, at least by novice counsellors, that supervisors possess more knowledge and serve as experts in the supervisory relationship. In turn, counsellors/supervisees are expected to be less knowledgable and less experienced and to look to the supervisor for direction and coaching. When counsellors/supervisees possess more knowledge and experience about multicultural counselling, a renegotiation of the terms of supervision seems warranted. This is not an unusual situation in cases where highly experienced counsellors return to school for the purpose of professional credentialing or when they seek supervision opportunities as a way to enhance their professional practices in community-based agencies or private practice. If supervisors are able to shift their perspectives about what their main roles in supervision are, this can open up many possibilities for collaborative learning. The supervisor might be better positioned to offer more knowledge about the therapeutic process and the process of supervision and be willing to engage counsellors/supervisees in sharing their culture-specific expertise. It is the active negotiation that is characteristic of a culturally sensitive working alliance.

It is also possible that, by virtue of life experience, some counsellors/supervisees may be more attuned to issues of culture in professional practice. Research has suggested that supervisors from nondominant racial/ethnic groups spend significantly more time discussing cultural issues in supervision than their White counterparts (Hird, Tao, & Gloria, 2005). The dynamics of supervision can be enhanced through exchanges with counsellors/supervisees about identity issues if supervisors who are of cultural minority status also consider such practices to be within their roles and responsibilities (Taylor, Hernandez, Deri, Rankin, & Siegel, 2006). Similarly, counsellors/supervisees who are members of nondominant groups will often have more culture-specific knowledge about how to relate to clients from those groups than a supervisor who is from a dominant group (Fukuyama, 1994).

Working With Cultural Expectations in Supervision

Despite the potential benefits of collaborative inquiry in culture-infused counselling supervision, supervisors must be mindful of cultural expectations that impact the supervisory relationship. For example, it should not be assumed that all counsellors/supervisees share a modernist world-view of supervision wherein meanings and understandings are mutually negotiated in a collaborative relationship (Gonzalez, 1997; Neufeldt, 1997). Depending on the academic or cultural backgrounds of the supervisor or supervisee, there may be expectations (implicit or explicit) about the supervisor's role as expert and the formal evaluative nature of the relationship.

There are rules of supervision that determine the roles of participants (Neufeldt, 1997), for example, supervisees and supervisors. The cultural norms of professional groups transmitted historically through education and supervision are powerful influences on contemporary practices (Hall, 2005). It is often difficult for supervisors who have been socialised within a particular professional context to break away from those traditions in socialising new supervisees.

The classic model of supervision is that the supervisor holds a position of authority in which expertise is shared with a supervisee who serves in a type of apprenticeship to the profession. Research confirms that most supervision unfolds in a top-down fashion in which the supervisor maintains relational control (Neufeldt, 1997). These findings are important considerations in culture-infused counselling supervision, where the sharing of multicultural expertise is presumably a major goal. Participants in a supervisory relationship may lack alternate models from which to tailor their relationship.

The supervision relationship differs depending upon the individuals involved. However, supervision rarely occurs in isolation and is heavily influenced by the organisational context in which supervision occurs (Holloway, 1995). The standards for supervisory relationships may be predetermined by cultural norms that have operated historically within an organisational context. Supervisors are encouraged to challenge those organisational norms that restrict the effectiveness of multicultural counselling supervision.

Rather than assuming that one way is the best way for all supervisory relationships, in a culture-infused model we challenge supervisors to tailor their supervisory styles to meet the cultural and learning needs of their supervisees. In turn, we try to support students to examine the expectations that they hold about supervision and enter into discussion with their supervisors about their learning needs. When this happens, there is a greater chance of matching styles of supervision with the needs of counsellors/supervisees.

Although this appears easily done, it requires both parties to consider cultural influences on their expectations of supervision. For example, supervisors who adopt a nondirective approach may be matched with supervisees who have been culturally socialised to listen to persons in authority and who wait to receive specific direction (Garret et al., 2001). Supervisees may be reluctant to bring up issues that challenge the expertise of the supervisor due to cultural upbringing about relationships of authority or fears about the evaluative components of supervision.

Toporek and colleagues (2004) point to the importance of open dialogue about the cultural influences on the supervisory relationship: '… the relationship may be a pivotal component of multicultural supervision that moderates how all other experiences are perceived' (p. 80). Within the supervisory relationship, trust must also be established in order to facilitate the mutual negotiation of supervisory goals and tasks. How trust and expertise are shared within the context of a supervisory relationship is bound by cultural expectations. Depending upon the degree of fit between supervisor and counsellor/supervisee expectations, the nature of the professional relationship may enhance or restrict the sharing of expertise.

Supervision Scenarios

In describing our approach to culture-infused supervision, we have provided four examples of how expectations about supervision are bounded by cultural beliefs and practices (Arthur & Collins, 2005a). These are adapted below in scenarios to illustrate multiple views of counsellor/supervisees regarding their experiences of supervision.

Scenario 1

Janet is a graduate student who is increasingly frustrated at her practicum site as she is disappointed by the quality of supervision. She chose the setting due to the reputation of the supervisor for excellent clinical practice. Yet, she is discouraged as the supervisor rarely gives his opinion and always asks her what she thinks. Janet is also very interested in discussing multicultural counselling. As the supervisor never brings up the topic, she does not believe it is an area of interest for the supervisor.

This scenario expands our consideration of mismatches when cultural influences and expectations in supervision are not discussed openly. The sense of frustration felt by the supervisee in this vignette may have been avoided through active negotiation of roles and expectations early in the supervisory relationship (Arthur & Collins, 2005a). In fact, to do so at the interview and selection stage may prevent mismatches in supervision preferences from occurring. Some supervisors or supervisees may self-select out of working together. However, such negotiation is more likely to open the door to working more effectively together.

Scenario 2

Michelle is very impressed with the clinical work of her supervisor but dreads their supervision sessions. Like many new supervisees, Michelle is reluctant to bring up any concerns or show areas of weakness for fear of being judged as incompetent. Yet, when Michelle asks for help, the supervisor gives her ideas that she always finds to be useful. When pressed to discuss what is 'missing' in the supervisory relationship, Michelle notes that she would like to have more informal discussion and have the supervisor show more interest in her as a person, rather than immediately launching into case consultation. The supervisee wonders if her experience might be different working with a female supervisor.

In this second vignette, a different kind of mismatch in supervisory relationship expectations is highlighted. Two of the key dimensions in counsellor supervision can be characterised as content needs (focus on case conceptualisation and intervention planning) and relational needs (developing a trusting working relationship between the supervisor and the supervisee). If we think about these dimensions on a continuum, Michelle's supervision needs at this time might be characterised as higher on relational needs; whereas the supervisor appears to be basing supervision strongly on content to improve counselling competencies. In reality, these two dimensions are not mutually exclusive. For supervisees whose world-view emphasises relationships as a primary component of learning, an immediate focus on the *business* of supervision will be unsettling. Supervisors may need to consider how to create a basis of comfort prior to structuring supervision time around case conceptualisation (Arthur & Collins, 2005a). It is also possible that gender issues may emerge as salient in negotiating the nature of the supervisory relationship. Gender dynamics are influential for counsellor/supervisee satisfaction with the supervisory relationship (Gatmon et al., 2001).

Scenario 3

Quan believes that there has been a high level of conflict with his supervisor, to the point that he fears a negative evaluation. Quan is concerned with the amount of supervision time taken on nonessential matters and a lot of time seems to be wasted when he really needs help with strategies for working with clients. Quan feels a lot of pressure to disclose about himself and this is not something he feels comfortable doing. He attempted to discuss his cultural values with his supervisor, but this only seemed to make a temporary difference in how supervision was approached. Quan is concerned that unless he shows more evidence of personal reflection, he will be penalised. This has resulted in a lot of anxiety about supervision and what he might need to do to meet the supervisor's expectations, despite his personal convictions.

The third scenario describes the experiences of a supervisee who felt that his cultural boundaries around privacy were violated through supervision. There is general agreement in the multicultural counselling literature on the importance of self-awareness and counsellors are encouraged to be continually reflective about the influence of their personal culture (Torres-Rivera, Phan, Maddux, Wilbur, & Garrett, 2001; Collins & Arthur, 2005b). Supervision approaches based on models of personal development also emphasise personal reflection and awareness as foundational to the development of higher level counselling skills. This can be a particularly sensitive area in multicultural supervision, as supervisees are encouraged to engage in personal reflection and disclosure with their supervisor about areas of potential vulnerability.

Underlying the process of gaining self-awareness are cultural norms about sharing personal information in public contexts. Depending upon the cultural backgrounds of either the counsellor/supervisee or the supervisor, there can be mismatches in expectations about the degree of disclosure expected and how that disclosure is managed. Without attention to expectations and the personal cultural identities of both the supervisor and the counsellor/supervisee, there is a risk that conflicting expectations will be detrimental to the supervisory relationship. In this scenario, the female supervisor who was trained in western perspectives was inadvertently challenging the gender role beliefs of a male who was socialised in a collectivist eastern culture. Rather than insisting on a high level of verbal disclosure, the supervisor may have expanded her methods for ascertaining this supervisee's level of reflective practice. This example underscores how conducting discussions about cultural variables in the supervisory relationship may be a necessary intervention (Gatmon et al., 2001).

Scenario 4

Nick was an experienced counsellor and he was very keen to enhance his multicultural counselling competencies through his graduate practicum. The instructor who coordinated his practicum placement encouraged him to discuss his interests with his site supervisor to see if it would be possible to place a greater emphasis on cultural influences on his work with clients. The supervisor was really interested in this idea, and they negotiated agreement that either of them could raise issues about culture in their supervision sessions. This openness motivated Nick to pay more close attention to the ways that he was approaching multicultural counselling and how his personal socialisation was potentially influential in the way that he worked with clients.

Discussions with his supervisor included aspects of Nick's cultural identity that were considerably different to the cultural identity of his supervisor. Through more open sharing of their world-views, their supervisory relationship was also strengthened.

The fourth scenario depicts a counsellor/supervisee who has high levels of multicultural competencies and who was proactive about pursuing his learning needs related to culture-infused supervision. A major contributing factor to Nick's positive experience of supervision was the openness of the supervisor to explore Nick's expressed learning needs. In this vignette, the receptivity of the supervisor to engage in a discussion of cultural identities provided an indication of support and acceptance.

These scenarios illustrate how culture-infused supervision is enhanced when supervisors are both open to and sufficiently skilled to address the learning needs of counsellors/supervisees. Ideally, supervisors respond to each counsellor/supervisee and each counsellor/client relationship in a unique way (Holloway, 1995; Neufeldt, 1997). In turn, when supervisors are responsive to discussions about cultural influences with their supervisees, they model appropriate behaviour for counsellors to initiate and follow with their clients (Hird et al., 2001).

Addressing Cultural Influences in Supervision

The previous discussion and supervision scenarios illustrate some of the ways that cultural factors influence expectations and behaviours in the supervisory relationship. Three positions were apparent in the scenarios: (a) supervisors avoid addressing cultural issues with supervisees, either intentionally or unintentionally; (b) supervisors wait for supervisees to bring up cultural issues and address them if they come up in the process of supervision; or (c) supervisors attempt to infuse cultural issues in supervision discussions from the beginning (Garrett et al., 2001).

When supervisors do not address culture in their supervisory practices, there are, at minimum, missed opportunities for deeper case conceptualisation and for enhancing the supervisory relationship and, at worst, examples of potential cultural oppression of either supervisees or clients. There have been strong positions taken that consideration of cultural influences for counselling goals and processes are essential for ethical practice (Sue & Sue, 1999; Pedersen, 1991). Developing cultural competence is now an integral part of standards of practice and codes of ethics in the field of counselling with clients (Pettifor, 2005). We are suggesting a similar mandate for culture-infused counselling supervision. Barnett (2007) identified attention to issues of diversity as a core requirement for effective and ethical supervision. We would argue that standards of practice for the supervision of multicultural counselling need to be addressed to enhance ethical practices.

Without discussion of the diversity/similarity within the supervisory dyad, unexamined cultural issues can adversely interfere with the development of a solid working alliance between supervisor and supervisee. The costs of not discussing cultural influences in supervision are most likely to be felt by supervisees and clients, as they typically hold the least amount of sociopolitical and contextual power (Hird et al., 2001). In most cases, supervisors are White and experience privilege in other areas of cultural identity (Brinson, 2004; Neville, Worthington, & Spanierman, 2001). This may make it more difficult for them to self-assess power differentials and appreciate the experiences of supervisees or clients from nondominant groups.

A layer of cultural complexity is added in dyads where the supervisor is from a nondominant group, including a nondominant racial group. The 'hierarchical difference' (McGoldrick et al., 1999, p. 203) is a sensitive issue that relates to matters of privilege and supervisor credibility. For supervision to be maximally effective, both supervisors and counsellors/supervisees need to be willing to explore the potential influences of their cultural background for the supervisory relationship. Discussion of cultural variables such as race, ethnicity, gender, sexual orientation, age, religion and socioeconomic status have been implicated for the strength of the supervisory working alliance and the supervisee's satisfaction with supervision (Brown & Landrum-Brown, 1995; Constantine, 1997, 2003; Gatmon et al., 2001).

In reviewing the literature on crosscultural supervision, an important recommendation is offered: the onus is on the supervisor to initiate discussions about culture in supervision (Estrada et al., 2004). Initiating discussions about personal culture can model to supervisees the importance of addressing difficult topics related to culture (Constantine, 2003). It opens the door for reflection about the influence of personal culture in supervisory relationships and in relationships with clients. The willingness of supervisors to initiate, take risks and show vulnerabilities to supervisees may support counsellors/supervisees to do the same through reflective practice. Supervision should provide a supportive foundation from which supervisees improve their multicultural counselling competencies. Research suggests a positive relationship between greater amounts of multicultural supervision and a supervisee's perceptions that they hold higher levels of multicultural counselling competence (Constantine, 2003).

The call for infusing culture into supervision and training requires an intentional approach to working with counsellors/supervisees. Divac and Heaphy (2005) emphasise experiential learning of supervisees in their model through regularly scheduled meeting for the purpose of facilitating cultural competence. The reflections offered in an article by Garrett and colleagues (2001) provide an excellent example of ways for supervisors to strengthen the supervisory relationship and, ultimately, the delivery of multicultural counselling. In keeping with our model of culture-infused counselling, however, the starting point is reflective learning about cultural biases and assumptions on the part of the supervisor (Brinson, 2004). The sharing of personal reflections by supervisors with supervisees may facilitate the imparting of multicultural counselling competencies. It has been suggested that self-disclosure about struggles with multicultural counselling may be comforting to supervisees and help them to address their own issues as they attempt to integrate multicultural perspectives into counselling (Hird et al., 2001). Through discussing their personal struggles and challenges, supervisors model the ongoing process of reflective practice and multicultural development (Chen, 2001; Helms & Cook, 1999). In this way, supervisors reveal themselves as lifelong learners interested in improving their understanding about the influences of culture in professional practice.

Tools for Reflective Practice

Although there is a growing body of literature attesting to the importance of multicultural counselling competencies, we have noted that there are few practical tools or concrete guidelines available in the literature that help counsellors translate concepts about multicultural counselling and supervision into practice (Estrada et al., 2004). Tools to facilitate exchanges about cultural influences in the supervision process are only beginning to appear. For example, Guanipa (2002) has developed a questionnaire for evaluating multicultural issues in marriage and family therapy supervision that is informative for multicultural counselling supervision. Supervisors and supervisees are invited to begin by reflecting about the way that culture is defined in supervision. Next, a series of questions have been designed for both supervisors and supervisees to support reflection on how culture is infused in supervision practices. In reviewing the items, supervisors and supervisees are invited to reflect upon cultural influences in their supervisory relationship and in the context of working directly with clients. Estrada and colleagues (2004) propose that both supervisor and supervisee create cultural genograms and complete racial identity inventories as a foundation for discussing their own cultural influences and the impact these may have on the supervision and counselling processes.

Cultural Auditing of Counselling Supervision

In addition to cultural auditing tools designed to enhance multicultural counselling competencies in direct client work and through organisational development (Arthur & Collins, 2005a; Collins & Arthur, 2005b), we have developed a cultural auditing tool for culture-infused counselling supervision (see Appendix B). This tool contains the steps and supervisory relationship considerations in conducting a cultural audit of supervision practices. We designed the cultural auditing process to provide practical points of reflection and discussion to be used in supervisor and supervisee relationships. The cultural auditing tool for supervision has been positively received by the counsellors/supervisees who we work with directly and by colleagues in Canada who are counsellor educators.

The *Conducting a Cultural Audit of Supervision Practices* (CCASP) tool is organised around 16 steps, or points of consideration for reflective practice. The steps are not intended to be followed in a linear order; rather they specify domains that are relevant at different stages and times of working together in multicultural counselling supervision. Not all steps may be relevant for every supervisory relationship; some may be more salient, and it may be beneficial to revisit certain stages as supervision unfolds. We have organised key content for reflection around six domains, which include: (a) relationship between supervisor and counsellor, (b) relationship between counsellor and client, (c) counselling and supervision conventions, (d) multicultural case conceptualisation, (e) goal-setting and intervention and (f) multicultural competency development. In each of the domains, content areas for reflection and discussion are suggested. We encourage supervisors to incorporate a cultural auditing process into their ongoing supervisory practices

Summary and Conclusions

Counselling students, graduates, more experienced counsellors, and those who hold supervisory roles need to consider how culture is infused into their professional roles and relationships. Culture impacts the reciprocal relationships between counsellors/supervisees, supervisors and clients. Supervision practices can support cultural learning during counsellor education programs or through ongoing professional practice in the workplace. We agree with other authors who take the position that cultural influences need to be examined within every aspect of the supervision process (Bernard & Goodyear, 1998; Torres-Rivera, Phan, Maddux, Wilbur, & Garrett, 2001). To that end, we have suggested the following strategies for strengthening culture-infused supervision practices (Arthur & Collins, 2005a):

1. Supervisors can become familiar with the applications of theoretical perspectives on supervision in crosscultural contexts. For a review of supervision theories and approaches and their crosscultural relevance, see Brown and Landrum-Brown (1995). In addition, a number of

models specifically address multicultural counselling supervision (e.g., Ancis & Ladany, 2001; Chen, 2001; Constantine, 1997; D'Andrea & Daniels, 1997; Garrett et al., 2001; Martinez & Holloway, 1997; Porter, 1994; Robinson, Bradley, & Hendricks, 2000; Stone, 1997).

2. Models and competency frameworks can be used by supervisors to help them gain insight into their level of multicultural supervision competencies (e.g., Allen, 2007; Ancis & Ladany, 2001; Constantine, 1997; D'Andrea & Daniels, 1997; Guanipa, 2002). These are helpful tools for supervisors to use in identifying their strengths and areas for continued professional development. In this chapter, we have additionally presented the CCASP tool as a new contribution to help supervisors and counsellors/supervisees translate ideas about culture into meaningful practices.

3. We have noted that there is a wide range of levels of exposure to multicultural competency training in counsellor education, and even less opportunity to gain competencies in multicultural counselling supervision (Arthur & Collins, 2005a). Workshop planning and attendance at presentations designed to address multicultural counselling and supervision are important directions for continuing education. Supervisors can lobby with conference planning committees to include content about multicultural counselling supervision (D'Andrea & Daniels, 1997).

4. Building a network of community resources is an important way to inform crosscultural understanding (Arthur & Collins, 2005a). Involvement in local communities helps strengthen supervisors' knowledge about cultural diversity. Bridging community resources also leads to important opportunities for counselling consultation to ensure culturally appropriate services (D'Andrea & Daniels, 1997).

5. Supervisors need to examine their professional strengths and limitations with counsellors/supervisees. It is reasonable to declare a scope of expertise, as supervisors cannot be expected to be experts in all areas of counselling practice. In reference to culture-infused counselling, supervisors should clarify their level of competence (Arthur & Collins, 2005a). For example, they may have a great deal of practical experience but lack the theoretical knowledge that is now available in counsellor education curriculum. In contrast, supervisors may be well informed about multicultural counselling competencies but lack the practical experiences that supervisees may have gained. This kind of discussion models ethical practice in establishing boundaries of expertise for culture-infused counselling (Chen, 2001).

6. We reiterate that responsibility for initiating discussions of cultural variables rests with the supervisor, 'to open the cultural door and walk

through it with the supervisee' (Bernard & Goodyear, 1998, p. 45). Discussions about cultural influences can ultimately strengthen the supervisory working alliance, enhance satisfaction with the quality of the supervisory relationship, facilitate a supportive learning environment and support the acquisition of culture-infused counselling competencies by both supervisor and supervisee (Constantine, 1997; Gatmon et al., 2001; Leach & Carlton, 1997; Ridley, Espelage, & Rubinstein, 1997).

In summary, the multicultural counselling field would benefit from expanding the focus of cultural influences on the counsellor–client dyad to also consider cultural influences on the supervisory relationship. Collaboration to enhance culture-infused counselling competencies through supervision can lead to rewarding ways of teaching and learning about culture together.

Educational Questions and Activities

1. Individual and Small Group Reflection Exercise

    The following reflection questions are intended to promote discussion about culture-infused supervision. Reflect about the way that you currently supervise students, or, if you are a student, the way that you are supervised during your practicum or field placement.

    • How are cultural influences about client issues introduced into supervision?

    • How are supervisor and supervisee cultures taken into account in the supervision process?

    • What cultural influences in the relationship between supervisors and supervisees have you experienced?

    • What are the cultural influences that you would like to discuss with your supervisor/supervisee?

    • What barriers do you experience in discussing culture with your supervisor/supervisee?

    • What helps you to discuss cultural influences with your supervisor/supervisee?

2. Some people argue that the multicultural counselling movement is directed towards racial and ethic minority clients. Others suggest that the focus of multicultural counselling be placed on a broader range of clients from nondominant groups who have experienced social oppression. Advocates of a generic position argue that every encounter with a client involves counselling across cultures. What are the relative strengths and limitations to each position? Which position do you support?

The field of multicultural counselling has grown from a focus on racial and ethic minorities to considering cultural influences on an expanded range of nondominant populations, such as religion, socioeconomic status, age, sexual orientation, gender and ability. However, it is not group membership alone that determines cultural influences; rather, it is the ways in which individuals internalise their identity, often based on multiple and intersecting notions of culture. Advocates of a universalistic approach argue that no two individuals are the same and that counselling always involves counselling across cultures. It is important to recognise that some groups continue to experience oppression in ways that require social advocacy on behalf of counsellors. It may be particularly important for counsellors to attend to the effect of culture on the experiences of clients from these groups.

3. Name three advantages of taking a culture-infused approach to supervision.
   - A culture-infused approach to supervision recognises the responsibility of supervisors and supervisees to acknowledge cultural influences on the ways in which counselling issues and interventions are determined.
   - The supervisory relationship provides a unique opportunity to integrate role modelling and discussion of cultural influences between supervisors and supervisees.
   - Through increasing competence and confidence about addressing cultural influences in supervision, supervisees develop competencies for service provision to all clients.

4. What are the potential barriers to infusing culture in counselling supervision?
   - Supervisors may lack knowledge about multicultural counselling and limit such discussions to specific clients, for example, racial minorities.
   - Supervisees may be interested in discussing cultural influences but may feel bound by cues from their supervisors about their level of interest and the perceived acceptability of doing so.
   - Perceived power differences between supervisees and supervisors may lead supervisees to remain silent about cultural differences that they believe impact the supervisory relationship.

5. Discuss three ways that supervisors foster a positive approach to infusing culture during multicultural counselling supervision.
   - Supervisors take the initiative to discuss their own sense of cultural identity and ways that they believe their identity impacts their pro-

fessional supervisory relationships, and they encourage supervisees to do the same.

- Supervisors take the initiative to discuss their own sense of cultural identity and ways that they believe their identity impacts their work with clients, and they encourage supervisees to do the same.
- Supervisors incorporate discussions about cultural influences on client issues and interventions as a regular agenda item for supervision sessions.

6. How does culture-infused counselling supervision potentially enhance the working alliance between counsellors and clients?

As noted in #3 above, positive role modelling in the supervisory relationship provides a forum for supervisees to explore their cultural identity and to develop multicultural counselling competencies to increase their awareness, knowledge and skills for practice. When discussions about culture are held in an open manner and considered 'everyday' practice, counsellors are more likely to incorporate reflective practice about culture into their work with clients. The supervisory relationship potentially offers a supportive forum for supervisees to learn about themselves, their clients, and ways to enhance the working alliance in multicultural counselling.

Selected Internet Resources

- American Psychological Association. (2002). *Guidelines on multicultural education, training, research, practice, and organizational change for psychologists.* Available at http://www.apa.org/pi/multiculturalguidelines.pdf

  These guidelines provide a framework and specific standards of practice for delivering services to racial and ethnic minorities, as well as guidelines for training, research, and organizational change.

- Home page of the Association of Counselor Education and Supervision, a division of the American Counseling Association. Available at http://www.acesonline.net/index.asp

  The Association for Counselor Education and Supervision (ACES) emphasises the need for quality education and supervision of counsellors in all work settings. The site contains news and information links to conferences and ongoing projects related to counsellor education and supervision.

- *Counselor Education and Supervision* is the official journal of the Association for Counselor Education and Supervision. The journal is dedicated to publishing manuscripts concerned with research, theory development, or program applications related to counsellor education and supervision. Available from http://chdsw.educ.kent.edu/ces/

- *The Clinical Supervisor* is a journal devoted exclusively to articles on the art and science of clinical supervision. An interdisciplinary, refereed publication, the journal facilitates the communication of ideas, experiences, skills, techniques, concerns and needs of supervisors in psychotherapy and mental health. Available from http://www.haworthpress.com/store/product.asp?sku=J001

Selected References for Further Reading

Arthur, N., & Collins, S. (2005). *Culture-infused counselling: Celebrating the Canadian mosaic.* Calgary, Canada: Counselling Concepts.

Bernard, J.M., & Goodyear, R.K. (2008). Fundamentals of clinical supervision (4th ed.). Needham Heights, MA: Allyn & Bacon.

Ponterotto, J.M. Casas, J.C., Suzuki,, C.A., & Alexander, C.M. (Eds., (2001). *Handbook of multicultural counselling* (2nd ed). Thousand Oaks, CA: Sage.

Pope-Davis, D.B., Coleman, H.L.K., Liu, W.M., & Torporek, R. (Eds.). (2003). *Handbook of multicultural competencies in counseling and psychology.* Thousand Oaks, CA: Sage.

References

Allen, J. (2007). A multicultural assessment supervision model to guide research and practice. *Professional Psychology: Research and Practice, 38,* 248–258.

American Psychological Association. (2002). *Guidelines on multicultural education, training, research, practice, and organizational change for psychologists.* Retrieved September 15, 2003, from http://www.apa.org/pi/multicultural guidelines.pdf

Ancis, J.R., & Ladany, N. (2001). A multicultural framework for counsellor supervision. In L.J. Bradley & N. Ladany (Eds.), *Counselor supervision: Principles, process, and practice* (3rd ed., pp. 63–92). Philadelphia, PA: Taylor & Francis.

Arredondo, P., & Perez, P. (2006). Historical perspectives on the multicultural guidelines and contemporary applications. *Professional Psychology: Research and Practice, 37*(1), 1–5.

Arredondo, P., Toporek, R., Brown, S.P., Jones, J., Locke, D., Sanchez, J., et al. (1996). Operationalization of the multicultural counseling competencies. *Journal of Multicultural Counselling & Development, 24,* 42–78.

Arthur, N. (1998). Counsellor education for diversity: Where do we go from here? *Canadian Journal of Counselling, 32,* 88–103.

Arthur, N., & Collins, S. (2005a). Expanding culture-infused counselling in professional practice. In N. Arthur & S. Collins, *Culture-infused counselling: Celebrating the Canadian mosaic* (pp. 151–212). Calgary, Canada: Counselling Concepts.

Arthur, N., & Collins, S. (2005b). Introduction to culture-infused counselling. In N. Arthur & S. Collins, *Culture-infused counselling: Celebrating the Canadian mosaic* (pp. 3–40). Calgary, Canada: Counselling Concepts.

Arthur, N., & Januszkowski, T. (2001). Multicultural competencies of Canadian counsellors. *Canadian Journal of Counselling, 35*(1), 36–48.

Barnett, J.E. (2007). In search of the effective supervisor. *Professional Psychology: Research and Practice, 38*(3), 268–272.

Bernard, J.M. (1992). Training master's level counselling students in the fundamentals of clinical supervision. *The Clinical Supervisor, 10,* 133–143.

Bernard, J.M., & Goodyear, R.K. (1998). Fundamentals of clinical supervision (2nd ed.). Needham Heights, MA: Allyn & Bacon.

Berkel, L.A., Constantine, M., & Olsen. E.A. (2007). Supervisor multicultural competence: Addressing religious and spiritual issues with counselling students in supervision. *The Clinical Supervisor, 26, 3–15.*

Brinson, J. (2004). Recognizing our cultural biases as counsellor supervisors: A reflective learning approach. *Guidance & Counseling, 19*(2), 81–91.

Brown, M.T., & Landrum-Brown, J. (1995). Counselor supervision: Cross-cultural perspectives. In J.G. Ponterotto, J.M. Casas, L.A. Suzuki, & C.M. Alexander (Eds.), *Handbook of multicultural counselling* (pp. 263–286). Thousand Oaks, CA: Sage.

Cary, D., & Marques, P. (2007). From expert to collaborator: Developing cultural competency in clinical supervision. *The Clinical Supervisor, 26,* 141–157.

Chen, E.C. (2001). Multicultural counselling supervision: An interactional approach. In J.G. Ponterotto, J.M. Casas, L.A. Suzuki, & C.M. Alexander (Eds.), *Handbook of multicultural counselling* (2nd ed., pp. 801–824). Thousand Oaks, CA: Sage.

Coleman, H.L.K. (2004). Multicultural counseling competencies in a pluralistic society. *Journal of Mental Health Counseling, 26*(1), 56–66.

Collins, S., & Arthur, N. (Eds.). (2005a). Enhancing the therapeutic alliance in culture-infused counselling. In *Culture-infused counselling: Celebrating the Canadian mosaic* (pp. 103–149). Calgary, Canada: Counselling Concepts.

Collins, S., & Arthur, N. (Eds.). (2005b). Multicultural counselling competencies: A framework for professional development. In *Culture-infused counselling: Celebrating the Canadian mosaic* (pp. 41–102). Calgary, Canada: Counselling Concepts.

Collins, S., & Arthur, N. (in press a). Culture-infused counselling: A fresh look at a classic framework of multicultural counselling competencies. *Counseling Psychology Quarterly.*

Collins, S., & Arthur, N. (in press b). Culture-infused counseling: A model for developing cultural competence. *Counseling Psychology Quarterly.*

Constantine, M. (1997). Facilitating multicultural competency in counselling supervision: Operationalizing a practical framework. In D.B. Pope-Davis & H.L.K. Coleman (Eds.), *Multicultural counselling competencies: Assessment, education and training, and supervision* (pp. 310–324). Thousand Oaks, CA: Sage.

Constantine, M. (2003). Multicultural competence in supervision. In D.B. Pope-Davis, H.L.K. Coleman, W.M. Liu, & R. Torporek (Eds.), *Handbook of multicultural competencies in counseling and psychology* (pp. 383–391). Thousand Oaks, CA: Sage.

Constantine, M., Warren, A.K., & Milville, M.L. (2005). White racial identity interactions in supervision: Implications for supervisee's multicultural counseling competence. *Journal of Counseling Psychology, 52,* 490–496.

D'Andrea, M., & Daniels, J. (1997). Multicultural counselling supervision: Central issues, theoretical considerations, and practical strategies. In D.B. Pope-Davis & H.L.K. Coleman (Eds.), *Multicultural counselling competencies: Assessment, education and training, and supervision* (pp. 290–309). Thousand Oaks, CA: Sage.

Divac, A., & Heaphy, G. (2005). Space for GRRAACCESS: Training for cultural competence in supervision. *Journal of Family Therapy, 27,* 280–284.

Estrada, D., Frame, M.W., & Williams, C.B. (2004). Cross-cultural supervision: Guiding the conversation toward race and ethnicity. *Multicultural Counseling and Development, 32,* 307–319.

Falender, C.A., & Shafranske, E.P. (2007). Competence in competency-based supervision practice: Construct and application. *Professional Psychology: Research and Practice, 38*(3), 232–240.

Fong, M.L., & Lease, S.H. (1997). Cross-cultural supervision: Issues for the White supervisor. In D.B. Pope-Davis & H.L.K. Coleman (Eds.), *Multicultural counselling competencies: Assessment, education and training, and supervision* (pp. 387–405). Thousand Oaks, CA: Sage.

Fukuyama, M.A. (1994). Critical incidents in multicultural counselling supervision: A phenomenological approach to supervision research. *Counselor Education & Supervision, 34*(2), 142–151.

Garrett, M.T., Borders, L.D., Crutichfield, L.B., Torres-Rivera, E., Brothertton, D., & Curtis, R. (2001). Multicultural superVISION: A paradigm of cultural responsiveness for supervisors. *Journal of Multicultural Counseling and Development, 29,* 147–148.

Gatmon, D. Jackson, D., Koshkarian, L., Martos-Perry, N., Molina, A., Patel, N., et al. (2001). Exploring ethnic, gender, and sexual orientation variables in supervision: Do they really matter? *Journal of Multicultural Counseling and Development, 29,* 102–113.

Gonzalez, R.C. (1997). Postmodern supervision: A multicultural perspective. In D.B. Pope-Davis & H.L.K. Coleman (Eds.), *Multicultural counselling competencies: Assessment, education and training, and supervision* (pp. 350–386). Thousand Oaks, CA: Sage.

Guanipa, C. (2002). A preliminary instrument to evaluate multicultural issues in marriage and family therapy supervision. *The Clinical Supervisor, 21*(2), 59–75.

Hall, P. (2005). Interprofessional teamwork: Professional cultures as barriers. *Journal of Interprofessional Care, 19*(Suppl.), 188–196.

Helms, J.E., & Cook, D.A. (1999). Using race and culture in therapy and supervision. In J.E. Helms & D.A. Cook (Eds.), *Using race and culture in counselling and psychotherapy: Theory and process* (pp. 277–298). Boston, MA: Allyn & Bacon.

Hird, J.S., Tao, K.W., & Gloria, A.M. (2005). Examining supervisor's multicultural competence in racially similar and different supervision dyads. *The Clinical Supervisor, 23,* 107–122.

Hird, J.S., Cavalieri, C.E., Dulko, J.P., Felice, A.A, & Ho, T.A. (2001). Visions and realities: Supervisee perspectives of multicultural supervision. *Journal of Multicultural Counseling and Development, 29,* 114–130.

Holloway, E.L. (1995). *Clinical supervision: A systems approach.* Thousand Oaks, CA: Sage.

Inman, A.G. (2006). Supervisor multicultural competence and its relation to supervisory process and outcome. *Journal of Marital and Family Therapy, 32,* 73–85.

Leach, M.M., & Carlton, M.A. (1997). Toward devising a multicultural training philosophy. In D.B. Pope-Davis & H.L.K. Coleman (Eds.), *Multicultural counselling competencies: Assessment, education and training, and supervision* (pp. 184–208). Thousand Oaks, CA: Sage.

Lowe, S.M., & Mascher, J. (2001). The role of sexual orientation in multicultural counseling: Integrating bodies of knowledge. In J.G. Ponterotto, J.M. Casis, L.A. Suzuki, & C.M. Alexander (Eds.), *Handbook of Multicultural Counseling* (2nd ed., pp. 755–778). Thousand Oaks, CA: Sage.

Martinez, R.P., & Holloway, E.L. (1997). The supervision relationship in multicultural training. In D.B. Pope-Davis & H.L.K. Coleman (Eds.), *Multicultural counselling competencies: Assessment, education and training, and supervision* (pp. 325–349). Thousand Oaks, CA: Sage.

MacDougall, C., & Arthur, N. (2001). Applying models of racial identity in counselling. *Canadian Journal of Counselling, 35,* 122–136.

McGoldrick, M., Almeida, R., Preto, N.G., Bibb, A., Sutton, C., Hudak, J. et al. (1999). Efforts to incorporate social justice perspectives into a family training program. *Journal of Marital and Family Therapy, 25*(2), 191–209.

Meissner, W.W. (2006). The therapeutic alliance: A proteus in disguise. *Psychotherapy: Theory, Research, Practice, Training, 43*(3), 264–270.

Messinger, L. (2007). Supervision of lesbian, gay and bi-sexual social work students by heterosexual field instructors: A qualitative dyad analysis. *The Clinical Supervisor, 26,* 195–222.

Neufeldt, S.A. (1997). A social constructivist approach to counselling supervision. In T.L. Sexton & B.L. Griffin (Eds.), *Constructivist thinking in counseling practice, research, and training* (pp. 191–210). New York: Teachers College Press.

Neville, H.A., Worthington, R. L., & Spanierman, L.B. (2001). Race, power, and multicultural counseling psychology: Understanding White privilege and color-blind racial attitudes. In J.G. Ponterotto, J. Manual Casas, L.A. Suzuki & C.M. Alexander (Eds.), *Handbook of multicultural counseling* (2nd ed., pp. 257–288). Thousand Oaks, CA: Sage.

Nilsson, J.E. (2007). International students in supervision: Course self-efficacy, stress, and cultural discussions in supervision. *The Clinical Supervisor, 26,* 35–46.

Norton, R.A., & Coleman, H.L.K. (2003). Multicultural supervision: The influence of race-related issues in supervision process and outcome. In D.B. Pope-Davis, H.L.K. Coleman, W.M. Liu & R. Torporek (Eds.), *Handbook of multicultural competencies in counseling and psychology* (pp.114–134). Thousand Oaks, CA: Sage.

Parham, T.A., & Whitten, L. (2003). Teaching multicultural competencies in continuing education for psychologists. In D.B. Pope-Davis, H.L.K. Coleman, W.M. Liu & R. Torporek (Eds.), *Handbook of multicultural competencies in counseling and psychology* (pp. 562–574). Thousand Oaks, CA: Sage.

Pedersen, P. (1991). Multiculturalism as a generic approach to counseling. *Canadian Journal of Counselling, 70,* 6–12.

Pettifor, J. (2005). Ethics and multicultural counselling. In N. Arthur & S. Collins (Eds.), *Culture-infused counselling: Celebrating the Canadian mosaic* (pp. 213–238). Calgary, Canada: Counselling Concepts.

Pope-Davis, D.B., Toporek, R.L., & Ortega-Villalobos, L. (2003). Assessing supervisors' and supervisees' perceptions of multicultural competence in supervision using the Multicultural Supervision Inventory. In D.B. Pope-Davis, H.L.K. Coleman, W.M. Liu, & R. Torporek (Eds.), *Handbook of multicultural competencies in counseling and psychology* (pp. 211–224). Thousand Oaks, CA: Sage.

Porter, N. (1994). Empowering supervisees to empower others: A culturally responsive supervision model. *Hispanic Journal of Behavioral Sciences, 16,* 43–56.

Priest, R. (1994). Minority supervisor and majority supervisee: Another perspective of clinical reality. *Counselor Education and Supervision, 34,* 152–158.

Ridley, C.R., Espelage, D.L., & Rubinstein, K.J. (1997). Course development in multicultural counselling. In H.L.K. Coleman (Ed.), *Multicultural counselling competencies: Assessment, education and training, and supervision* (pp. 131–158). Thousand Oaks, CA: Sage.

Robinson, B., Bradley, L.J., & Hendricks, C.B. (2000). Multicultural counselling supervision: A four-step model toward competency. *International Journal for the Advancement of Counselling, 22,* 131–141.

Roysircar, G., Hubbell, R., & Gard, G. (2003). Multicultural research on counselor and client variables. In D.B. Pope-Davis, H.L.K. Coleman, W.M. Lui & R.L. Toporek (Eds.), Handbook of multicultural counseling and psychology (pp. 247–266). Thousand Oaks, CA: Sage.

Silverstein, L.B. (2006). Integrating feminism and multiculturalism: Scientific fact or science fiction. *Professional Psychology: Research and Practice, 37*(1), 21–28.

Steward, R.J., Morales, P.C., Bartell, P.A., Miller, M., & Weeks, D. (1998). The multiculturally responsive versus the multiculturally reactive: A study of perceptions of counsellor trainees. *Journal of Multicultural Counseling & Development,* 26(1), 13–28.

Stone, G.L. (1997). Multiculturalism as a context for supervision: Perspectives, limitations, and implications. In D.B. Pope-Davis & H.L.K. Coleman (Eds.), *Multicultural counselling competencies: Assessment, education and training, and supervision* (pp. 263–289). Thousand Oaks, CA: Sage.

Sue, D.W., Arredondo, P., & McDavis, R.J. (1992). Multicultural counseling competencies and standards: A call to the profession. *Journal of Counseling and Development, 70,* 477–483.

Sue, D.W., & Sue, D. (1999). *Counseling the culturally different: Theory and practice* (3rd ed.). New York: Wiley.

Taylor, B., Hernandez, P., Deri, A., Rankin, P., & Siegel, A. (2006). Integrating diversity dimensions in supervision: Perspectives of ethnic minority AAMFT supervisors. *The Clinical Supervisor, 25,* 3–21.

Toporek, R.L., Ortega-Villalobos, L., & Pope-Davis, D.B. (2004). Critical incidents in multicultural supervision: Exploring supervisees' and supervisors' experiences. *Journal of Multicultural Counseling and Development, 32,* 66–83.

Torres-Rivera, E., Phan, L.T., Maddux, C., Wilbur, M.P., & Garrett, M.T. (2001). Process versus content: Integrating personal awareness and counselling skills to meet the multicultural challenge of the twenty-first century. *Counselor Education & Supervision, 41*, 28–40.

Weinrach, S.G., & Thomas, K.R. (2002). A critical analysis of the multicultural counseling competencies: implications for the practice of mental health counseling. *Journal of Mental Health Counseling, 24*(1), 20–35.

chapter eighteen

Supervision of Applied Specialties: Unique Aspects

Gary H. Bischof, Mary L. Anderson, C. Dennis Simpson,
Eric M. Sauer and Stephen E. Craig

This chapter focuses on unique aspects of supervision in five specialisation areas. These areas include marriage and family therapy, school counselling, alcohol and drug abuse counselling, supervision in university-based training clinics and supervision in community agencies. The authors are faculty members of Western Michigan University in Kalamazoo, Michigan, United States of America (USA). Each author possesses expertise in a particular specialisation area and has written that section of the chapter as follows: Marriage and Family Therapy — Bischof; School Counselling — Anderson; Alcohol and Drug Counselling — Simpson; University Training Clinic — Sauer; Community Mental Health Counselling — Craig. Each section below highlights some of the key issues and unique features of providing supervision within that specialisation area.

Marriage and Family Therapy Supervision

This section addresses unique aspects of supervision in the area of marriage and family therapy (MFT). MFT is both an established mental health discipline and an area of specialisation within other mental health professions, such as social work, counselling or psychology. Supervision within the discipline of marriage and family therapy is the primary focus here. This section contains three subsections, one on the family systems background and core values of the field of MFT and how these have informed supervision practices, and a second on emphases in supervision that have flowed from this family systems base. A third subsection addresses unique supervision strategies that have evolved within MFT, such as live supervision, reflecting teams and the use of genograms. A brief discussion of current trends and future developments in MFT supervision concludes this section.

MFT Historical Development and Core Values

A primary and unifying factor in MFT is the conceptual and theoretical base of family systems theory. Family systems theory was embraced by the early pioneers in MFT and also by those who were assisting couple and families from an atheoretical perspective (e.g., early marriage counsellors) (Nichols & Schwartz, 2007). MFT adopted ideas espoused by general systems theory, which included the notion that the whole is greater than the sum of its parts, that an open system continuously interacts with its environment and that mechanisms exist in systems that both maintain homeostasis and seek creative change, or morphogenesis. Also influential in the development of family systems theory was cybernetics, the study of feedback mechanisms in self-regulating systems. Concepts such as circular causality and feedback loops, maintaining homeostasis, family rules and sequences of interaction were derived from cybernetics.

MFT, drawing from these roots, created a radical, new approach to the understanding and treatment of behavioural symptoms and human problems, shifting the focus from within, which had been the prevailing view at the time, to relationships and context and making sense of one's behaviours based upon the overall dynamics of the family system. Intervention shifted from a focus on the individual, the past and insight into the *why* of problems, to an active, directive approach that focused on the *what* and *how* and altering present interactions within the family system (Nichols & Schwartz, 2007).

Todd and Storm (1997), in their introductory chapter in a prominent text on systemic supervision, note that three values permeated the early development of MFT that have significantly influenced MFT supervision. The first involves the tradition of showing one's clinical work to others. Initially, marriage and family therapists (MFTs) showed their work to one another out of their enthusiasm and a desire to learn about the clinical innovations of MFT. Visual instruction and family observation fit well with family therapy's focus on relationships and interactions, and was a radical departure from the private, confidential supervision involved in psychoanalysis. Early supervisors frequently demonstrated MFT to their supervisees, worked with them as co-therapists and formed teams to assist trainees in becoming MFTs. This 'show and tell' value has informed the emphasis upon the use of raw data in MFT supervision. MFT supervisors routinely employ video and live supervision, and many believe that simple case consultation is inadequate as the primary mode of supervision.

Indeed, this value is reflected in the emphasis on the use of raw data in the American Association for Marriage and Family Therapy's Approved Supervisor Handbook (AAMFT, 2007).

A second value described by Todd and Storm (1997) was that early MFTs invited comment and feedback on their work. Supervisors asked supervisees to notice particular aspects of their therapy and were interested in receiving feedback. The use of one-way mirrors enhanced this capability, and this technology facilitated a way to see, from a bit more removed distance, the interactions among family members and between the therapist and family. Behind the mirror supervisors and supervisees would discuss their observations, often building synergistically upon one another's comments. This value further promoted the use of raw data and also encouraged MFT supervisors to supervise in dyads, groups and teams, which enhanced the opportunity for commenting on one another's work.

The third and final value flowed naturally from a family systems perspective. This value involved the supervisors' recognition of themselves as an integral part of the therapeutic system (Todd & Storm, 1997). The questioning of supervisor objectivity led supervisors to look at themselves and their contributions to the supervisory process as key players in the overall family–therapist–supervisor system. This value led to the appreciation of supervision as an endeavour in its own right and the later establishing of training guidelines and qualifications for supervisors. Interestingly, in the US, of all the mental health disciplines' professional organisations, only the AAMFT and the American Association of Pastoral Counseling designate supervisors, define supervisors' qualifications and require supervisor training. Recently, the AAMFT also added an every 5-year continuing education requirement for their designated Approved Supervisors (AAMFT, 2007).

Family Systems-Informed Emphases in MFT Supervision

Isomorphism. Another idea that flows from a family systems perspective as applied to supervision is isomorphism. Isomorphism can be defined as interactional patterns that replicate themselves and are transferred across various subsystems of the overall therapeutic system, that is, from treatment to supervision or from supervision to therapy (Liddle, 1988). For example, GB was involved in a supervision training group and it was observed that 'niceness' seemed to be isomorphically occurring in the therapist–client relationship, and also in the therapist–supervisor relationship, and both were feeling somewhat stuck. Both therapist and supervisor had been employing a supportive and encouraging style when more gentle challenge seemed to be called for. When this observation was shared with the supervisor, it freed him up to be more challenging to the therapist, who in turn became more appropriately challenging to the client. Thus, such systemic recognition of parallel processes across levels can serve to help alter and shape interactions in the therapeutic system.

Therapy/Supervision in stages and the family life cycle. Thinking in stages has been a useful organising scheme for family therapy. Haley (1976) purported early on that therapy progressed in stages, and that family dynamics often shift from the presenting issues and patterns to another dysfunctional pattern before settling into healthier, sustainable family processes. Seeing human dilemmas through the lens of family life cycle stages and transitions has been identified as one of the enduring concepts in MFT (Carter & McGoldrick, 2005; Nichols & Schwartz, 2007). Reframing presenting problems as understandable and expected difficulties associated with transitions between life cycle stages have contributed significantly to the prevailing notion in MFT that clients or families are *stuck* rather than pathological or sick. This attitude has permeated supervision in MFT, with the framework of life cycle stages playing a prominent role both in conceptualising clients and appreciating how the therapist's own life cycle stage and experiences might interface with those of one's clients. This developmental perspective has also informed the articulation of stages in the supervision process and enhanced the understanding that supervisees at different career stages will likely have differing needs and preferences in supervision (Liddle, 1988).

Multiple layers of context: Multiculturalism and diversity. As the field of MFT has evolved, the early focus on immediate and extended families has been expanded to include other layers of context, such as the neighbourhood, community and various sociopolitical forces. Early models of MFT, developed primarily by males, were exposed to a feminist critique that took into account the influence of patriarchy and constrained gender roles for both men and women. Over time, the field has also embraced an appreciation for the impact of race, ethnicity, religion and spirituality, sexual orientation and other aspects of culture on both clients and therapist–client interaction. A wide range of diverse family forms are acknowledged and celebrated. MFT supervision has reflected these trends, too. Efforts have been made to recruit as supervisors racial and ethnic minorities, and to include overt discussion in training and supervision on the potential influence of multiculturalism and diversity in the therapeutic process. Supervisees are encouraged to sensitively and responsibly address the influence on families of issues such as racism, heterosexism, classism, sexism, ageism, and so forth.

MFT-Informed Strategies in Supervision

Genograms. Murray Bowen's foundational idea about the transmission of relational patterns across generations is another key concept in MFT.

A map depicting the family tree and relationships among three or more generations of one's family of origin, the genogram grew out of Bowen's work and his presentation of his own genogram was a watershed moment in the development of MFT (Braverman, 1997). Genograms are widely used in MFT, with some models (e.g., intergenerational, experiential) using them more than others (e.g., MRI brief strategic, solution-focused). Genograms aid clinicians in seeing the client and family in context and enhancing a family systems perspective. Genograms have also become increasingly used by supervisors of many theoretical orientations. Some supervisors use client genograms to teach systemic thinking and to organise large amounts of family data. Others use them to assist supervisees to become more sensitive to issues of culture or spirituality or other issues in client families. Refer to the latest edition (2008) of the classic text on genograms by McGoldrick, Gerson and Petry for details on current symbols and a variety of uses of genograms.

In addition to the benefits of using client genograms, supervisors who are particularly interested in the development of the self of the therapist have supervisees create and share their own genograms in supervision. Caution should be taken in this use of supervisee genograms as clarity needs to be maintained between doing supervision that is related to clinical cases and therapist development and doing personal therapy, which is beyond the realm of supervision. The supervisor should secure permission from the supervisee to address family of origin issues of the supervisee as they might be influencing one's clinical work, as well as permission to address such issues in a group format. Supervisees' genograms can be used to increase supervisee differentiation, enhance awareness about how one's family of origin experiences might impact clinical work and to promote resolution of 'stuckness' in the therapeutic system (Braverman, 1997). Next, the use of double and triple genograms in supervision is discussed.

The double genogram approach is recommended for supervisees who seem to be thwarted in clinical cases by negative experiences or roles in the supervisee's family of origin (Braverman, 1997). The client's genogram is presented simultaneously with the therapist's and a discussion is generated about the quality of the relationships in each genogram with an eye to uncovering possible links between the two families. The genograms help supervisees to gain some distance from the material, using an intellectual process to master emotional reactivity.

The triple genogram approach occurs in supervision-of-supervision, that is, in the supervisor's own training and development as a supervisor (Braverman, 1997). This approach has two parts. In the first, the supervisor utilises the double genogram with a supervisee while being observed by the supervisor's mentor. The supervisor mentor then meets privately with the supervisor, whose genogram is also added to the two from the double genogram approach, and likewise, a similar discussion and search for patterns and links ensues, making connections between interventions used by the supervisor and his or her family of origin. Braverman (1997) recommends that supervisors do not share their genograms with supervisees, due to issues around not making things too complicated for the supervisee and upsetting the supervisor–therapist hierarchy. Given a growing postmodern emphasis on collaborative relationships and flattening hierarchies, it might be appropriate for supervisors to share their genograms with supervisees, especially for more experienced supervisors and supervisees.

Live supervision. Live supervision was briefly discussed above related to the value of MFTs showing their work to others and seeking feedback from colleagues. Live supervision involves *observation* of live therapy sessions, typically from behind a one-way mirror or through remote feed to the supervisor's office or central location, and *intervention* during the session that may take the form of phone-ins, mid-session breaks, or the supervisor joining the session. Live supervision has been termed the sine qua non of supervision in MFT, and nearly half of the literature on MFT supervision is about live supervision (Montalvo & Storm, 1997).

Jay Haley, Salvador Minuchin and Braulio Montalvo developed live supervision as a method of supervision in the early 1950s (Montalvo & Storm, 1997). They broke many of the traditional rules of supervision by observing and guiding clinicians' work in the moment; they were active, directive and intervened in the ongoing therapeutic interaction. Montalvo (1973) authored a now classic article on the ground rules for this new mode of supervision. Clear expectations and agreement about items such as phone-ins and mid-session breaks are made beforehand, and the supervisor adapts interventions to the therapist's style and preferred ways of working. All supervisory input is viewed as a suggestion unless supervisors say supervisees 'must do something', which is usually done to manage risk or comply with ethical standards. Montalvo sees live supervision 'as a symbol of family therapy's strong traditional respect for the immediacy of the family's presenting problem, for what's observable and has to be empirically addressed in order to be helpful' (Montalvo & Storm, 1997, p. 289). Live supervision has had its proponents and detractors; a summary of key benefits and limitations follow.

Live supervision affords the opportunity of access to more and direct information that is not filtered by therapists' descriptions as would be true in case consultation. Supervisors can intervene in the immediate moment, when it is most therapeutically appropriate, thus enhancing the quality of the therapeutic interaction. Supervisors are able to pick up more of the tone and systemic interaction among the family members and between the therapist and clients. Learning is also enhanced for other trainees who may be observing and commenting along with the supervisor behind the mirror. Supervisees in research studies have reported they are excited by the intense involvement of supervisors in live supervision, that they like the sense of having a safety net, and that live supervision allows them to be more creative and comfortable in trying on new behaviours (Montalvo & Storm, 1997).

Critics of live supervision view it as 'intrusive, pushy and dehumanizing' for supervisees and clients (Montalvo & Storm, 1997, p. 285), or believe that it violates therapist–client privacy and negatively affects the client–therapist relationship. Some supervisors have reported concerns that they feel overly responsible for their supervisees' therapy and that it might limit the development of the therapist's own style. Some supervisees have remarked that they feel like 'puppets' and may become overly reliant on live supervision. One study by Liddle, Davidson and Barrett (1988) found differences in the responses of novice and experienced supervisees. Novice therapists worried about being judged or seen as incompetent, but this typically rapidly disappeared after some positive experience with live supervision. More experienced clinicians were more apprehensive about power and control issues, but these feelings dissipated once they felt respected. Both groups viewed mid-session breaks favourably, wanted to be active participants in intervention planning, and preferred therapist-initiated over supervisor-initiated consults as time went on. A unique innovation of live supervision, the use of reflecting teams is addressed next.

Reflecting teams. Developed initially by Tom Andersen and colleagues in Norway (Andersen, 1987, 1990), reflecting teams have been used primarily with narrative and social constructionist-informed models of family therapy. Reflecting teams involve making the previously secretive discussions by the team observing behind the mirror open and visible to clients. Rather than a team message being delivered by the therapist to the family, the family is privy to the multiple perspectives of the team members. This can be accomplished by the family and team switching places, so that the family and therapist go behind the mirror and listen to the team discuss the family's situation and the therapeutic conversation that had just occurred. Following this, the family and therapist return to the therapy room and the family shares their reactions to what they observed from the team. 'By coming in front of the mirror and letting each of their individual voices be heard, reflecting team members put the postmodern notions of multiple perspectives, horizontal, collaborative relationships, and transparency into action' (Freedman & Combs, 1996, p. 171).

Supervision using reflecting teams can take place in a number of ways. Simply by using reflecting teams with cases, supervisees can see in action the value of offering multiple perspectives and empowering clients. Therapists and team members learn to focus on clients' strengths and resources, often the focus of team reflections, and appreciate the dilemmas clients are encountering. Supervisees learn to pay closer attention to the nuances of therapeutic conversation. Because team members are directly contributing to the treatment conversation, they have a higher level of involvement with cases. An essential role of the supervisor using reflecting teams is to instil an attitude of curiosity and respect for one another and for clients. The supervisor facilitates the creative exploration of structures and keeps an open dialogue going about what is working and not working in supervision. Indeed, this approach challenges the hierarchical nature of the supervisor and supervisee roles. The same curious attitude and use of multiple perspectives can be employed in group supervision outside the therapy hour, with various members of the group offering alternatives on what may be going on with the family and with the interaction among the family, therapist, and team or within the team itself (Roberts, 1997).

Current Trends and Future Developments

Current developments in the field of MFT are reflected in MFT supervision. A couple of key trends are addressed here. One is the move away from singular allegiance to a particular model of MFT to embracing more integrative approaches. Foy and Breunlin (2001) describe supervision from a metaframeworks perspective, a popular integrative approach. Integrative supervision involves learning the model, doing thorough assessment and determining interventions for dynamics at various levels of the overall system. Attention to common factors is another area of growing interest in MFT and supervision. Unique facets of common factors in MFT include a relational focus, and working with multiple members of a family that leads to an expanded direct treatment system and expanded therapeutic alliances (Sprenkle & Blow, 2004). Morgan and Sprenkle (2007) offer a common factors approach to supervision that focuses upon three general dimensions: (1) emphasis upon clinical vs. professional competence; (2) specificity, ranging from particular to general and (3) relationship, from collaborative to directive. They detail the benefits of taking a common factors approach to supervision and contend that it synthesises common practices from current knowledge about supervision. Doing supervision from postmodern (Unger, 2006), feminist (Prouty, Thomas, Johnson, & Long, 2001), and social justice (McGeorge, Carlson, Erickson, & Guttormson, 2007) perspectives have also received recent attention.

Finally, supervisory experts have identified several areas that warrant future attention in MFT supervision (Lee, Nichols, Nichols, & Odom, 2004; Storm, Todd, Sprenkle, & Morgan, 2001). These authors thoughtfully address some of the commonly held assumptions about MFT supervision, offer challenges to these and make recommendations for the future practice of and research on supervision. Indeed, the lack of empirical support for common assumptions and practices is highlighted, and they recommend expanding research on supervision. Other key recommendations include continuing attention to multicultural and diversity issues and recognition of the influence of the various contexts in which MFT is practiced. The use of explicit contracts, considering power dimensions and the potential enhancements and complications of multiple relationships in the supervisor–supervisee relationship, weighing the strengths and limitations of various modalities of supervision, and tailoring supervision strategies to supervisees' goals and styles are also encouraged.

School Counselling Supervision

Quality supervision is crucial as school counsellors face increasingly complex counselling situations, along with escalating expectations and demands (Protivnak, 2003; Wood & Rayle, 2006). Supervision is especially important for school counsellors today, given the evolving nature of the profession. Reform initiatives put forth in the US through the American School Counselor Association National Model (ASCA, 2003), and the Transforming School Counseling Initiative (The Education Trust, 2003) have created a new vision for the school counsellor role (Milsom & Akos, 2005). The profession of school counselling is in transition, from a responsive, crisis-oriented approach, to comprehensive programs with clearly defined functions and goals (Gysbers & Henderson, 2006). Supervision is an effective means of increasing competency and enhancing professional development, yet the supervision needs of school counsellors go largely unmet (Herlihy, Gray, & McCollum, 2002). In this section, the issues impacting school counsellor supervision will be discussed, along with current supervision models specific to school counselling.

Current Status and Unique Challenges

Historically, the lack of clinical supervision has been an expressed concern (Dollarhide & Miller, 2006), and this deficit has been confirmed by several research studies (Agnew, Vaught, Getz, & Fortune, 2000; Benshoff & Paisley, 1996; Crutchfield & Borders, 1997; Page, Pietrzak, & Sutton, 2001; Roberts & Borders, 1994; Sutton & Page, 1994). In a study conducted by Page et al. (2001), 24% of participants reported receiving supervision, 57% indicated that they desired supervision in the future and 33% responded that they had no need for supervision. Across studies, Miller and Dollarhide (2006) determined that between 21% and 37% of school counsellors reported that they did not desire supervision. Herlihy et al. (2002) suggested that there may be a generalised perception that school counsellors do not need clinical supervision, and that this belief has been reinforced by a lack of state mandated post-degree supervision for school counsellors. Luke and Bernard (2006) hypothesised that there is a gap between supervision models that focus on individual counselling, and the multiple roles and responsibilities of school counsellors. It has also been proposed that few school counsellors are trained as supervisors, and that training at the master's level could encourage appreciation and desire for supervision (Henderson, 2000; Herlihy et al., 2002; Miller & Dollarhide, 2006; Studer, 2005).

Another key factor influencing supervision is that school counsellors operate within multiple systems relating to diverse groups of individuals, including students, parents, teachers, administrators and community members. Each of these groups exerts role expectations and demands on the school counsellor, and this varies by each group's perceptions and needs (Wood & Rayle, 2006). School administrators, in particular, may view the school counsellor's role as primarily administrative, with responsibilities such as academic advising and scheduling. The assignment of clerical duties creates confusion about the function and value of the supervisory role, and may lead school counsellors to view administrative supervision as equitable to clinical supervision (Herlihy et al., 2002; Henderson & Lampe, 1992; Wood & Rayle, 2006). This perception could be reinforced by other factors impacting school counsellor supervision, including district funding shortages, concern about taking away from direct services and a generalised lack of understanding regarding the benefits of supervision (Paisley & McMahon, 2001). Although the value of clinical supervision is evident in the literature, the most common type of supervision offered to school counsellors is administrative, provided by a school administrator with a focus on topics like job performance and staff relationships (Dollarhide & Miller, 2006; Herlihy, et al., 2002; Studer, 2005).

The expectations and responsibilities for school counsellors in the US have expanded, due to the reform initiatives developed by the American School Counseling Association (ASCA, 2003), and The Education Trust (2003). The ASCA National Model (2003) is based on three counselling domains: academic, career and personal/social. Each domain has associated standards and benchmarks that are implemented through four types of delivery systems: school guidance curriculum, individual student planning, responsive services and system support. A central goal of comprehensive school counselling programs is achievement for all students, and school counsellors are now expected to be leaders in advocacy, collaboration and systematic change (Dollarhide & Miller, 2006; Gysbers & Henderson, 2006; Studer, 2005).

An important issue for supervisors to consider is the *degree of transformation*, that is, the extent to which the school counselling program has moved to compliance with the ASCA National Model (ASCA, 2003; Miller & Dollarhide, 2006). Transformed school counselling programs are preventative, developmental and aligned with the educational mission of the school (Gysbers & Henderson, 2001). In her study, Studer (2005) found that approximately 50% of school counsellors reported working under a traditional model, and approximately 49% were either in a transformed model or were in the process of making this change. A problem for many school counsellor trainees is that they are initially introduced to a comprehensive model of counselling, and then are supervised by school counsellors performing under a traditional model. It is possible, however, that as the process of transformation and implementation of the ASCA National Model (2003) continues, supervision could serve to enhance the clarity and functions of the school counsellor role (Dollarhide & Miller, 2006; Miller & Dollarhide, 2006). As more counsellors become familiar with the benefits of a comprehensive, developmental school counsellor program, and supervise accordingly, those whom they train will likely assume a greater leadership role in advocating for systematic change (Studer & Oberman, 2006).

Models of School Counselor Supervision
Those asked to supervise may find the task daunting, yet the opportunity to influence the development of a new colleague can be an enjoyable and profound experience (Magnuson, Black, & Norem, 2004). Documented benefits of supervision for school counsellors include increased effectiveness, enhanced professional development and confidence (Agnew et al., 2000; Crutchfield & Borders, 1997; Herlihy et al., 2002). To provide quality supervision, it is important for supervisors to choose an approach that will most benefit the development of the counsellor supervisee (Stoltenberg, 1981). Although excellent models of supervision exist, many are inadequate for the supervision of school counsellors, due to the broader scope and diversity of their responsibilities (Magnuson, Black, & Norem, 2004; Wood & Rayle, 2006).

In response to the unique supervision needs of school counsellors, Luke and Bernard (2006) proposed the School Counseling Supervision Model (SCSM). The SCSM combines Bernard's (1997) Discrimination Model with the most common components of comprehensive school counselling programs: large group guidance, responsive counselling and consultation, individual advisement, and programmatic planning, coordination and evaluation (Gysbers & Henderson, 2001). Luke and Bernard (2006) developed a matrix for the model that includes Bernard's (1979, 1997) supervisor roles (teacher, counsellor and consultant), and supervisor foci (intervention, conceptualisation and personalisation), along with the four comprehensive counselling domains above. The Discrimination Model has had wide applications as a clinical supervision model, and the purpose of the SCSM is to adapt the model to the specific supervision needs of school counsellors (Luke & Bernard, 2006).

Wood and Rayle (2006) created a model for school counsellors-in-training called The Goals, Functions, Roles and Systems Model (GFRS). The authors stated that they developed the model to provide some 'attention and direction to the neglected area of specialised school counseling supervision' (p. 265). The GFRS Model is designed to reflect the systems and contexts of school counselling, and address the multiple responsibilities school counsellors are expected to fulfil. The model is theoretically based, drawing upon the Working Alliance Model of Supervision (Bordin, 1983), the Discrimination Model (Bernard, 1997), and the Systems Approach to Supervision Model (SAS; Holloway 1995). According to the authors (Wood & Rayle, 2006), the GFRS Model emphasises the shared agreement of supervisor and trainee, the constructivist process of supervision and the context of multiple, dynamic systems. General goal areas include: leadership; advocacy; assessment and use of data; system support; responsive services; and the planning, development and delivery of a guidance curriculum. Within the context of the GFRS Model, the supervisor's role is to facilitate the accomplishment of co-constructed supervision goals and support the goals and functions of supervision within multiple systems. The five primary aspects of the supervisory role are: evaluator, adviser, coordinator, teacher and mentor. The authors suggest that, due to the theoretical nature of the model, further research is needed to determine the actual roles and functions of supervision in school counselling (Wood & Rayle, 2006).

Protivnak (2003) presented a framework for using a variety of supervision modalities in relation to the four stages of school counsellor development as proposed by Littrell, Lee-Borden, and Lorenz (1979): dependent, pseudodependent, interdependence and independence. Protivnak (2003) identified the supervision modalities appropriate for each of the four developmental levels. Stage 1, the *dependent* stage was described as most often occurring during practicum and internship. This first stage is characterised by feelings of anxiety and a reliance on directives provided by the supervisor (Stoltenberg, 1981). For this stage, Protivnak (2003) suggested a structured approach, with a focus on clear expectations, tasks and responsibilities of supervisors and trainees (Drapela & Drapela, 1986; Nelson & Johnson, 1999). In Stage 2, *pseudodependence*, school counsellor supervisees desire independence, yet become aware of their deficits and strengths (Littrell et al., 1979). According to Protivnak (2003), an appropriate approach for this stage is the Northside Independent School District (NISD) Model (Henderson & Lampe, 1992). This model provides the supervisor with a highly structured format that includes supervision conferences, pre-observation, observation, postobservation and analysis of postobservation. Identified benefits for supervision with the NISD model are: feedback regarding counselling skills, learning new techniques and receiving support from other professionals. In Stage 3, *interdependence*, school counsellors desire to work consultatively as an equal professional, and exhibit increased confidence and independence (Nelson & Johnson, 1999). Protivnak (2003) cited peer group supervision (Crutchfield & Borders, 1997) as a desired modality for this stage of counsellor development, providing feedback and collegial support. He also recommended The Structured Peer Consultation Model for School Counselors (Benshoff & Paisley, 1996) for developing consultation skills, counselling skills and support (Protivnak, 2003). In Stage 4, *independence,* counsellors are capable of working independently (Littrell et al., 1979), and for this level, Protivnak (2003) suggested that counsellors may continue to benefit from peer supervision, along with self-supervision continuing education.

Peer supervision has been widely implemented as a strategy to address counsellors' need for supervision (Agnew et al., 2000; Benshoff & Paisley, 1996; Crutchfield & Borders, 1997; Peace & Sprinthall, 1998), and survey data reveal that many school counsellors are participating in this form of supervision (Page et al., 2001; Sutton & Page, 1994). At the core of peer supervision is case presentation, and some supervision models provide a structure for this process (Benshoff & Paisley, 1996; Remley, Benshoff, & Mowbray, 1987). Reported benefits of participation in peer supervision include: feedback from multiple sources, vicarious learning, support and encouragement, sense of community, enhanced collective self-esteem, improved case conceptualisation skills and effectiveness (Bradley & Kottler, 2001; Butler & Constantine, 2006; Crutchfield & Borders, 1997; Roberts & Borders, 1994; Starling & Baker, 2000). Although more statistical evidence is needed regarding the effectiveness of peer group supervision (Wilkerson, 2006), this approach could prove to be a useful format for school counsellors.

Murphy and Kaffenberger (2007) proposed a model of supervision for site-supervisors of practicum and internship students. The format of the model was specifically developed to align with the framework of the ASCA National Model (2003), in combination with the supervisor roles and foci of the Discrimination Model (Bernard, 1997). In their model, Murphy and Kaffenberger (2007) also included Benshoff's (2003) process variables (supervision stages, gender, age, race, ethnicity and personality characteristics) that influence the supervisor/supervisee relationship. Their model includes a training component, with a detailed description of how to use the model when training site-supervisors with the ASCA National Model (2003) as a foundation for supervision. Murphy and Kaffenberger (2007) suggested that continued supervision training for on-site supervisors is the best way to assure that student counsellors receive quality supervision.

While this is not an exhaustive overview, this selection of school supervision models represents the types of models that are becoming available for school counsellor supervisors. The development of school-specific models is in its early stages and a general deficit exists. The need is apparent for further research, models, and strategies designed to address the supervision needs of school counsellors (Wood & Rayle, 2006).

Supervisor Competency

Supervisor competency is a key ethical concern for school counsellor supervision, due to the prevalence of a lack of training (Henderson, 2000; Herlihy et al., 2002; Miller & Dollarhide, 2006; Murphy & Kaffenberger, 2007). It is unfortunate that standards regarding supervision are not explicitly detailed in the ethical guidelines of the American School Counselor Association (ASCA, 2004). However, the American Counseling Association Code of Ethics (2005) includes standards mandating that supervisors must be adequately trained in supervision methods and techniques (Standard F.2.a.), and must practice within the scope of their competence (Standard C.2.a.). The Ethical Guidelines for Counseling Supervisors (ACES, 1995) state that supervisors must have training in supervision prior to becoming supervisors (2.01), and must also continue with educational activities, courses, seminars and conferences on an ongoing basis (2.02).

It is imperative for practicing school counsellor supervisors to actively pursue training and ongoing professional development in supervision (Herlihy et al., 2002; Miller & Dollarhide, 2006). This is especially important as reform initiatives continue to transform the profession of school counselling, and school counsellors strive to establish a new, consistent professional identity (Milsom & Akos, 2005). The specialised expectations and demands of school counsellors require supervisors that are prepared to provide school-specific supervision in a competent, holistic and ethical manner (Wood & Rayle, 2006). It is also imperative that school counsellors-in-training have a clear understanding of supervision. This would help them to make the most of their supervisory experiences and to provide supervision for other school counsellors in the future (Dollarhide & Miller, 2006).

Guidelines for school counsellor supervisors have been proposed by Herlihy, (2002) that are congruent with the ethical guidelines of professional counselling associations. She recommended training and ongoing professional development in supervision to avoid ethical and legal pitfalls, and to become a more effective supervisor. She also suggested that school counsellor supervisors work diligently to protect the confidentiality of minors and to maintain appropriate boundaries with supervisees. She stressed actively pursuing administrative support for supervision, along with collaborating with counsellor educators at nearby universities to provide professional development opportunities for practicing school counsellors. Herlihy (2002) underscored that school counsellor supervisors should have their own liability insurance and have a plan in place for handling legal situations. On-site supervisors are responsible for all of the supervisee's actions at the school site. This is a direct liability for supervisors, yet a surprising number of school counsellor supervisors rely solely on their school district's liability insurance (Murphy & Kaffenberger, 2007).

Summary

The status of school counselling supervision is far from ideal (Herlihy, 2002), yet the stakes are high for the profession of school counselling. Providing quality supervision is both a responsibility and a challenge and is essential in preparing school counsellors to meet the demands of the 21st century (Murphy & Kaffenberger, 2007). The number of new school counsellors is increasing, and these school counsellors are facing the same complex problems, ethical dilemmas, and demands that are placed on more experienced counsellors (Henderson, 2000). While the importance of supervision for school counsellors is gaining momentum in the literature (Crutchfield & Borders, 1997), further research, models and training are needed. Increasing opportunities for clinical supervision will require systemic change, beginning with school counsellors' perceptions regarding the value of supervision (Dollarhide & Miller, 2006). It is hoped that as the profession of school counselling moves forward, the supervision provided to school counsellors will serve to enhance their competency, clarify their professional identity and encourage them as leaders and advocates for change.

Supervision of Alcohol and Drug Counselling

Professional treatment for alcohol and other drug disorders is in a rapid state of change. Monthly new evidence-based strategies for treatment are being published and treatment has expanded to include the complex nature of co-occurring disorders. Additionally, the client population for treatment of alcohol and other drug disorders poses the unique aspects of extensive client denial of the disorder and significant other enabling for continuance of the disorder.

A challenge to those providing clinical supervision in alcohol and other drug abuse treatment is the aging of the treatment workforce and the diversity of direct treatment counselling skills in the workforce. Further, the alcohol and other drug abuse counselling profession includes recovering and nonrecovering counsellors (Powell, 2004).

The recovery, or nonrecovery dynamic of the counsellor is complex, in that it also includes extreme differences in the professional education of the counsellor. Some governmentally certified alcohol and other drug abuse authorities certify counsellors with only a high school diploma who may practice in parallel with professionals having a terminal graduate degree in counselling (Mann, 1973; Valle, 1984). While both the recovering and nonrecovering counsellors tend to provide equitable treatment outcomes (Aiken & LoSciuto, 1985; LoSciuto, Aiken, Ausetts, & Brown, 1984) they tend to have differing styles of counselling clients (Lawson, Petosa, & Peterson, 1982).

While a number of articles and books (Machell, 1987; Powell, 2004) have been published regarding the clinical supervision of alcohol and other drug abuse counselling, there has been little evidence-based research on the supervision of counselling for substance abuse disorders. Based upon the diverse backgrounds of alcohol and other drug abuse counsellors, multiple entities have produced models of competencies for these counsellors (Center for Substance Abuse Treatment, 2006) as well as models of competencies for clinical supervisors of those counsellors (Center for Substance Abuse Treatment, 2007). Each of those definitional competency documents was a result of consensus of the international certification and reciprocity consortium, role delineation studies and meetings of international experts.

Alcohol and Other Drug Abuse Counsellor Competencies

The basis for all alcohol and other drug abuse counsellor competencies are the trans-disciplinary foundations of knowledge, skills and attitudes of understanding addiction, treatment knowledge, professional readiness and application to practise (Center for Substance Abuse Treatment, 2006).

In order to meet the competency of understanding addiction the counsellor must: (1) understand a variety of models and theories of addiction and other problems related to substance abuse; (2) recognise the social, political, economic, and cultural context within which addiction and substance abuse exists, including risk and resiliency factors that characterise individuals and groups and their living environments; (3) describe the behavioural, psychological, physical health and special effects of psychoactive substances on the person using and significant others and (4) recognise the potential for substance use disorders to mimic a variety of medical and mental health conditions and the potential for medical and mental health conditions to co-exist with addiction and substance abuse (Center for Substance Abuse Treatment, 2006; Lawson, Lawson, & Rivers, 1996).

The competency of treatment knowledge demands the counsellor must: (1) describe the philosophies, practices, policies and outcomes of the most generally accepted and scientifically supported models of treatment, recovery relapse prevention and continuing care for addictions and other substance-related problems; (2) recognise the importance of family, social network and community systems in the treatment and recovery process; (3) understand the importance of research and outcome data and their application in clinical practice and (4) understand the value of an interdisciplinary approach to addiction treatment (Center for Substance Abuse Treatment, 2006, Heather & Miller, 1998).

The application to practise focuses on counsellor competencies to: (1) understand the established diagnoses criteria for substance use disorders and describe treatment modalities and placement criteria within the continuum of care; (2) describe a variety of helping strategies for reducing the negative effects of substance use, abuse and dependence; (3) tailor helping strategies and treatment modalities to the client's stage of dependence, change and recovery;(4) provide treatment services appropriate to the personal and cultural identity and language of the client; (5) adapt practice to the range of treatment settings and modalities; (6) be familiar with medical and pharmacological resources in the treatment of substance use disorders; (7) understand the variety of insurance and health maintenance options available and the importance of helping clients to access those benefits; (8) recognise that crisis may indicate an underlying substance use disorder and may be a window of opportunity for change and (9) understand the need for and use of methods for measuring treatment outcomes (Center for Substance Abuse Treatment, 2006; Lewis, 1994; Miller, Gold & Smith, 1997).

To achieve the competencies of professional readiness the counsellor must: (1) understand diverse cultures, and incorporate the relevant needs of culturally diverse groups, as well as people with disabilities, into clinical practice; (2) understand the importance of self-awareness in one's personal, professional and cultural life; (3) understand the alcohol and other drug abuse counsellor's professional obligations to adhere to ethical and behavioural standards of conduct in the helping relationship; (4) understand the importance of ongoing supervision and continuing education in the delivery of client services; (5) understand the obligation of the alcohol and other drug abuse counsellor to participate in prevention and treatment activities and (6) understand and apply setting-specific policies and procedures for handling crisis or dangerous situations, including safety measure for clients and staff (Center for Substance Abuse Treatment, 2006; Lowinson & Ruiz, 2004).

Using these competencies as the base for alcohol and other drug abuse counselling, the clinical supervisor is able to focus supervision on the strengths and weaknesses of counsellors, both as evaluation and to enhance knowledge, skills and attitude.

Alcohol and Other Drug Abuse Clinical Supervision

Of great importance in the clinical supervision of alcohol and other drug abuse counsellors is the clinical supervisor having met all competencies of the counsellor role and being able to demonstrate these competencies as required in the clinical supervision process. Further, clinical supervision in the alcohol and other drug abuse treatment profession must acknowledge, and adapt to, three unique aspects of this profession: (1) a significant number of alcohol and other drug abuse treatment providers are paraprofessionals, (2) many alcohol and other drug abuse professional counsellors and paraprofessionals providing treatment strongly believe the client must be in recovery to provide effective treatment and (3) alcohol and other drug abuse treatment providers can be influenced by personal issues (Juhnke & Culbreth, 1994).

The supervision of alcohol and other drug abuse counsellors involves the traditional aspects of leadership, supervisory alliance, critical thinking, organisational management and administration, counsellor development, professional and ethical standards, program development and quality assurance, performance evaluation and administration (Center for Substance Abuse Treatment, 2007).

Leadership focuses on the multidirectional social influence process through which clinical supervisors seek voluntary participation of supervisees to achieve clinical and organisational goals (Powell, 2004). Supervisory alliance addresses the mutual understanding of the goals and tasks of supervision and a rigorous professional binding of the clinical supervision and supervisee (Muse-Burke, Ladany, & Deck 2001).

Critical thinking refers to the multiple cognitive processes of conceptualising, analysing, applying information, synthesising and evaluating (Robinson, 2001). Organisational management and administration is the process of working with and through others to achieve organisational objectives in an efficient, legal and ethical manner (Falvey & Bray, 2002). Counsellor development consists of the multifaceted process involving teaching, facilitating, collaborating, and supporting counsellor self-efficiency (McMahon & Simons, 2004). Professional and ethical standards specify those activities for protecting the public, clients, counsellors, and staff members (Borders & Brown, 2005).

Program development and quality assurance are the processes of guiding the evolution of the service delivery organisation to maximise its effectiveness and designing, implementing, monitoring and improving a program's activities to ensure maximum effectiveness (Lindblaum, TenEyck, & Gallon, 2005). Performance evaluation is to regularly monitor the quality of supervisee's performance, facilitate improvement in supervisee's clinical competence and to assess supervisee's readiness to practise with increasing autonomy (Falender & Shafranske, 2004). Administration in clinical supervision focuses on following the organisation's policies and procedures, ensuring maintenance of case records, monitoring case documentation and developing relationships with referral sources in the community (Bernard & Goodyear, 2004). Overarching within the clinical supervision of alcohol and other drug abuse is the clinical supervisor's demonstrated competence in the assessment, diagnosis and treatment of substance use disorders through knowledge, skill and attitude. Through this the clinical supervisor obtains the respect of the supervisee.

Summary

The clinical supervision of counsellors providing alcohol and other drug abuse services have great similarities to the knowledge, skills and attitudes required of all clinical supervisors. In the provision of clinical supervision of alcohol and other drug abuse counselling the supervisor must also be able to demonstrate the knowledge, skills and attitudes incorporated in the extensive specific competencies expected of the counsellor. Further, the clinical supervisor must be adept at applying supervision to both professional and paraprofessional counsellors, counsellors with strong (nonevidence-based) beliefs in recovery and treatment, and able to assist the counsellor in eliminating personal issues from professional practice.

Supervision in University Training Clinics

For the past 7 years, I (ES) have been a counselling psychology faculty member and director of a departmental training clinic at Western Michigan University (WMU). In this time, I have learned that supervision in a training clinic is unique and multifaceted. The overarching supervision goals of teaching and monitoring client welfare (Bernard & Goodyear, 1998) are the same as in other clinical settings, however, several aspects of training clinics makes supervision in this setting distinct. Keeping with the goal of this chapter, which is to describe supervision of applied specialties, this next section will illustrate the process of clinical supervision in an academic departmental training clinic. To begin, I will first provide an overview of departmental training clinics in the United States. Second, to situate my own experiences, I will provide some background about the department that houses our two training clinics and then describe my uncommon faculty appointment. Third, I will outline the structure of supervision for our master's students enrolled in counselling practica and internships. Fourth, I will provide a brief description of my work supervising the therapy provided by the counselling psychology doctoral students. Finally, I will introduce the Association of Directors of Psychology Training Clinics (ADPTC) and then describe two important documents that clinical supervisors in similar applied settings may find particularly helpful.

Overview of University Training Clinics
Psychology labs have existed in the United States for more than 100 years — dating back to Lightner Witmer's first psychology lab at the University of Pennsylvania. The original goal of Witmer's lab was to combine the discoveries of science and practice (Witmer, 1996). In the modern era, psychology training clinics have expanded and are now associated with other professional training programs including counsellor education and counselling psychology programs. These training clinics are becoming increasingly more important to graduate training, and are especially utilised for predoctoral practicum training in clinical psychology programs. Despite their expansion, training clinics have held firmly to the longstanding tri-part mission of providing affordable counselling and psychological services to the community, enhancing the clinical training of graduate students and promoting clinical research. The relative emphasis placed on each of these three areas varies across training clinics (ADPTC, 2006).

Overview of the Department of Counselor Education and Counseling Psychology at WMU
The Counselor Education and Counseling Psychology (CECP) Program at Western Michigan University offers seven master's degree programs and two doctoral degree programs. Three master's programs (i.e., College Counseling, Community Counseling, and School Counseling) and the doctoral program in Counselor Education are accredited by Council for Accreditation of Counseling and Related Programs (CACREP). Similarly, our doctoral program in Counseling Psychology is fully accredited by the American Psychological Association (APA). Finally, our master's program in Counseling Psychology is not accredited (the APA does not accredit master's programs) but the curriculum has been designed so that students get necessary educational and clinical training experiences to meet the requirements to be a Limited Licensed Psychologist in the state of Michigan. These licen-

sure and accreditation issues have a significant impact on the structure and process of supervision, which will be articulated in the following sections.

Our department houses two training clinics or education/counselling laboratories called the Centers for Counseling and Psychological Service. One centre is located on the main university campus and the other is located 55 miles north in a regional graduate centre. The graduate centre clinic is centrally located in a large metropolitan area and provides a range of low cost psychological services to a diverse community population.

An Uncommon Faculty Appointment

I am currently serving as director of the clinic located in the regional centre and thus I will focus my comments on my personal experiences directing this particular clinic. As clinic director, I am responsible for administrative leadership, oversight of clinic operations, supervision of trainees and staff and expansion of the scope of clinical services. My fiscal-year faculty appointment is unusual in that I am a tenured associate professor *and* clinic director. Although I am responsible for typical faculty duties (e.g., scholarship and research, graduate advising, dissertation chairing, and committee work), my teaching load has been reduced to give time to direct the centre. Thus, instead of the regular teaching load of four courses per academic year, I am assigned to teach/supervise one section of a master's-level internship each semester.

In-House Supervision of Master's-Level Practica and Internships

At the master's level, the nature of clinical supervision in our training clinic is largely driven by the 2009 CACREP standards. Specifically, supervision of our master's level students occurs in two primary courses. First, as part of the 100-hour Counseling Practicum, students are required to accrue 40 hours of direct service with clients, including individual and group counselling. As part of this experience, students attend a 4-hour practicum each week. Within this time frame, 1½ hours are allocated for group supervision and 2 hours are typically allocated for counselling clients. Four to five practicum groups are assigned to the centre each semester. To maintain the required six-to-one faculty to student ratio, the size of practicum groups are restricted to five to six students. A typical master's student caseload is two clients, although students can take on additional clients with supervisor approval. All students also attend 1 hour of individual and/or triadic supervision weekly from their faculty instructors *outside* of the regular practicum class meeting

At the master's level, all counselling sessions must be videotaped and faculty supervisors are required to be in the centre when students are working with their clients. A primary benefit of supervision in this on-campus setting includes the physical space and technology for careful monitoring and direct observation. One-way mirrors and TV monitoring allow students to be directly observed by their clinical supervisors and peers. The videotaping and TV monitoring equipment can simultaneously record eight different counselling sessions. The tapes of trainees' counselling sessions are used for individual, triadic and group supervision. Some practicum instructors also use training models that employ co-therapy with supervisors, and/or phone calls directly into counselling sessions. To my knowledge, the technology and structure that allows for these varied forms of observation and careful monitoring is not typically available at our off-campus placements. Given that the practicum students are typically in the earliest stages of development as helping professionals, this high level of monitoring is necessary.

The second way that master's students receive clinical supervision in the departmental training clinic is during the internship, which is called Field Practicum. As part of this 600-hour internship, students are required to accrue 240 hours of direct service with clients in an off-campus community setting. As part of the internship experience, clinical supervision has two primary components: on and off campus. Students in CACREP accredited program are required to average 1 hour of individual and/or triadic supervision with his or her on-site supervisor per week. These students are also required to attend 1½ hours of group supervision, which is conducted by a program faculty member each week in the training clinic on campus. Counselling psychology master's students who are on internship must follow different administrative rules for clinical supervision based on the Michigan Board of Psychology supervision requirements. In particular, counselling psychology students must receive 8 hours of supervision per month from a fully licensed psychologist (LP). Of these required 8 hours, our program requires students to receive 1 hour of individual supervision on site. Typically, these students also choose to attend the weekly group supervision sessions in the training clinic to get their 8 hours of supervision in each month. In rare cases, counselling psychology students are able to secure all 8 hours of LP supervision on site and are thus not required to attend the faculty-led supervision groups on campus.

Since coming to WMU, in my role as psychology clinic director, I have been teaching and supervising internships. Essentially, this process involves overseeing students' professional development in a group setting of ten or fewer. Our students work with their academic advisors and me to find internship placements in a variety of community settings (e.g., public and private schools, community mental health centres, private practices, psychiatric hospitals, college and university counselling centres). Some of our students are placed in more than one location.

In reflecting upon Bernard's (1997) discrimination model of supervision roles (i.e., teacher, counsellor, consultant), I commonly find myself more aligned with the role of consultant in these supervision groups, although certainly counsellor and teacher roles emerge during the semester as well. My higher reliance on the consultant role seems to be related to a number of structural factors. First, our CECP faculty expects students at this level to be somewhat more autonomous on internship. Thus, students do not typically need the same level of monitoring and oversight that is provided in practicum. Second, I generally do not have direct access to client files or counselling sessions — via live observation or videotapes. Instead, the CECP program relies on a number of different on-site supervisors to provide direct supervision of our interns.

As faculty supervisor, my primary goal for group supervision is to cultivate the development of a sound supervisory alliance with each student. With strong supervisory working alliances, the group can serve as a secure base from which students can explore various aspects of their clinical work. I continually invite them to bring their clinical struggles to group for help and then try to let the group supervision process develop naturally. To be most effective, I have developed a largely nondirective stance. I can create a tentative plan for group but typically the interns take me where they need to go each week. Analogous to a nondirective counselling session, from week to week, it is often quite difficult to predict what a supervisee's most pressing needs will be. Moreover, I agree with Neufeldt (2007) and others who have argued that too much structure in early practicum training may promote passive learning and inhibit professional development. The structure of group has evolved over the years but it typically starts with students checking in each week by reporting to the group how things are going at their internship sites. For example, are students getting enough direct contact hours? Are they experiencing a variety of professional activities? During 'check-in' time students can request 'time' or ask for 'help' if they have important topics or clinical issues to bring to group. Following the check-in, we then take stock of how many students have requested time and then estimate about how much time should be allocated to each student. We also triage by giving precedence to students who have more pressing concerns or cases. Students then take turns presenting important concerns related to their clinical work and receiving feedback from the group. Students are encouraged to tell the group what type of feedback they are looking for before their case presentations begin. As we hear cases, I try to make sure that students are giving and receiving detailed and constructive feedback and that we are balancing support with respectful challenging. As a faculty supervisor, I help students to develop a scientific mindset in their case conceptualisations and encourage them to use the counselling literature to guide practice.

Supervision of Doctoral Students

Each year, four counselling psychology doctoral associates (students receiving paid assistantships) are assigned to work in the centre. These 20-hour per week assignments offer students rich opportunities to provide a wide range of (supervised) clinical services to a diverse community clientele. For instance, our doctoral associates conduct intake assessments with all prospective clients, provide counselling, and administer psychological tests and assessments. As clinic director, I supervise all of the psychological services provided by our doctoral associates. A full discussion of these doctoral associateship duties has been provided elsewhere (Sauer & Huber, 2007) and is beyond the scope of this chapter. Consequently, I will centre my comments below on my experiences providing group supervision of the doctoral students' therapy cases.

Each semester, a portion of the doctoral associate hours (2 to 6) are allocated for counselling clients. The doctoral students in the centre have more clinical experience and are assigned to the centre for a full fiscal year — sometimes their contracts are renewed for more than 1 year. Given these factors, they can be assigned more difficult clients and/or clients who may need relatively longer-term therapy. Although the structure of supervision is similar to how I work with master's students, it is important to highlight how these processes are similar and different. Similarities include that this group also meets for 1½ hours of weekly group supervision. Parallel to the intern supervision groups, the group begins with a check-in during which each student gives a general sense of how things are going with each client. In this case as direct supervisor, however, I need to hear about every client each week. Students can report this in a general way: 'client X continues to attend therapy and is making progress towards goals and I have no current concerns about my work with her'. Once the check-in process is complete we take stock of who asked the group for help and begin discussing the most pressing clinical concerns. However, unlike my supervision with the master's-level interns, supervision with the doctoral students is more direct. Since they are working with clients in the clinic, I have direct access to their clinical work. For instance, they can either bring videotapes of counselling sessions to group supervision or I can watch sessions live. I also monitor and sign their clinical paperwork such as electronic progress notes, supervision notes and terminations summaries. On occasion, doctoral students will ask me to sit in on part of a counselling session when significant concerns or emergencies arise.

The Association of Directors of Psychology Training Clinics

Beyond my direct experiences working with graduate students in the centre, one national group in the US has been extremely helpful in my development as a clinic director. In the final section, I will introduce this group and describe two important resources for directors and clinical supervisors. The Association of Directors of Psychology Training Clinics (ADPTC) is the organisation for directors of psychology training clinics in the United States and Canada. Part of the mission of the organization reads: '... directors are typically associated with pre-doctoral graduate training programs in professional psychology — clinical, community, counseling, child clinical, and school psychology at regionally accredited universities' (ADPTC, web site home page).

In addition to providing critical support and mentoring for training clinic directors, this organisation has developed two indispensable resources related to clinical supervision. First, Hatcher and Lassiter (2007) recently identified the 'domains and levels of competence that should be the focus of practicum training' (p. 49). In fact, these core practicum competencies are now being adopted by graduate programs in professional psychology in the US. Hatcher and Lassiter provide a competencies outline that clearly summarises core skill areas that can be expected to be obtained during practicum across three competencies levels: novice, intermediate and advanced. Related directly to supervision, there is a list of competencies that are expected in the formation of supervisory relationships, which include: (a) working collaboratively with a supervisor, (b) being prepared for supervision, (c) accepting and implementing supervisory feedback, and negotiating autonomy and dependence on supervisors and (d) demonstrating the ability to 'self-reflect' and 'self-evaluate' clinical work and use supervision. As part of the training process, clinical supervisors can use or modify the Competency Review form that is provided in the Hatcher and Lassiter article to evaluate a student's current skill level in each core area and then modify training goals accordingly. A downloadable copy of the complete Practicum Competencies Outline is available at the ADPTC website: http://www.adptc.org.

ADPTC (2006) has also developed clear guidelines for psychology training clinics. Beyond providing descriptive information about training clinics in general, clinical supervisors may find the subsection on clinical supervision to be helpful. In this section, there is information about best practices for supervision, which may be especially relevant to those who may be developing clinic policies related to clinical supervision. For example, to ensure high quality supervision, all clinical supervisors (a) should be 'licensed and qualified' to practise in the areas they supervise in the clinic; (b) need to 'understand and adhere' to ethical guidelines, as well as state and federal laws related to practice and supervision; (c) should use written supervision contracts with supervisees that outline clear goals and objectives for practicum and (d) should make certain that clinic policies are followed.

Community Mental Health Supervision

The literature that informs clinical supervisor training has focused predominantly on supervision-related issues for student interns (i.e., pregraduates). However, the supervision that occurs after students graduate from training programs and start entry-level positions in community mental health settings has often been overlooked. For purposes of this section, a *community mental health organisation* will be defined as Corey, Corey and Callanan (2007) suggested including 'any institution-public or private, nonprofit or for-profit-designed to provide a wide range of social and psychological services to the community' (p. 486).

Helping professionals from many disciplines, including counselling, counselling psychology, clinical psychology, marriage and family therapy and social work are involved in service delivery to the broadly defined community mental health system. The purpose of this section is to heighten the beginning supervisor's awareness of supervision-related issues that have some unique relevance in the postgraduate practice of supervision, especially for supervisees who are working in the community mental health system. After all, it has been well documented that supervision is among the most frequent activities of community mental health professionals (Bernard & Goodyear, 2004) and, at some point in one's career, the likelihood that one will provide clinical supervision to more junior members of the profession is high. This section will highlight the work of clinical supervisors of community mental health professionals.

Unique Challenges for the Community Mental Health Supervisor

Supervision in community mental health settings is a unique endeavour. Community mental health directors often employ professionals from various disciplines with diverse educational and training backgrounds. Mental health counselling professionals work with some of the most high-risk populations in the mental health system. Clients of community mental health organisations often face significant mental health issues, including thought disorders, mood disorders and personality disorders.

Pre-graduate interns and entry-level counselling professionals may be easily stressed by the complexity of client needs in community mental health settings (Ginsburg, 2000). Ginsburg suggests that clinical psychology interns who are working on medical inpatient settings for the first time '... are often unprepared ...' and 'may feel overwhelmed by the intensity of their patients' needs as well as the pressure associated with clinical work within a constricted time frame' (p. 201). Bradley and Olson (1980) conducted a survey of 183 clinical psychology students and their perceived competence as psychotherapists. Although they examined many different variables for their relationship to felt competence, two variables were the best predictors: (1) the total number of supervisors that a trainee had and (2) the total number of hours spent in supervision. Thus, community mental health professionals are best served when opportunities for practice are matched with adequate levels of clinical supervision.

In this author's (SEC) experience supervising community mental health professionals, I have learned many valuable lessons that are not always elaborated on through most of the traditional supervision literature. The remainder of this section focuses on some of the most prevalent issues that I have experienced in the practice of supervision with community mental health professionals:

1. organisation of the supervision experience

2. evaluation

3. protocol for handling emergencies and crisis situations.

These areas should not be considered distinct from one another, but rather, should be viewed as a series of tasks that have considerable overlap. For example, organising the supervision experience will, by necessity, include a discussion about evaluation. While these are not necessarily an exhaustive list of the challenges associated with the supervision of community mental health professionals, supervisors who consciously attend to these broadly defined considerations will be prepared to handle most situations well.

Organisation of the Supervision Experience

Bernard and Goodyear (2004) devote an entire chapter on the organisation of the supervision experience in their foundational text on supervision. In particular, they remind supervisors of the importance of clearly establishing the boundaries and expectations of supervision. This, they contend, will support a more 'intentional' (p. 180) brand of supervision. In community mental health settings where supervisors may serve in multiple roles, organising the supervision experience can be particularly challenging and thus, of critical importance.

One issue that is consistently raised within community mental health agencies is the question of who is responsible for what facet of the supervision experience. In essence, this involves making the distinction between *administrative* supervisors and *clinical* supervisors. Bernard and Goodyear (2004) describe the administrative supervisor as someone who is not only concerned about service delivery and staff's professional development, but they 'must also focus on matters such as communication protocol, personnel concerns, and fiscal issues' (p. 180). Clinical supervisors, on the other hand, have the primary responsibility of ensuring client welfare while promoting the professional development of the supervisee. While some supervisors will simultaneously serve as both administrative and clinical supervisor for the same supervisee, some agencies will have different individuals, each of whom is responsible for either the administrative or the clinical supervision role. Bernard and Goodyear noted that in many organisations, 'there is no distinction between clinical supervision and administrative supervision' (p. 181).

The Association for Counselor Education and Supervision (ACES, 1995) has a set of ethical guidelines that discourage the same individual from serving in both an administrative and clinical supervisory capacity. In fact, they suggest that when possible, the roles should be appropriately divided among several supervisors to avoid potential areas of conflict. Tromski-Klingshirn (2006) reported that, while the practice of simultaneous service as clinical and administrative supervisor is discouraged, the reality is that approximately 50% of practicing counsellors receive their administrative and clinical supervision from the same person. When supervisors have the responsibility for serving in both capacities, the blurring of roles can become a potential problem, thereby emphasising the importance of role clarification and the minimisation of potential conflicts (ACES).

The beginning phase of the clinical supervision relationship is the time when role clarification must take place. However, the supervisor and supervisee must remain vigilant and continually monitor and reassess the roles throughout the supervision process. There are two primary strategies that may assist with role delineation or role clarification: (1) role induction and (2) the supervision contract (Bernard and Goodyear, 2004).

Role induction. Role induction has been defined as, 'teaching about the role that one is about to adopt' (Bernard & Goodyear, 2004, p. 195).The potential benefits of role induction on supervisee readiness are noteworthy. Specifically, Bahrick, Russell, and Salmi (1991) discovered that, following role induction, supervisees reported a clearer understanding of what was expected of them in the supervision experience as well as a greater likelihood to freely disclose concerns to their supervisors.

For many community mental health professionals who have recently left the highly structured supervision environment provided in most graduate training programs, they may experience considerable discomfort when faced with weekly supervision in which there is a predominant reliance on supervisee self-report to determine the agenda for supervision. In less structured supervision environments, like those often found in postgraduate training experiences, supervisors are responsible for establishing clear expectations.

During the initial supervision session, whether it is group supervision or individual supervision, supervisees are informed that they must bring an agenda to each supervision session (Fall & Sutton, 2004). This helps ensure that the responsibility for the supervision experience is a mutual one and does not rest solely on the supervisor or supervisee. Role induction also includes a discussion about who else may have a supervisory role with them in their employment setting and how the specific responsibilities of each person will be delineated.

In the situation where an on-site person is serving in an administrative supervisory role and another supervisor outside the agency is serving as the clinical supervisor, it is recommended that the outside clinical supervisor request an opportunity to meet conjointly with the administrative supervisor and supervisee. This permits all parties to discuss, among other items, the parameters for supervision, including the responsibilities for evaluation, responsibilities for client welfare and how crises or emergencies will be handled. A conjoint meeting is not always possible, however, so at a minimum, a letter from the administrative supervisor is requested, at least confirming awareness of the role of the clinical supervisor and acknowledging receipt of a copy of the supervision contract. The following section details the recommended elements in a supervision contract.

Supervision contract. Supervision contracts have been accepted as a best-practice for articulating the roles that will be honoured by clinical supervisor and supervisee. There is general consensus in the literature that supervisees, both inexperienced and experienced alike, are most likely to benefit from a supervisory experience that is structured (Osborn & Davis, 1996; Ronnestad & Skovholt, 1993). A structured supervision experience that values the collaborative input from both supervisor and supervisee is preferred. Osborn and Davis, in an effort to provide structure and the 'joint effort' (p. 127) of supervisor and supervisee, have provided a series of guidelines to facilitate the development of a supervision contract. These guidelines have proven very helpful to the author's supervision of community mental health professionals. The guidelines and a brief description of each follow:

1. Purpose, Goals, and Objectives. This section of the contract spells out in written format the mutual expectations of both supervisor and supervisee. Questions that should be addressed include, (a) What is the purpose of the supervision for the supervisee? (i.e., 'to fulfil requirements towards licensure'); and (b) What is the supervisor's purpose? (i.e., 'to ensure client welfare and promote the professional competence of the supervisee').

2. Context of Services. This section should include the proposed dates, times, and durations of the supervision meetings. The context of services should also include a description of the methods used (e.g., group versus individual supervision) and theoretical approach to supervision, including intervention strategies most commonly used.

3. Method for Evaluation. For purposes of the contract, this section should include how evaluations will be conducted, how often, and if a particular instrument is going to be used, it should also be disclosed here. Supervisors and supervisees should have a clear sense of how competence and growth will be assessed. A fundamental question that must be written out here is, 'How will we know when supervision is no longer needed or necessary?' This may be influenced by a couple of factors, including number of clinical hours needed and whether or not established criteria of competence have been met.

4. Duties and Responsibilities of Supervisor and Supervisee. In this section, the duties of supervisor and supervisee are clearly articulated. In cases where the administrative supervisor and clinical supervisor are different persons, it is recommended to include in supervision contracts the responsibilities of not only the clinical supervisor and supervisee but also the administrative supervisor. It may also prove helpful to have the administrative supervisor sign on to the same supervision contract, though this may not always be possible. Some common responsibilities of the clinical supervisor may be (a) to review case notes and treatment plans, (b) to teach counselling skills when appropriate and (c) to monitor the basic attending skills of the supervisee. For supervisees, some typical responsibilities include (a) adherence to relevant ethical codes and applicable laws, (b) to have a prepared agenda for each supervision meeting and (c) to attend all supervision meetings on time.

5. Procedural Considerations. In the procedural considerations section, Sherry (as cited in Osborn & Davis, 1996) suggests including the type of information that will be shared in supervision (e.g., skills used in sessions, diagnosis and treatment plans), how the information will be shared (e.g., case notes, live observation, videotape or digital recordings), and the types of record-keeping that the supervisee will be required to maintain. Supervisees may also maintain a log of their current case load and document each date and time that client is discussed in supervision to ensure that all clients are periodically reviewed.

6. Supervisor's Scope of Competence. Much like the information included in a professional disclosure statement, this section calls for supervisors to disclose their background as it relates to training and professional areas of expertise.

Evaluation

Evaluation has been described as a central process to clinical supervision; however, supervisors report that the role of evaluation is among the most challenging (Bernard & Goodyear, 2004; Borders & Brown, 2005; Bradley, 1989). One of the reasons that evaluation has proved challenging relates to the difficulty in establishing clearly defined criteria for assessing competence. Robiner, Fuhrman and Ristvedt (as cited in Bernard & Goodyear, p. 19) describe clinical competence as a 'moving target with an elusive criterion'. The process of evaluation in postgraduate supervision is often more problematic than in pregraduate training, due to a lack of access to recorded sessions and other means for direct observation of the supervisee's skills. As a result, the author suggests a multifaceted process for evaluation that includes formative feedback, summative evaluations, live supervision methods, case-note review and the encouragement of self-assessment, all methods that have been recommended by Bernard and Goodyear.

Quality of supervision has been associated with the amount and quality of feedback received (Magnuson, Norem, & Wilcoxon, 2000). Feedback need not always be given in written form, though it is helpful to give supervisees some tangible feedback throughout the supervision process. The inability to use videotaping in many community mental health settings has led to the creation of alternative methods to evaluate competency. One form of evaluation that has proven particularly helpful is the establishment of co-therapy opportunities whereby the author co-leads a group or individual session with a supervisee. While such an approach can create some logistical challenges, namely the assurance that clients have been previously informed and consented to this potential method, it can provide some rich opportunities for evaluation. Such co-therapy experiences afford the opportunity to directly observe supervisee skill level. Co-therapy or direct observation also provides material for future supervision sessions, which might include highlighting supervisee strengths or skill deficiencies or an opportunity to realign goals for supervision.

Other less intrusive forms of evaluation may be used, including role-plays, case note evaluation, and having supervisees complete written and oral case conceptualisations. Another often forgotten vehicle for evaluation is the supervision relationship itself. Most counselling professionals recognise the benefits of using immediacy in the counselling relationship. However, supervisors often overlook the potential benefit of using conflict and other dynamics in the supervision relationship to evaluate how supervisees utilise problem-solving skills to negotiate such challenges.

Protocol for Handling Emergencies and Crisis Situations

Given that community mental health professionals are among the frontline of service providers for a population that has the potential for high-risk behaviour, it is imperative that supervisors and supervisees establish a plan for how emergencies (e.g., suicidal/homicidal clients, suspected reports of child abuse or neglect, how to document following a suicide risk assessment, following through with documentation that is required by various local and state agencies, etc.) will be handled. As indicated earlier, this emergency protocol should not only be discussed verbally but should be confirmed in writing through the supervision contract.

Osborn and Davis (1996) have suggested that the emergency protocol should be included in the procedural considerations section of the supervision contract. Essentially, supervisees should know who to contact, under what circumstances to contact and the method for communicating with the supervisor. Supervisees should understandably become more confident with their abilities to handle crisis situations with time and feedback. However, the supervisor also shares 'vicarious liability' (Bernard & Goodyear, 2004, p. 68; Magnuson et al., 2000, p. 179) for the actions or inaction of supervisees, and thus supervisees are expected to keep the supervisor well informed of any potential or actual risk issues promptly.

Summary

This section has highlighted some of the unique elements for those who supervise community mental health professionals. While some of the issues themselves may also appear relevant for other areas of the counselling profession, they take on a unique form in the postgraduate supervision practice for community mental health professionals. This section has reviewed some of the primary issues for consideration, including ways to help organise the supervision experience, challenges and strategies related to evaluation, and ways of establishing protocols for handling emergencies and crisis situations.

Concluding Statement

This chapter has offered an overview of the unique aspects of supervision in five specialty areas. The authors have described historical developments as well as current trends and issues regarding supervision in the areas of marriage and family therapy, school counselling, alcohol and drug counselling, and the unique settings of university training clinics and community mental health organisations. One can readily see the influences of treatment context and setting on clinical supervision in these diverse specialty areas. As supervision in these specialisations has developed over time, professional organisations have increasingly established standards and guidelines for best practices of supervision. This trend is likely to continue in the future as increased attention is paid to the important role of supervision in various disciplines and settings.

Marriage and Family Therapy
Educational Questions and Activities

1. Consider the three strategies mentioned in MFT supervision (i.e., genograms, live supervision, and reflecting teams). Identify the strengths and limitations of each. Address your personal reaction to each strategy and discuss how supervisees and clients might respond to the use of each strategy.

   Answer: Genograms: Strengths: promotes therapist self-awareness, help with stuck cases, can assist supervisor in understanding context of therapist and client; Limitations: some might be reluctant to share personal information, might be inconsistent with preferred style, could stir up emotional issues. Live supervision: Strengths: Immediacy and unfiltered information, can intervene in actual session, therapist feels supported; Limitations: therapist can become overly dependent and can limit development of therapist's own style, client or therapist might feel watched and dislike interruptions, technology might not be available. Reflecting teams: Strengths: can help teach value of multiple perspectives, observers are more involved and attentive, clients hear directly from team members; Limitations: multiple views could be overwhelming or confusing for client or therapist, competition among team members could develop, can be challenging for therapist or supervisor to take a more challenging and hierarchical position if needed.

2. Select a clinical case for discussion. Identify how isomorphism, family life cycle issues and multicultural and diversity issues might be at play in the therapeutic system. Be sure to include attention to various levels (i.e., the client, therapist, and supervisor levels) and note any significant interactions among these levels.

   Answer: Isomorphism addresses patterns or processes that exist at various levels of a system and might include things like interpersonal dynamics, denial, emotional tone, taking responsibility, etc. Family life cycle stages or experiences for the client(s), therapist and supervisor might be relevant here, and could enhance or hamper therapeutic effectiveness. One could also consider other developmental factors, such as experience level of the therapist and supervisor and the client's previous experience in therapy. Multicultural and diversity issues of the client(s), therapist, and supervisor could include differences or similarities in race, ethnicity, gender, sexual orientation, class, age, disability, etc. One might also consider the degree of awareness and knowledge of multicultural and diversity issues at the client, therapist and supervisor levels.

Selected Internet Resources

- http://www.aamft.org/

  Website of the American Association for Marriage and Family Therapy, the primary professional organisation for MFT in the US and Canada. Includes guidelines for Approved Supervisors, the AAMFT Approved Supervisor Handbook, and a service for finding Approved Supervisors.

- http://www.aifs.gov.au/afrc/

  Website of the Australian Institute of Family Studies (Australia's foremost centre for research and information on family wellbeing) and the Australian Family Relations Clearinghouse (an informational and advisory unit focused on the enhancement of family relations across the lifespan).

- http://www.aft.org.uk/

  Website of the Association for Family Therapy & Systemic Practice in the UK, the leading body representing those working with families in the UK.

Selected References for Further Reading

Liddle, H.A., Breunlin, D.C., & Schwartz R.C. (Eds.) (1988). *Handbook of family therapy training and supervision.* New York: Guilford Press.

Storm, C.L., & Todd, T.C. (Eds.) (1997). *The reasonably complete systemic supervisor resource guide.* Boston: Allyn & Bacon.

Todd, T.C., & Storm, C.L. (Eds.) (1997). *The complete systemic supervisor.* Boston: Allyn & Bacon.

School Counseling

Educational Questions and Activities

1. Supervision is a transformational process designed to support personal and professional growth. Consider a metaphor to describe a supervisory experience, from the supervisor and/or supervisee perspective. Use words and/or pictures to depict this. Process in small groups. What supervisory concepts, models, and/or applications might serve to transform the metaphor?

   (a) This activity provides an opportunity for participants to discuss supervisory experiences, from less than optimal to excellent. Transforming the metaphor gives substance to the discussion around improved supervision strategies.

2. Discuss the ASCA National Model (2003) as a format for school counsellor supervision. What specific strategies would be appropriate for supervision in each of the four domains: Foundation, Delivery System, Management, and Accountability?

(a) This activity provides an opportunity to discuss the role of the school counsellor supervisor using the ASCA National Model as a structural basis. Supervision strategies, ideally, will relate to leadership, advocacy, collaboration, and systematic change within the four domains indicated above.

Selected Internet Resources

- http://www.schoolcounselor.org

  The American School Counselor Association (ASCA) supports school counsellors in working with students to achieve academic success and in preparing them to lead fulfilling lives as responsible members of society. ASCA's website is an international resource for school counsellors, providing professional development, publications and resources, research and advocacy to more than 24,000 professional school counsellors from around the world.

- http://www2.edtrust.org/EdTrust/Transforming+School+Counseling/main/

  The Education Trust advocates for academic achievement for all students at all levels, pre-kindergarten through college. The central goal is to close the achievement gaps that separate low-income students and students of colour from other young people. This website provides a wealth of information for professionals and general audiences on policies designed to improve education. The website contains articles, research, and data identifying achievement patterns among different groups of students. This is a valuable website for school counsellors.

Selected References for Further Reading

American School Counselor Association. (2003). *The ASCA national model: A framework for school counseling programs.* Alexandria, VA. Author.

Gysbers, N.C., & Henderson, P. (2006). *Developing and managing your school guidance programs* (4th ed.). Alexandria, VA: American Counseling Association.

Roberts, W.B., Morotti, A.A., Herrick, C., & Tilbury, R. (2001). Site supervisors of professional school counseling interns: Suggested guidelines. *Professional School Counseling, 4,* 208–215.

Studer, J. (2005). Supervising counselors-in-training: A guide for field supervisors. *Professional School Counseling, 8,* 353–359.

Alcohol and Drug Counselling

Educational Questions and Activities

1. Why do clinical supervisors need to have skills in administration?

   Answer: To assure policies and procedures are followed and standard practices are maintained for case record-keeping.

2. What are the areas of competencies the clinical supervisor must address with the alcohol and other drug abuse counsellor?
   Answer: Knowledge, skills and attitude.

3. Why is critical thinking a major component of the clinical supervision of alcohol and other drug abuse counsellors?
   Answer: Because clinical supervisors must be adept in applying skills, and train the counsellor to adapt to varying situations posed by clients.

Selected Internet Resources
- Clinical Supervision in Addiction Treatment
  http://www.unodc.org/ddttraining/treatment/VOLUME%20D/Topic%202/1.VoID_Clinical_Supervision.pdf
- TAP 21-A, Clinical Supervision
  http://www.nattc.org/resPubs/tap21/clinicalsupervisioncompetencies.html
- Competencies for Supervisors in the Treatment of Addictions
  http://www.cas.utulsa.edu/pshcy/2007%20update/supervision_in_addictions%5Bl%5D.pdf

These websites contain the actual annotated competencies for alcohol and other drug abuse counsellors as well as the actual annotated competencies for clinical supervisors of alcohol and other drug abuse counsellors.

Selected Reference for Further Reading
Powell, D. J. (2004). *Clinical supervision in alcohol and drug abuse counseling: Principles, models, methods* (3rd ed.). San Francisco: Jossey-Bass.

University Training Clinics
Educational Question
You are assigned to supervise a practicum group in a departmental training clinic. The supervision will be done in groups of ten students or fewer. As you imagine preparing for the orientation meeting, reflect on the following core areas that you would want to be prepared to discuss with your students: What are the main goals and objectives for the course? What are your hopes and expectations for the practicum students? What do you expect the students will be hoping for and expecting from this course? What are some of the advantages and disadvantages of group supervision? What are the ground rules for supervision? Where, when, and how often will the group be meeting?

Selected Internet Resource
- http://www.adptc.org
  This site of the Association of Directors of Psychology Training Clinics will provide important internet resources for training clinic directors

and clinical supervisors including downloadable copies of the complete Practicum Competencies Outline and Guidelines for Psychology Training Clinics.

Selected References for Further Reading

Meyer, J. (1994). *Developing and directing counselor education laboratories.* Alexandria, VA: American Counseling Association.

Neufeldt, S.A. (2007). *Supervision strategies for the first practicum.* Alexandria, VA: American Counseling Association.

Community Mental Health Counselling
Educational Questions and Activities

As a clinical supervisor of pre-licensed professionals, you must know the applicable laws and regulations pertaining to such practice. Visit your web-based governmental or regulatory site. Search for the public health code or its equivalent which contains relevant licensure laws, administrative rules for licensed health professions and other relevant documents. Respond to the following:

1. What is the 'scope of practice' for your profession or for that of your supervisee? The scope of practice will be defined in the licensing or regulatory law.

2. What does the public health code, or its equivalent, say about supervision? How much supervision must be face-to-face?

3. What are the regulations regarding duty to warn, confidentiality and privileged communication, mandated reporting of suspected child abuse and neglect, etc.?

4. What steps do you need to take as a clinical supervisor to become more informed of the legal and ethical dimensions for supervising community mental health professionals?

Selected Internet Resources

* http://www.acesonline.net/ethical_guidelines.asp

    This site provides the ethical guidelines for counselling supervisors, put forth by the Association for Counselor Education and Supervision.

* http://listserv.kent.edu/archives/cesnet-1.html

    This site allows the user to search for discussion topics that have been featured on CESNET, an international list-serve of counsellor educators and supervisors, counselling psychologists and other helping professionals who provide clinical and administrative supervision. While not all topics are supervision-related, this link allows the user to enter 'search-strings' on supervision related topics to see what others in the profession are saying.

- http://www.amhca.org/
This is the host-site for the American Mental Health Counselors' Association (AMHCA) and has information pertinent to those supervising in community mental health professions.

Selected References for Further Reading

Bernard, J.M., & Goodyear, R.K. (2008). *Fundamentals of clinical supervision* (4th ed.). Boston: Allyn & Bacon. (see also 2004 3rd ed.)

Campbell, J.M. (2006). *Essentials of clinical supervision.* Hoboken, NJ: John Wiley & Sons.

Falvey, J.E., & Cohen, C.R. (2003). The buck stops here: Documenting clinical supervision. *The Clinical Supervisor, 22,* 63–80.

Osborn, C.J., & Davis, T.E. (1996). The supervision contract: Making it perfectly clear. *The Clinical Supervisor, 14,* 121–134.

References

Agnew, T., Vaught, C.C., Getz, H.G., & Fortune, J. (2000). Peer group clinical supervision program fosters confidence and professionalism. *Professional School Counseling, 4,* 6–12.

Aiken, L.S., & LoSciuto, L.A. (1985). Ex-addict versus non-addict counselor's knowledge of drug use. *International Journal of the Addictions, 20,* 417–433.

American Association for Marriage and Family Therapy (AAMFT). (2007). *Approved supervisor designation standards and responsibilities handbook.* Alexandria, VA: Author.

American Counseling Association. (2005). *ACA code of ethics.* Alexandria, VA: Author.

American School Counseling Association (ASCA). (2004). *Ethical standards for school counselors.* Retrieved June 11, 2008, from www.schoolcounselor.org/content.asp?contentid=173

American School Counselor Association (ASCA). (2003). *The ASCA national model: A framework forschool counseling programs.* Alexandria, VA. Author.

Andersen, T. (1987). The reflecting team: Dialogue and meta-dialogue in clinical work. *Family Process, 26,* 415–428.

Andersen, T. (Ed.). (1990). *The reflecting team: Dialogues and dialogues about the dialogues.* Kent, England: Borgmann Publishing.

Association for Counselor Education and Supervision (ACES). (1995). Ethical guidelines for counseling supervisors. *Counselor Education and Supervision, 34,* 270–276.

Association of Directors of Psychology Training Clinics (ADPTC). (n.d.). *Mission statement.* Retrieved July 2, 2008, from: http://www.ADPTC.org

Association of Directors of Psychology Training Clinics (ADPTC). (2006). *Guidelines for training clinics.* Retrieved July 2, 2008, from: http://www.ADPTC.org

Bahrick, A.S., Russell, R.K., & Salmi, S.W. (1991). The effects of role induction on trainees' perceptions of supervision. *Journal of Counseling and Development, 69,* 434–438.

Benshoff, J.M. (2003, September). *Introduction to supervision. Supervision workshop.* George Mason University, Fairfax, VA. As cited in Murphy, S. & Kaffenberger, C.

(2007). ASCA national model: The foundation for supervision of practicum and internship students. *Professional School Counseling, 10,* 289–296.

Benshoff, J.M., & Paisley, P.O. (1996). The structured peer consultation model for school counselors. *Journal of Counseling and Development, 74,* 314–318.

Bernard, J.M. (1979). Supervisor training: A discrimination model. *Counselor Education andSupervision, 19,* 60–68.

Bernard, J.M. (1997). The discrimination model. In C.E. Watkins, Jr. (Ed.), *Handbook of psychotherapy supervision* (pp. 310–327). New York: Wiley.

Bernard, J.M., & Goodyear, R. K. (1998). *Fundamentals of clinical supervision* (2nd ed.). Needham Heights, MA: Allyn & Bacon.

Bernard, J.M., & Goodyear, R.K. (2004). *Fundamentals of clinical supervision* (3rd ed) Boston: Allyn & Bacon.

Borders, L.D., & Brown, L.L. (2005). Ethical issues in supervision. In L. B. Borders (Ed.) *The new handbook of counseling supervision* (pp. 49–72). Mahwah, NJ: Lawrence Erlbaum.

Borders, L.D., & Brown, L.L. (2005). *The new handbook of counseling supervision.* Mahwah, NJ: Lawrence Erlbaum.

Bordin, E.S. (1983). A working alliance based model of supervision. *The Counselling Psychologist, 11,* 35–42.

Bradley, L. (1989). *Counselor supervision* (2nd ed.). Bristol, PA: Accelerated Development.

Bradley, L.J., & Kottler, J.A. (2001). Overview of counselor supervision. In L.J. Bradley & N. Ladany (Eds.), *Counselor supervision: Principles, process, and practice* (3rd ed., pp. 3–27). Philadelphia: Brunner-Routledge.

Bradley, J.R., & Olson, J.K. (1980). Training factors influencing felt psychotherapeutic competence of psychology trainees. *Professional Psychology, 11,* 930–934.

Braverman, S. (1997). The use of genograms in supervision. In T.C. Todd & C.L. Storm (Eds.), *The complete systemic supervisor* (pp. 349–362). Boston: Allyn & Bacon.

Butler, S.K, & Constantine, M.G. (2006). Web-based peer supervision, collective self-esteem and case conceptualization ability in school counselor trainees. *Professional School Counseling, 10,* 146–152.

Carter, B., & McGoldrick, M. (Eds.) (2005). *The expanded family life cycle: Individual, family, and social perspectives* (3rd ed.). Boston: Allyn & Bacon.

Center for Substance Abuse Treatment. (2006). Addiction counseling competencies: The knowledge, skills and attitudes of professional practice. *Technical Assistance Publication (TAP) Series 21. DHHS Publication No. (SMA) 06–4171.* Rockville, MD: Substance Abuse and Mental Health Services Administration.

Center for Substance Abuse Treatment. (2007). Competencies for Substance Abuse Treatment Clinical Supervisors. *Technical Assistance Publication (TAP) Series 21-A. DHHS Publication No. (SMA) 07–4242.* Rockville, MD: Substance Abuse and Mental Health Services Administration.

Council for the Accreditation of Counseling and Related Education Programs (CACREP). (2009). *2009 Standards.* Retrieved August 25, 2008, from: http://www.cacrep.org/2009standards.pdf

Corey, G., Corey, M.S., & Callanan, P. (2007). *Issues and ethics in the helping professions* (7th ed.). Belmont, CA: Thomson Brooks/Cole.

Crutchfield, L.B., & Borders, L.D. (1997). Impact of two clinical peer supervision models on practicing school counselors. *Journal of Counseling and Development, 75,* 219–230.

Dollarhide, D.T., & Miller, G.M. (2006). Supervision for preparation and practice of school counselors: Pathways to excellence. *Counselor Education and Supervision, 45,* 242–252.

Drapela, V.J., & Drapela, G.B. (1986). The role of the counselor in intern supervision. *The School Counselor, 34,* 93–99.

Falender, C.A., & Shafranske, E.P. (2004). Evaluation of the supervisory process. In *Clinical supervision: A competency-based approach* (pp. 195–226). Washington, DC: American Psychological Association.

Fall, M., & Sutton, J. M. (2004). *Clinical supervision: A handbook for practitioners.* Boston: Pearson.

Falvey, J.E., & Bray, T.E. (2002). *Managing clinical supervision: Ethical practice and legal risk management.* Pacific Grove, CA: Brooks/Cole-Thomson Learning.

Foy, C., & Breunlin, D. (2001). Integrative supervision: A metaframeworks perspective. In S. McDaniel, D. Lusterman, & C. Philpot (Eds.), *Integrating family therapy: An ecosystemic approach* (pp. 387–394). Washington, DC: American Psychological Association.

Freedman, J., & Combs, G. (1996). *Narrative therapy: The social construction of preferred realities.* New York: Norton.

Ginsburg, R.D. (2000). Challenges for trainees on inpatient units. *The Clinical Supervisor, 19,* 199–204.

Gysbers, N.C., & Henderson, P. (2001). Comprehensive guidance and counseling programs: A rich history and a bright future. *Professional School Counseling, 4,* 246–256.

Gysbers, N.C., & Henderson, P. (2006). *Developing and managing your school guidance programs* (4th ed.). Alexandria, VA: American Counseling Association.

Haley, J. (1976). *Problem solving therapy.* San Francisco: Jossey-Bass.

Hatcher, R.L., & Lassiter, K.D. (2007). Initial training in professional psychology: The practicum competencies outline. *Training and Education in Professional Psychology, 1,* 49–63.

Heather, N., & Miller, W.R. (Eds.). (1998). *Treating addictive behaviors* (2nd ed.). New York: Plenum Press.

Henderson, P. (2000). *Supervision of school counselors.* Greensboro, NC: ERIC Clearinghouse on Counseling and Student Services. (ERIC Document Reproduction Service No. ED372353).

Henderson, P., & Lampe, R.E. (1992). Clinical supervision of school counselors. *The School Counselor, 39,* 151–158.

Herlihy, B. (2002). Legal and ethical issues in school counselor supervision — Special issue: Legal and ethical issues in school counseling. *Professional School Counseling, 6,* 1–8.

Herlihy, B., Gray, N., & McCollum, V. (2002). Legal and ethical issues in school counselor supervision. *Professional School Counseling, 6,* 55–60.

Holloway, E.L. (1995). *Clinical supervision: A systems approach.* Thousand Oaks, CA: Sage.

Juhnke, G.A., & Culbreth, J.R. (1994). Clinical supervision in addictions counseling: Special challenges and solutions. *ERIC Digest*. Available at http://www.ericdigests. org/1995-1/clinical.htm

Lawson, A.W., Lawson, G.W., & Rivers, P.C. (1996). *Essentials of chemical dependency counseling* (2nd ed.). Gaithersburg, MD: Aspen Publishers

Lawson, G., Petosa, R., & Peterson, J. (1982). Diagnosis of alcoholism by recovering alcoholics and by non-alcoholics. *Journal of Studies on Alcohol, 43*, 139–154.

Lee, R., Nichols, D., Nichols, W., & Odom, T. (2004). Trends in family therapy supervision: The past 25 years and into the future. *Journal of Marital and Family Therapy, 30*, 61–69.

Lewis, J.A. (Ed.). (1994). *Addictions: Concepts and strategies for treatment*. Gaithersburg, MD: Aspen Publishers.

Lindblaum, G., TenEyck, T.G., & Gallon, S.L. (2005). *Clinical supervision: Building chemical dependency counselor skills* (3rd ed.). Salem, OR: Northwest Addiction Technology Transfer Center.

Liddle, H.A. (1988). Systemic supervision: Conceptual overlays and pragmatic guidelines. In H.A. Liddle, D.C. Breunlin, & R.C. Schwartz (Eds.), *Handbook of family therapy training and supervision* (pp. 153–171). New York: Guilford Press.

Liddle, H.A., Davidson, G., & Barrett, M (1988). Outcomes of live supervision: Trainee perspectives. In H.A. Liddle, D.C. Breunlin, & R.C. Schwartz (Eds.), *Handbook of family therapy training and supervision* (pp. 386–398). New York: Guilford Press.

Littrell, J.M.; Lee-Borden, N., & Lorenz, J.A. (1979). A developmental framework for counseling supervision. *Counselor Education and Supervision, 19*, 119–136. As cited in Protivack, J. (2003). *Supervision modalities developmentally appropriate for school counselors.* (ERIC Document Reproduction Service No ED474587).

LoSciuto, L.A., Aiken, L.S., Ausetts, M.A., & Brown, B.S. (1984). Paraprofessional versus professional drug counselors and their clients. *International Journal of the Addictions, 19*, 233–252.

Lowinson, J.H., & Ruiz, P. (Eds.). (2004). *A comprehensive textbook* (4th ed.). Baltimore, MD: Lippincott, Williams & Wilkins.

Luke, M., & Bernard, J. (2006). The school counseling supervision model: An extension of the discrimination model. *Counselor Education and Supervision, 46*, 282–295.

Machell, P.F. (1987). Obligation of a clinical supervisor. *Alcoholism Treatment Quarterly, 4*, 105–108.

Magnuson, S., Black, L., & Norem, K. (2004). Supervising school counselors and interns: Resources for site supervisors. *Journal of Professional Counseling: Practice, Theory and Research, 32*, 4–15.

Magnuson, S., Norem, K., & Wilcoxon, A. (2000). Clinical supervision of prelicensed counselors: Recommendations for consideration and practice. *Journal of Mental Health Counseling, 22*, 176–188.

Mann, M. (1973). *Attitude: Key to successful treatment*. Springfield, IL: Charles C. Thomas.

McGeorge, C., Carlson, T., Erickson, M. & Guttormson, H. (2007). Creating and evaluating a feminist-informed social justice couple and family therapy training model. *Journal of Feminist Family Therapy, 18*, 1–38.

McGoldrick, M., Gerson, R., & Petry, S. (2008). *Genograms: Assessment and intervention* (3rd. ed.). New York: Norton.

McMahon, M., & Simons, R. (2004). Supervision training for professional counselors: An exploratory study. *Counselor Education and Supervision, 43*, 301—309.

Miller, G., & Dollarhide, C. (2006). Supervision in schools: Building pathways to excellence. *Counselor Education and Supervision, 45*, 296–303.

Miller, N.S., Gold, M.S., & Smith, D.E. (Eds.). (1997). *Manual of therapeutics for addiction*. New York: Wiley–Liss.

Milsom, A., & Akos, P. (2005). CACREP's relevance to professionalism for school counsellor educators. *Counselor Education and Supervision, 45*, 147–158.

Montalvo, B. (1973). Aspects of live supervision. *Family Process, 12*, 343–359.

Montalvo, B., & Storm, C.L. (1997). Live supervision revolutionizes the supervision process. In T.C. Todd & C.L. Storm (Eds.), *The complete systemic supervisor* (pp. 283–297). Boston: Allyn & Bacon.

Morgan, M., & Sprenkle, D. (2007). Toward a common-factors approach to supervision. *Journal of Marital and Family Therapy, 33*, 1–17.

Murphy, S., & Kaffenberger, C. (2007). ASCA national model: The foundation for supervision of practicum and internship students. *Professional School Counseling, 10*, 289–296.

Muse-Burke, J.L., Ladany, N., & Deck, M.D. (2001). The supervisory relationship. In L.J. Bradley & N. Ladany (Eds.), *Counselor supervision: Principles, process and practice* (pp. 28–57). New York: Brunner–Routledge.

Nelson, M.D., & Johnson, P. (1999). School counselors as supervisors: An integrated approach for supervising counseling interns. *Counselor Education and Supervision, 39*, 89–101.

Neufeldt, S.A. (2007). *Supervision strategies for the first practicum*. American Counseling Association: Alexandria, VA.

Nichols, M.P., & Schwartz, R.C. (2007). *Family therapy: Concepts and methods* (8th ed.). Boston: Pearson/Allyn & Bacon.

Osborn, C.J., & Davis, T.E. (1996). The supervision contract: Making it perfectly clear. *The Clinical Supervisor, 14*, 121–134.

Page, B.J., Pietrzak, D.R., & Sutton, J.M. (2001). National survey of school counsellor supervision. *Counselor Education and Supervision, 41*, 142–150.

Paisley, P.O., & McMahon, G. (2001). School counseling for the 21st century: Challenges and opportunities. *Professional School Counseling, 5*, 106–115.

Peace, S.A., & Sprinthall, N.A. (1998). Training school counselors to supervise beginning counselors: Theory, research, and practice. *Professional School Counselor, 1*, 2–8.

Powell, D.J. (2004). *Clinical supervision in alcohol and drug abuse counseling: Principles, models, methods*. San Francisco: Jossey–Bass.

Protivnak, J. (2003). *Supervision modalities developmentally appropriate for schoolcounselors*. (ERIC Document Reproduction Service No ED474587).

Prouty, A., Thomas, V., Johnson, S., & Long, J. (2001). Methods of feminist family therapy supervision. *Journal of Marital and Family Therapy, 27*, 85–97.

Remley, T.P., Jr., Benshoff, J.M., & Mowbray, C.A. (1987). A proposed model for peer supervision. *Counselor Education and Supervision, 27,* 53–60.

Roberts, E.B., & Borders, L.D. (1994). Supervision of school counselors: Administrative, program, and counseling. *The School Counselor, 41,* 149–158.

Roberts, J. (1997). Reflecting processes and 'supervision': Looking at ourselves as we work with others. In T.C. Todd & C.L. Storm (Eds.), *The complete systemic supervisor* (pp. 334–348). Boston: Allyn & Bacon.

Robinson, C.R. (2001). The role of critical thinking skills in counselor supervision inquiry: Critical thinking. *Across the Disciplines, 20*(3), 19–25.

Ronnestad, M. H., & Skovholt, T. M. (1993). Supervision of beginning and advanced graduate students of counseling and psychotherapy. *Journal of Counseling and Development, 71,* 396–405.

Sauer, E.M., & Huber, D.M. (2007). Implementing the Boulder Model of training in a psychology training clinic. *Journal of Contemporary Psychotherapy, 37,* 221–228.

Sprenkle, D., & Blow, A. (2004). Common factors and our sacred models. *Journal of Marital and Family Therapy, 30,* 113–129.

Starling, P.V. & Baker, S.B. (2000). Structured peer group practicum supervision: Supervisees' perceptions of supervision theory. *Counselor Education and Supervision, 39,* 163–176.

Stoltenberg, C. (1981). Approaching supervision from a developmental perspective: The counselor complexity model. *Journal of Counseling Psychology, 28,* 59–65.

Storm, C. L., Todd, T. C., Sprenkle, D. H., & Morgan, M. M. (2001). Gaps between supervision assumptions and common practice: Suggested best practices. *Journal of Marital and Family Therapy, 27,* 227–239.

Studer, J. (2005). Supervising counselors-in-training: A guide for field supervisors. *Professional School Counseling, 8,* 353–359.

Studer, J., & Oberman, A. (2006). The use of the ASCA national model in supervision. *Professional School Counseling, 10,* p. 82–87

Sutton, J.M., & Page, B.J. (1994). Post-degree clinical supervision of school counselors. *The School Counselor, 39,* 23–33.

The Education Trust. (2003). *National center for transforming school counseling.* Retrieved June 23, 2008, from http://www2.edtrust.org/EdTrust/Transforming+School+Counseling/main

Todd, T.C., & Storm, C.L. (Eds.) (1997). *The complete systemic supervisor.* Boston: Allyn & Bacon.

Todd, T.C., & Storm, C.L. (1997). Thoughts on the evolution of MFT supervision. In T.C. Todd & C.L. Storm (Eds.), *The complete systemic supervisor* (pp. 1–16). Boston: Allyn & Bacon.

Tromski-Klingshirn, D. (2006). Should the clinical supervisor be the administrative supervisor? The ethics versus the reality. *The Clinical Supervisor, 25,* 53–67.

Unger, M. (2006). Practicing as a postmodern supervisor. *Journal of Marital and Family Therapy, 32,* 59–71.

Valle, S.K. (1984). Supervision in alcoholism counseling? *Alcoholism Treatment Quarterly, 1,* 101–114.

Wilkerson, K. (2006). Peer supervision for the professional development of school counselors: Toward an understanding of terms and findings. *Counselor Education & Supervision, 46,* 59–67.

Witmer, L. (1996). Clinical psychology. *American Psychologist, 51,* 248–251. (Reprinted from *The Psychological Clinic,* 1907, *1,* 1–9).

Wood, C., & Rayle, A. (2006). A model of school counseling supervision: The goals, functions, roles, and systems model. *Counselor Education and Supervision, 45,* 253–266.

———++++———

chapter nineteen

The Use of Technology in Supervision

DeeAnna Merz Nagel, Stephen Goss and Kate Anthony

Technology has been used to enhance clinical supervision — to some extent at least — for several decades. While we will offer a cursory overview of assistive technologies that have been in the counsellor educator mainstream for some time, our primary focus will address clinical supervision that is delivered via technology developed largely since the late 1980s and early 1990s. In short, we will move past what by now may be considered traditional uses of technology in supervision to more advanced ways in which technology can be utilised to deliver clinical supervision.

Technology Assisted Supervision

Transcription, tape recorders, 'bug-in-the-ear', audiovisual recordings, and videotaping are all terms that, historically, have encompassed the use of technology in supervision. For instance, we have used one form of technology or another to capture verbatim transcripts or other recordings of counselling sessions for later review by supervisors. Transcription is still used in clinical and university settings to capture the actual interview or counselling session. So much can be processed and discussed with the actual transcript in hand. Studies (e.g., Arthur & Gfroerer, 2002) have supported the use of transcription as a method for feedback during supervision. The actual session is transcribed through transcription apparatus or word processing. Thus, the spoken word is captured and can be analysed for content and therapeutic style, and even pauses are accounted for in the transcript. The use of technology for transcription purposes has been in place for decades.

Along with transcription devices, audio and visual technological assistance can be used to capture para-linguistic cues. Historically, this has been accomplished by using a tape-recorder or by what may now seem like even more archaic technology such as phonographic discs. As long ago as 1942, when record players were still something of a rarity, Carl Rogers noted with enthusiasm the (then) remarkable benefits of being able to actually hear the words and tone used by both counsellor and client in sessions:

> These recorded interviews have proven extremely valuable in the training of advanced students ... they give a vivid and clear-cut picture of various client attitudes which is much more meaningful than anything the counselor can obtain through abstract descriptions ... Probably the most significant use of our recordings is in the process of supervision. It is the unanimous testimony of counselors that they have gained a great deal and have been able to correct many mistakes ... [allowing] the inexperienced and experienced counselor alike a new understanding of the therapeutic process. (Rogers, 1942, pp. 429–431)

Rogers concluded that,

> ... the use of these relatively new mechanical devices provides for the first time a sound basis for the investigation of therapeutic processes, and the teaching and improvement of therapeutic techniques. Therapy need no longer be vague, therapeutic skill need no longer be an intuitive gift. (p. 434)

Today we use digital technology to record such 'priceless raw material' (Rogers, 1942, p. 431) and have a plethora of technologies from which to choose, all of which are far simpler to use than acetate-covered metal discs. With the advent of video recorders, we have added visual components as well. In most cases, transcription and audio/visual recording can be used to capture the supervisee's session with a client and afterwards, the written word and/or the audio/visual recording can be used in clinical supervision to discuss the supervisee's abilities, strengths and areas requiring improvement. With the advent of video CD, DVD or hard disk, instant review is available. The use of technology has allowed supervisors to guide and teach supervisees in ways that were not possible decades ago. Properly used, technology can add to the supervisor's skill set and enhance his or her theoretical orientation. The supervisor who is guided by theory should use adjunctive technology such as videotaping in a purposeful manner (Pelling & Renard, 1999) and in such a way as not to interrupt the rich process between supervisor and supervisee.

Recordings of therapy sessions, and supervisory ones, allow detailed analysis of critical moments in the process. Since the excitement surrounding audio recording noted in 1942, specialist supervisory techniques have been developed extending the depth and detail available to practitioners. An example is Interpersonal Process Recall (IPR; Kagan, 1980; Gimmestad & Greenwood, 1974), a recording-based technique that has in itself led to significant enhancements of the supervisory process and, in research settings, notable refinements of our understanding of even the most fundamental elements of counsellor competence, such as the meaning of congruence or transparency (Grafanaki, 2003; Grafanaki & McLeod, 2002). IPR requires counsellor and client, or supervisor and supervisee, to revisit critical moments in their sessions by reviewing video or audio recordings. The supervisor's role is to function as a source of support and expertise to both parties by inquiring about their experience and facilitating their exploration and description of each moment or segment of a session selected for in-depth examination. As a result of what Kagan (1980) identified as a tendency among counsellors to be overly diplomatic, their unassisted account of their work may be incomplete or inaccurate, whether through behaving as though they had not properly understood the depth of implications in client statements by 'feigning clinical naivety' so as to avoid areas towards which they are aversive, or simply by 'tuning out', which Cashwell (2001) describes as being the result of the counsellor becoming 'engrossed in their own thought process [while] trying to decide what to do next. The result is that the counsellor misses messages from the client, some of which may seem obvious to the supervisor' (p. 1) when reviewing the recorded session. Although now very familiar to many counsellors and supervisors, and well established, such extensions of supervision that would otherwise rely on the practitioner's more or less biased or selective clinical memory have proved highly effective in extending and enhancing the process of learning from clinical experience that is the basis of supervisory work. The relative objectivity achievable through any systematic use of audio or video recordings offers a clear advantage.

Enhancing Use of Video and Audio through Analytical and Research Software

Increasingly, software tools have been developed that allow analysis of audio or recordings of sessions in more sophisticated ways than simply watching or listening to them as they occurred. Despite being primarily intended and developed for research purposes, tools such as NVIVO™ (Richards, 1999; Walsh 2003) allow supervisors and supervisees to take on a more sophisticated role as investigators of clinical practice. Audio or video recordings of sessions can be replayed while a transcript and annotations scroll by on screen, synchronised with the recording as it plays. Once segments of the session have been coded according to content, affective expression or, indeed, to highlight any other features of particular interest, specific sections can not only be retrieved for targeted review, but also similarly coded sections of other recordings can be collated and their themes and characteristics studied at whatever level of detail may be required.

Thus, a counsellor or supervisor could readily examine the practitioners' habitual responses to, say, expressions of anger or aggression, discussions of specific family dynamics, examples of transference/countertransference, interpersonal processes or problematic emotional expression and so on. Where aspects of practice have been identified as requiring particular attention, it is a relatively straightforward, if time-consuming, process to build a library of recorded segments for comparison and more detailed review and to demonstrate developing counsellor competence over time. In this way, the benefits of supervision can be extended well beyond the time available for direct contact between supervisor and supervisee.

This is, perhaps, especially appropriate for trainee counsellors who may be expected to invest more time in examining aspects of their work in detail whether in preparation for supervision sessions, or to examine problematic areas of practice or particular aptitudes and successes. However, there is perhaps much potential in their use for qualified practitioners as a routine part of their continuing professional development.

As software becomes both more readily available, less costly and easier to use, this kind of detailed processing of sessions becomes increasingly accessible for practitioners as an extension of their practice as a matter of routine, wherever supervisory or developmental needs warrant the time and effort involved. Tools such as VideoPaper (Concord Consortium, 2005) are now available free of charge, and while affording less sophisticated analysis than programs developed for research purposes their relative ease of use makes them commensurately more readily used by nonspecialists, requiring very little more expertise than a word processor. Such applications have been used in counsellor training with some notable successes (Trahar, 2008) and can be readily applied in supervisory settings throughout a practitioner's career.

Extending Direct Observation

While observation of practice is commonplace in training settings, direct access to counselling sessions in routine practice is generally both impractical and, in many circumstances, may be considered unacceptably intrusive. However, where it is appropriate, it is not necessary for an observer to remain in the same room with counsellor and client, immensely reducing the impact of such observation. Originally, supervision methods using technology involved the use of two-way mirrors to view the supervision session while the supervisor wore headphones to listen actively. The supervisor intervened by knocking on the door. The supervisee answered the door, received the verbal input and implemented the strategy with the client. This technique has been enhanced with what is known as 'bug-in-the ear' technology, involving more advanced headsets and transmitters for both the supervisor and the supervisee. This has allowed for better continuity during the session and does not alert the client to the supervisor's immediate presence (Borders & Brown, 2005).

Miller, Miller and Evans (2002) summarise another form of technology that is used during live monitoring of the counselling session known as BITE or 'bug-in-the-eye'. This computer equipment is used to provide instant feedback during the session. A computer is located about a metre from the supervisee and another computer is available to the supervisor who is in another room. When the supervisor desires to interject a comment or suggestion, he/she uses text that appears on the supervisee's computer and is not visible to the client. Budget constraints have caused universities to avoid costly BITE systems, but today a similar process could be simulated utilising encrypted instant messaging between the supervisor and supervisee. The supervisee would place the computer screen at such an angle so that the client could not view the messages coming in or use a privacy screen that would not allow viewing of the text on the screen from different angles.

Delivering Clinical Supervision via Technology

Regardless of theoretical orientation, clinical supervisors are trained first as counsellors and understand the importance of the relationship. Rapport-building, trust and positive regard are universal components in establishing a counselling relationship with a client. Likewise, these components are essential in establishing the supervisory relationship as well. We will discuss several ways clinical supervision can be delivered via technology. It is important to understand that clinical supervision via technology, referred to as cybersupervision, online supervision, e-supervision and other similar terms, is not a theory or a technique, but rather delineates other pathways for the relationship to be experienced.

As a helpful framework, consider that counsellors now offer counselling and psychotherapeutic services via distance technology as either adjunct or as a stand-alone service. Counsellors may use phone, email, instant messaging, chat, videoconferencing or virtual world platforms to deliver services. The counsellor may choose one delivery method or combine several forms of technology to accommodate the client's needs. For instance, a counsellor may see a client face-to-face and offer intermittent between-session emails. Or a counsellor may offer text-based services that are through email, instant messaging or a combination. The use of webcams has also enhanced the online counselling process. With platforms that are increasingly available and with some actually tailored to the counselling profession, secure instant messaging, document and link sharing and the sharing of digital media during a videoconferencing session is now available as part of the suite of services a counsellor may offer. These varied examples illustrate the use of technology in counselling but may certainly extend to the provision of clinical supervision as well. We will summarily discuss each method of delivery as applied to the clinical supervision relationship.

Phone

The telephone, whether formally or not, has been used in clinical supervision and direction in many settings throughout the years. Many mental health practitioners have worked in settings whose direct or clinical supervisor was either available at regularly scheduled times or during cases requiring immediate or as-needed consultation. Mobile phones (also known as cell phones or handy phones in some parts of the world) have replaced pagers and beepers for many professionals and are used for similar purposes with regard to supervision and consultation.

Formal use of the phone for purposes of clinical supervision requires an understanding of the therapeutic and supervisory relationship without visual cues. While excellent listening skills are necessary in traditional counselling and supervision settings, the need for listening skills is heightened with the lack of visual cues. The supervisor must listen attentively without the benefit of facial expressions or body gestures that might further confirm an emotion. The tone of voice and pacing of the conversation, as well as the moments of silence, require more attention than traditional face-to-face settings. The ability to ask for clarification to avoid misunderstandings is essential. Creating an atmosphere that is conducive to phone conversations without the interruption of outside noises from either party's environment must be considered.

Additionally, the differences in the use of mobile phones versus landline phones must be understood. When the supervisor or supervisee uses mobile phones, each party may encounter differences in voice cadence and tone such as echo, tenor, buzzing and other static noises. When more than two people are on the line, as in a conference call, the same concerns may apply. It should also be considered that the same conversation via landline phones may cause different interpretations in the emotionality of the parties than when carried out on mobile telephones, not least because of the relative levels of privacy available, quality of connection and issues relating to ensuring use of telephones in circumstances appropriate to the needs of the conversation (Monk et al. 2004; Walsh & White, 2006).

Consider also that scheduled phone calls allow for forethought and intentionality with both parties having time to prepare. Impromptu phone calls involving a crisis or immediate supervisory issue may leave the supervisor and supervisee feeling unprepared for the interaction. Being caught 'off guard' may change the person's tone of voice. One party may hear an element of surprise in the other's voice. Tendencies to rush conversation or end the communication in cases of emergencies must be understood and not misinterpreted as either abrupt or casual responses to a situation.

Supervisors and supervisees may also use text messaging as an added form of communication using a mobile phone. While texting is often a brief form of communication, some may find the immediacy of a text message useful.

E-mail

Delivering clinical supervision via e-mail is not a new concept. While many clinical settings incorporate e-mail into traditional forms of clinical supervision, still other settings use e-mail casually, and use this delivery method to staff cases and offer feedback to supervisees. A supervisor may see a supervisee face-to-face and add e-mail as an adjunct between supervision sessions. Adjunct e-mails may be used so that the supervisee can write about his or her experience in between supervision sessions. The supervisor may send additional information for the supervisee to consider via e-mail at the close of a session. The supervisor may also utilise e-mail as a way to check-in with supervisees, particularly regarding difficult cases. The use of e-mail has become so common that most people understand e-mail etiquette. Still, a basic understanding of the components of an e-mail will assist both the supervisor and supervisee. All aspects of e-mail communication should be considered. From the e-mail subject line to the body of the e-mail to the e-mail closure, each part of the e-mail has the potential to carry expression and meaning. Conveying empathy and emotion through e-mail text using emoticons, parenthetical expression, emotional bracketing and quoted text are but examples of the richness of communicating in this medium (Suler, 2003).

Supervisors may construct e-mails differently and with different purposes depending from which theoretical orientation the supervisor is operating. E-mail is akin to letter writing in that both parties have a chance to be reflective and think through thoughts and suppositions during the composition. Because e-mail is an asynchronous form of communication, an immediate response should not be expected. Supervisors have an opportunity to posit questions to the supervisee and the supervisee can answer with researched or spontaneous thought.

Bulletin Board/Forum/Listserv

Bulletin boards and forums are similar in set-up and are usually hosted on a web page wherein parties can log in with a user name and password. The moderator of the forum can determine who has access to it and offer a prescreening/registration process or allow individuals to sign up at will. Listservs are similarly moderated. While forums are viewed by topic and each topic may have a thread of responses, listservs are generally delivered as an e-mail response or as a group of responses at the end of the day. Preferences for either forums or listservs vary. Forums and listservs can be useful to the clinical supervision process offering asynchronous group supervision or peer consultation. A forum can be set up to be moderated by a clinical supervisor who may choose to 'screen' each post before allowing the post to appear on the forum. The supervisor may alternatively allow postings by supervisees without prior screening and intercede as necessary to redirect or correct. Most listservs have fewer moderator features.

It should be noted that with e-mail and forums, the supervisee may have the opportunity to state in rather bold terms, what is on his or her mind; in this way, the asynchronous nature allows for emotional venting. The emotion can be released and the writer of the message can simply 'walk away' with no expectation of an immediate response. Munro (2002) accurately refers to this phenomenon as 'emotional hit and run'. The message may be particularly critical or may appear to have been written without forethought. The supervisor in turn has the opportunity to engage the supervisee in processing this material.

IM/Chat

Utilising Instant Messaging and Chat (internet relay chat) is an effective way to process clinical supervision issues either as a stand-alone experience or as adjunct to face-to-face supervision and/or other technology delivery methods. Supervisors can schedule formal sessions with supervisees weekly, replicating the typical clinical supervision hour familiar in most face-to-face settings. Supervisors who are offering direction and supervision in an agency setting may choose to be available for immediate contact, using symbols that are offered in most chat programs to signify availability (e.g., Available, Away, Busy, Do Not Disturb). Boundaries for impromptu contact should be established between the supervisor and supervisee so that a clear understanding exists regarding the need for immediate contact. Supervisees, with the proper established boundaries, may experience comfort knowing their supervisor is accessible regardless of the supervisee's intent or need to make immediate contact.

IM/Chat is synchronous, occurring in real-time. The tendency for the supervisee to use text for emotional venting as with asynchronous forms of communication is less likely. Still, the lack of visual and auditory cues may prompt a supervisee to state information of a personal nature that is not relevant or that might be more detailed than he or she would ordinarily share in a face-to-face session. The supervisor should be aware of this possibility and assist the supervisee in remaining focused on issues pertaining to clients and the therapeutic work setting.

Similar to the use of phone, IM/Chat can be different to face-to-face sessions in terms of pacing and moments of silence. While many IM/Chat programs offer a prompt that alerts the person that a response is forthcoming (e.g., *Sally is typing a response . . .*) other programs do not offer a textual cue to alert that the person is typing. Silences should be expected and, with proper pacing, addressed. In the context of a therapeutic chat session, the supervisee might benefit from the use of emotional bracketing to describe to the supervisor what feelings have been evoked during the clinical supervision session. This technique is certainly beneficial during psychoanalytic/psychodynamic supervisory sessions.

Videoconferencing/Webcam

Videoconferencing as a supervision training tool is being utilised in counsellor education programs and other allied health programs to enhance clinical insight. When visual and paralinguistic tools are considered necessary, the use of videoconferencing for group or individual supervision is a viable alternative. Many formal education programs and internships require a face-to-face component and, in lieu of the literal face-to-face meetings, the use of video technology can be a viable substitute. This solution also accommodates rural internship sites when face-to-face meetings are not feasible due to travel costs and time. Greater flexibility in scheduling and enhanced collaboration between the university program and the off-campus setting are also benefits (Dudding & Justice, 2004).

For clinical supervisors who do not work in an educational setting, the use of webcams can be added as a way to offer supervision with a visual component. The clinical supervisor can use a webcam with a supervisee for scheduled or impromptu appointments and can combine webcam with chat and e-mail as previously discussed.

Virtual Worlds

Virtual worlds such as Second Life™ are being used for many purposes including entertainment, education and psychotherapy. With this in mind, it is not too difficult to imagine a clinical supervision session taking place in a virtual world.

Virtual worlds offer the ability to create a different 'self' referred to as an avatar. The avatar is how a person presents themselves in the virtual world. For some people, the presentation is a representation of the person's perceived self. For others, the avatar is a representation of how the person would wish to be perceived. To provide clinical supervision in a virtual world is to add a visual component that is enhanced by imagination. The opportunity may simply provide a visually appealing component for the supervisor and supervisee or, depending on the theoretical orientation of the supervisor, avatar supervision may add more information to the process. For instance, a supervisor may have a better understanding of the supervisee after seeing and experiencing an avatar that is based on the supervisee's preference of perception.

Virtual world counselling and supervision offers Instant Messaging and chat and platforms like Second Life™ allow for blocking off a space, property or in this case, virtual office from anyone who may 'teleport' to the location. Additionally, proprietary software exists to allow for higher levels of secure communication. The supervisor's office can be created in the likeness of the supervisor's real-life office, or the supervisor can create a different ambience with the option of offering educational materials and web links from within the virtual world setting.

Considerations for the use of Technology in Supervision
Review of Current Standards

In 2001, the British Association for Counselling and Psychotherapy (BACP) published their first *Guidelines for Online Counselling and Psychotherapy* (Goss et al., 2001). In 2005 these were updated to include guidance for online supervision (Anthony & Jamieson, 2005) and further updated these with a 3rd edition after only another four years (Anthony & Goss, 2009). While the pace of change in the uses of technology in supervision and therapy is likely to continue to require such relatively frequent redrawing of ethical guidance, at the time of writing, the authors are unaware of any other formal standards, guidelines or ethical codes related to online clinical supervision.

In the United States, the National Board of Certified Counselors (NBCC) has created a document that contains a statement of principles for guiding the evolving practice of internet counselling, and offers a certification designation of Approved Clinical Supervisor (ACS) with its own code of ethics; however, neither document addresses specific ethical issues related to online supervision.

Also applicable in the United States, the National Association of Social Workers and the Association of Social Work Boards (2005) has developed standards for the use of technology in social work practice. This document briefly addresses supervision issues regarding acquired technological skill through supervision or consultation and awareness of pertinent laws that may restrict or allow the use of technology.

The Association for Counselor Education and Supervision (ACES), a division of the American Counseling Association, has established a Code of Ethics but reference is not made to technology or online supervision. ACES has, however, established Technical Competencies for Counselor Education with the latest revision completed in 2007 by the Technology Interest Network.

These are but three examples of various organisations that, while addressing clinical supervision and technology, have not yet addressed the delivery of clinical supervision via technology with formal standards, guidelines or codes of ethics.

Contracting/Informed Consent

Anthony and Goss (2009) address the following issues warranting negotiation in the contracting/informed consent process.

- Various methods of delivery exist and the mode of communication should be agreed upon prior to beginning supervision.
- Technical breakdowns, while not common, are unavoidable. Therefore, clearly established steps should be implemented when technological glitches occur.
- Boundaries regarding scheduling of sessions and immediate availability should be established.
- Record-keeping methods including storage and disposal should be stated.
- Misunderstandings are inevitable and the contract should state how misunderstandings will be negotiated.
- Clearly established rules and sanctions for group supervision should be stated in the contract.

Confidentiality should be addressed and specifics related to the use of technology should extend to the client of the supervisee. While the supervisee may not be utilising technology with his or her client, the client has a right to be informed about whether or not case details will be discussed with a supervisor via distance technology applications. As reflected in the new BACP guidelines and later in this chapter, encryption or equivalent levels of security should be incorporated into transmission of communication via the internet. In addition, supervisors should also be aware of confidentiality issues when using mobile phones for conversation or SMS texting.

Ethical/Legal Concerns

Clinical supervisors must practise within their realm of expertise. The primary purpose for clinical supervision is to teach, assist and mentor a mental health practitioner who requires guidance in order to provide the best standard of care to his or her clients. If the clinical supervision process is one that is fraught with technological glitches, pauses and general unease due to a lack of proficiency, the richness of the supervisory process will be lost. It is incumbent upon the supervisor to ensure that the supervisor and the supervisee possess the competencies necessary to engage in online clinical supervision. Following such standards as the aforementioned Technical Competencies for Counselor Education assures that within college and university settings, supervisors and supervisees have an expected level of competency with regard to the use of technology. These competencies will be discussed later in this chapter.

In addition to competency and proficiency with the technology, Dudding and Justice (2004) suggest that issues related to portability, versatility, ease of use and cost-effectiveness should be addressed. By attending to these concerns prior to implementing technology into the supervision process, the integrity of clinical supervision and the quality of care to the client can be maintained.

Beyond ease of use, other ethical concerns relate to the authentication of the supervisor and supervisee. If the supervisor is practicing in a university setting this issue may not be as relevant, but for independent clinical supervisors who may practice with people with whom a face-to-face relationship has not been established, authentication of identity is paramount. Likewise, the supervisee should be able to verify the supervisor's credentials and experience (Anthony & Goss, 2009). Supervisors can provide information on their web sites that delineate experience by posting a curriculum vitae and providing links to credentialing and licensing bodies. Supervisors can verify a supervisee's identity by asking for a copy of school transcripts, a driver's license number and other information during the informed consent and contractual process.

Consideration should be given to the supervisor's licensing laws and scope of practice. Laws may dictate who may provide clinical supervision in certain jurisdictions. Along with legal concerns and risk management, supervisors should consider carrying liability (malpractice) insurance and enquire from the insurance provider about coverage when the service is delivered via technology.

Encryption/Confidentiality

In supervision, training and counsellor education, we have become accustomed to 'blinding the record'; ensuring that identifying information is revealed on a 'need to know' basis. Clinical supervisors may discuss cases with other peer professionals. During group supervision and supervisees may come from various and different clinical settings to discuss cases. Most group supervision practice involves the understanding that case information is to remain confidential. The same concept applies to supervision delivered via technology. Encrypted services should be considered for all clinical supervision sessions involving the technology discussed within this chapter. Encryption, while not required by any set of laws, has been incorporated into guidelines and codes of ethics as best practice regarding the transmission of confidential client information. If encryption is not possible, and provided your code of ethics allows for exceptions, the lack of encryption and risk to confidentiality should be made a component of the informed consent process.

Verbatim Material

Verbatim written records of counselling or supervision sessions can be generated by transcription or from e-mail, chat or other text-based forms of distance provision (Anthony, 2003; Chechele & Stofle, 2003; Colon & Friedman, 2003; Goss & Anthony, 2003, Anthony and Goss, 2009). The ease with which records of any kind can be copied, distributed and redistributed simultaneously opens the possibility of consulting for routine supervision or to access specialist expertise across any distance. However, there is a significantly increased need to pay attention to data protection issues and issues of confidentiality. Such detailed records must, of course, be treated with immense care and their creation brings clear risks and responsibilities for those affected. Transmission of any verbatim records, even when carefully and thoroughly anonymised, must always preserve privacy for both client and counsellor and any others directly related to the matter under discussion and, indeed, the supervisor where relevant. It is essential, for example, that any records sent over the internet are securely encrypted. Now that encryption software is widely available, can be free of charge and is easy to use (see Hushmail.com, for example), this should be considered a basic and required extension of the usual ethical requirement to protect the content of therapy from unwarranted intrusion. Failing to take sufficient measures to protect confidentiality may now be considered a basic lapse in the ethical judgment of the practitioner or supervisor. Ruled out, for example, is the use of publicly accessible or unencrypted web sites, blogs, chat or e-mail for detailed case discussion or supervision, just as it does for the provision of distance counselling itself.

Nonetheless, the potential value of verbatim records of therapeutic encounters should not be underestimated. The same applies, of course, to supervisory relationships conducted via any text-based means. Given suitable protection, it is possible for a supervisor to have access to the entire content of the therapeutic process. Both client and counsellor, or supervisor and supervisee, can readily review whole therapy or supervision sessions. The verbatim record can also be subjected to detailed textual analysis. A number of methods exist for this, often developed originally for qualitative research purposes, from grounded theory (Glaser, 1992; Glaser & Strauss, 1967; Mey & Mruck 2007; Strauss & Corbin, 1990) to stanza analysis (Gee, 1986, 1991, 2005; McLeod, 2001) to narrative techniques (Angus & McLeod, 2004; McLeod, 1997). The potential utility of such analysis, whether relatively straightforward and impressionistic or more detailed and sophisticated, suggests that there is much that could be gained by individual practitioners willing to invest the time required and, by extension, for supervision and the counselling profession as a whole, especially where themes in case material can be collated and generalised conclusions drawn. Text-based therapy and supervision could open up whole new areas of research, as well as increasing the level of oversight of practice available.

With the advent of technology and the ability of the supervisee to access actual verbatim material such as chat transcripts and e-mails, the supervisor is well advised that ownership of the clinical record be stated clearly in the informed consent process. This ownership agreement applies to client/therapist relationships as well. An example of the ownership inclusion is provided here:

> All information disclosed within sessions and the written records pertaining to those sessions are confidential and may not be revealed to anyone without your written permission, except where disclosure is required by law. Likewise, you are expected to keep our communications confidential and you understand that all records of communication between [CLIENT/THERAPIST or SUPERVISOR/SUPERVISEE] remain the property of [NAME OF THERAPIST OR SUPERVISEE] … I make every effort to keep all information confidential. Likewise, I ask that you determine who has access to your computer and electronic information from your location. This would include family members, co-workers, supervisors and friends. I encourage you to only communicate through a computer that you know is safe i.e. wherein confidentiality can be ensured. Be sure to fully exit all online counselling sessions and emails … Due to the nature of the therapeutic process and the fact that it often involves making a full disclosure with regard to many matters which may be of a confidential nature, it is agreed that should there be legal proceedings … neither you nor your attorney, nor anyone else acting on your behalf will call on me to testify in court or any other proceeding, nor will disclosure of the psychotherapy records be requested … (excerpt from http://www.deeannamerznagel.com)

By including such provisions in the informed consent process, the supervisee gains an understanding about the importance of guarding the client record; verbatim material is less likely to be carelessly used in litigation and the client's confidentiality is maintained. It is advised that counsellors and supervisors check with a legal authority within their country or jurisdiction to determine the applicability of such a clause as stated above.

Transference/Countertransference

Transference/counter-transference issues that develop during clinical supervision are often the sentinel moments supervisors and supervisees reflect upon. These moments are no less pivotal when they occur via distance using technology. One must first embrace the concept that the modalities we have discussed in this chapter all hold different but powerful characteristics and possibilities. Certainly, text-based clinical supervision is different to clinical supervision that takes place via phone or videoconference. Synchronous versus asynchronous supervision engage the supervisor and supervisee in different ways. However different each delivery method may be, transference/countertransference issues are no less remarkable, offering to the supervisory relationship an opportunity for growth and exploration. Fenichel (2003) relates as myth the idea that one cannot or does not develop strong feelings in online therapeutic relationships much like traditional transference and countertransference relationships.

The disinhibition effect should be considered as an influence to the transference and countertransference processes that occur in online supervisory relationships. The disinhibition effect can occur in both therapeutic and nontherapeutic relationships particularly with text-based communication. While the following is a rather condensed summary of a complex theory (Munro, 2002; Suler, 2004), one can begin to appreciate the different subtleties that might even magnify transference/countertransference issues seen in face-to-face supervisory relationships.

- While the parties may be known to each other, without visual and/or auditory cues, a sense of anonymity still exists.
- Without paralinguistic cues, one can feel invisible, with no worry of how a facial expression or tone of voice may be interpreted.
- With asynchronous communication, either party can state a feeling in the moment with no regard for what the immediate response might be.
- Without sensory cues, either party may begin to imagine the relationship as occurring inside one's head or imagining the relationship as unreal.
- When parties communicate online, a neutrality exists, with no perceived hierarchy.
- Personality tendencies and communication styles may be enhanced online via text-based communication.

As with online counselling, pacing, moments of silence, use of netiquette, emoticons and avatars, as well as how different forms of technology are combined will effect the supervisory relationship. How issues are interpreted, and how the supervisor perceives the supervisee and likewise, the supervisee perceives the supervisor are also considerations.

Suitability of the Supervisor
Technical Competencies
The Association for Counselor Education and Supervision's Technical Competencies for Counselor Education (Jencius, Poynton, & Patrick, 2007) includes 12 competencies that students and counsellor educators should possess. These competencies are reasonable expectations for students and educators who are working within a college/university setting that allows for acquisition of these skills. In summary, technological expectations are as follows:

- Ability to use productivity software to develop web pages, word processing documents, databases, spreadsheets and other forms of documentation.
- Ability to use audiovisual equipment such as video recorders, audio recorders, projection equipment and videoconferencing equipment.
- Ability to acquire, use and develop multimedia software for use in presentations, training and practice.
- Ability to use statistical software to organise and analyse data.
- Ability to use computerised and/or internet-based testing, diagnostic, and career decision-making programs with clients.
- Ability to use e-mail.
- Ability to help clients search for and evaluate various types of counselling-related information via the internet.
- Ability to subscribe, participate in, and sign off related listservs and other Internet-based professional communication applications.
- Ability to access and use counselling-related research databases.
- Ability to use the internet to locate, evaluate and use continuing education, professional development and supervision options in counselling.
- Ability to perform basic computer operation and maintenance tasks.
- Knowledge of legal, ethical and efficacy issues associated with the delivery of counselling services via the internet.

These competencies help ensure that counsellor educators and mental health practitioners in training possess the necessary skills to enhance their ability to assist clients in this technological age. With these competencies as the foundation, additional skills can be developed. As we have discussed, each form of distance technology comes with its own set of nuances from text without paralinguistic cues, to differences in synchronous and asynchronous communication, to the subtleties of combining different forms of technology. Additional training and education will aid the clinical supervisor in determining which form of distance technology best suits a certain work setting, theory or supervisee. As with online counsellors, online supervisors may choose to limit their area of expertise to a certain form method and style of delivery.

Training and Education

Training of clinical supervisors varies from country to country. In the United Kingdom, training and a qualification is required to become an accredited supervisor with BACP, which also applies to becoming an accredited counsellor via a counselling course. In Australia, all practising counsellors registered with the Australian Counselling Association (ACA) and the Psychotherapy and Counselling Federation of Australia (PACFA) are required to undergo ongoing clinical supervision to maintain their registration (ACA, 2009; PACFA, 2009). In regard to supervisor registration, ACA has the only register for counsellor/psychotherapist supervisors in Australia. ACA requires all its registered supervisors to meet clinical membership requirements and to have undergone formal supervision training through an ACA-approved supervisor's course. PACFA do not have a register for supervisors nor do they have any set standards for supervisors at this time. In the United States, uniform methods of training clinical supervisors do not exist in most of the counselling disciplines (Falvey, 2002). For instance, most licensed mental health practitioners are authorised to provide clinical supervision under his/her scope of practice. Some states require that the clinician who offers clinical supervision has held a license for an average of 3 years but not necessarily with any additional training. Theories and methods of clinical supervision vary across disciplines as well.

With regard to the use of technology in supervision, when determining whether a requirement for additional training and education should exist, we should look to our codes of ethics as our standard for best practice. Most codes of ethics offer guidelines to practitioners, stating that therapeutic services should only be rendered if the practitioner has the appropriate training and level of competence in a particular practice area. One might extend this concept to all areas of clinical supervision, including the use of technology. Nagel (2007) suggests key components to becoming a seasoned distance counsellor. These components, slightly modified, may be extended to the concept of becoming seasoned as a clinical supervisor who uses technology:

- Acquire knowledge, both rudimentary and advanced, via formal training such as continuing education courses (offered face-to-face and online), professional journals and other written materials.
- Integrate existing knowledge and skills with newly acquired knowledge and skills.

- Consider ongoing clinical supervision, peer supervision, or case consultation.
- Join organisations that offer peer support and/or disseminate new knowledge and advances in the use of technology and supervision.
- Once skill and experience are acquired, contribute to the field of clinical supervision about the use of technology by mentoring other supervisors, adding to the existing body of quantitative and qualitative literature, and educating licensing boards, legislative bodies and counsellor educators in university settings.

Other Suitability Considerations

Use of technology to provide counselling or counselling supervision raises great opportunities for those with the skills to make use of the potential it affords. However, it is not always suitable for all practitioners and some important caveats will generally apply to their use.

Firstly, it is essential that sufficient training is undertaken to ensure that the pitfalls that exist for the unwary (such as the disinhibition effect, the potential damage of misunderstandings, and issues of acting out, etc.) are avoided, and training programs are available through web sites (such as http://www.onlinecounsellors.co.uk or http://www.onlinetherapyinstitute.com).

All but the most established forms of technology are notorious for their potential to fail, at least until they are sufficiently familiar and their use routine (Adams, 1999). Sufficient technical knowledge must exist on both sides of the relationship to ensure that both parties can make adequate use of it and that trouble-shooting, for example where the technology fails and connection is lost, can be offered by the supervisor. Alternative means of contact should be available in such circumstances and local support for use in emergency situations is as important as in any clinical situation. Some casework requires particularly close supervision and consideration should always be given to the adequacy of the supervisory relationship that can be provided. It is also worth noting that, at present, much research remains to be done to establish clearly the limitations of at least the more novel forms of technological enhancements of routine supervisory practice. However, this is far from suggesting that supervision provided via any technological interface is less likely to be adequate than face-to-face consultation. Indeed, there are likely to be distinct advantages, not least from the supervisory equivalent of disinhibition and the advantages of being afforded opportunities for both parties to reflect on their communications in detail, which would suggest that counsellors might be more willing to discuss the more problematic areas of their work when consulting at a distance.

Conclusion

Technological developments will, inevitably, continue to occur. Despite the skills and insights of those specialising in the study of the future of innovation predicting the direction that these will lead us in, they will always be, to some extent, uncertain. What is obvious already, however, is that existing technologies have the potential to significantly extend the benefits of supervision for practitioners of all forms of counselling. With the caution appropriate for all innovations in clinical practice and support we can expect continued progression in the value, use and acceptance of technology in providing for the support and development needs of counselling practitioners.

Educational Questions and Activities

1. What level of specialist training and experience in online relating and online therapy is necessary in order to offer supervision online, whether for online therapy or face-to-face? Readers may wish to reflect on which forms of technology they would be comfortable using for supervision or other clinical applications.

   A. It is an ethical requirement that anyone offering online therapy receives suitable and sufficiently in-depth training in order to equip them to do so. The same is true for offering online supervision. It is essential that both therapists and their supervisors are aware of the issues involved in online relating in general and online therapy in particular, including the issues particular to the modality used, such as disinhibition when working with text-only formats. Online work is *not* a specialism that is recommended for inexperienced practitioners at any level, especially those in training, and competence in face-to-face work must be assured before progressing to translating the practitioner's skills to the online environment. Furthermore, it must then be remembered that competence in one medium does not necessarily indicate competence in another. For example, communication via face-to-face modalities draws on verbal and nonverbal social communication skills whereas online work requires a more literary aptitude such as the ability to communicate with clarity in order to avoid misunderstandings while retaining the natural expression and spontaneity of any other form of communication. Specialist postqualification training for online supervision should be sought wherever available. Further advice is available through a number of websites such as http://www.onlinetherapyinstitute.com.

2. What concerns are there for therapists and supervisors in maintaining an online presence in social or professional networking facilities?

A. Social and professional networking facilities can be an excellent way of maintaining and creating relationships online. However, practitioners should be aware that their friends and acquaintances, or indeed their colleagues or clients, may post material or comments about them without their consent or control that will be visible by clients, supervisees and others online and that may be open to interpretations that they would not want. Mental health practitioners should ensure that all their activities online are consistent with the professional persona they wish to project and that they may need to remind others of the importance of this. It is especially important to ensure that when contracting for online supervision (or therapy) that the supervisee (or client) is aware that the content of sessions should be treated as confidential, probably remaining the property of the practitioner offering the service. For example, while it can be entirely appropriate to write blog entries regarding one's experiences of supervisions or in therapy in general, any specific or identifiable reference to any individual (including those providing services as well as their clientele) should be avoided. You may also wish to consider what other boundary issues arise in online supervision.

3. What back-up procedures should be in place for use in the event of technological breakdown or crisis/emergency situations and who is responsible for ensuring that they are adequate?

A. A back-up system is required for when either person's computer crashes, or one or both parties lose their internet connection, or the online tool being used fails during supervision. In such an eventuality, or if for any other reason either party to online supervision using synchronous communication tools loses their connection during the course of the meeting, there should be a pre-agreed procedure for reconnecting/rescheduling the meeting, for example the other party might wait five minutes for a reconnection to happen, and then use a telephone call or mobile text message in order to assess the problem and reschedule the meeting while any technology problems are addressed and rectified. It should be the supervisor's responsibility for ensuring the systems are adequate and understood as part of the contracting process.

4. Is online supervision important for online therapy provision?

A. There is ongoing debate as to whether online supervision should be a requirement for online work, or whether face-to-face supervision would be preferable in giving a wider perspective of the issues and therapeutic process.

5. What issues arise in cutting and pasting client material from online sessions for the purposes of supervision and what safeguards are required?

   A. Supervisors and supervisees should agree whether and how communications will be stored or logged. Communications of any sort should not be forwarded, Cc'd (courtesy copied) or Bcc'd (blind courtesy copied) to anyone, either in their entirety or in part, without the explicit consent of all those involved in that communication. If consent for use of communications is obtained for supervision purposes, the safeguards that should be in place should be at least the use of passwords and encryption, the latter of which must be used whenever information not suitable for the public domain (e.g., details of any casework not in a form suitable for publication) are communicated over the internet by any means.

Selected Internet Resources

- Online Therapy Institute
  http://www.onlinetherapyinstitute.com
  Designed for individuals and organisations who wish to enrich their knowledge about online counselling, clinical supervision and the impact of technology on mental health. Topics and issues of interest extend to internet and cybersex addictions, gaming, virtual worlds, social networking, SMS texting and online peer support.

- DeeAnna Merz Nagel
  http://www.deeannamerznagel.com
  Clinical supervision and consultancy available regarding online counselling and the impact of technology on mental health.

- OnlineCounsellors.co.uk
  http://www.OnlineCounsellors.co.uk and
  http://www.KateAnthony.co.uk
  Offers training and consultancy on online counselling and online supervision designed for clinicians and organisations who wish to enrich their knowledge about the impact of technology on mental health.

- International Society For Mental Health Online
  http://www.ISMHO.net
  A multi-disciplinary association of students, teachers, researchers, clinical practitioners, online mental health professionals and other people interested in the field of mental health who meet online to discuss current issues in the field.

References Related to the Internet and Psychology

- http://construct.haifa.ac.il/~azy/refindx.htm
  Annotated references related to the internet and psychology.

Selected References for Further Reading

Anthony, K., & Goss, S.P. (2009), *Guidelines for online counselling and psychotherapy* (3rd ed.): Including guidelines for online supervision. Rugby, UK: BACP Publishing.

Goss, S., & Anthony, K. (2003). *Technology in counselling and psychotherapy A practitioner's guide.* Houndmills, UK: Palgrave Macmillan.

Nagel, D.M., & Anthony, K. (in press). *Clinical supervision in mental health: Best practice for online applications.* Springfield, IL: Charles C Thomas Publishing.

References

Adams, D. (1999). *How to stop worrying and learn to love the Internet.* Retrieved July 4, 2008, from http:www.douglasadams.com/dna/19990901–00-a.html

Angus, L., & McLeod, J. (2004), *The handbook of narrative and psychotherapy: Practice, theory and research.* London: Sage.

Anthony, K. (2003). The use and role of technology in counselling and psychotherapy. In S. Goss & K. Anthony (Eds.), *Technology in counselling and psychotherapy: A practitioner's guide* (pp. 13–36). Houndmills, England: Palgrave Macmillan.

Anthony, K., & Jamieson, A. (2005), *Guidelines for online counselling and psychotherapy: Including guidelines for online supervision* (2nd ed.). Rugby, England: BACP Publishing.

Anthony, K., & Goss, S.P. (2009), *Guidelines for online counselling and psychotherapy: Including guidelines for online supervision* (3rd ed.). Rugby, England: BACP Publishing.

Arthur, G.L., & Gfroerer, K.P.(2002). Training and supervision through the written word: A description and intern feedback. *The Family Journal, 10*(2), 213–219.

Australian Counselling Association (ACA). (2009). *Professional supervision.* Brisbane, Australia: Author. Retrieved January 22, 2009, from http://www.theaca.net.au

Borders, L.D., & Brown, L.L. (2005). *The new handbook of counseling and supervision.* Mahwah, NJ: Lawrence Erlbaum Associates, Publishers.

Cashwell, C.S. (2001, October), IPR: Recalling thoughts and feelings in supervision. *Reading for Child and Youth Care Workers, 33.* Retrieved Jan 12, 2009 from http://www.cyc-net.org/cyc-online/cycol-1001-supervision.html

Chechele, P.J., & Stofle, G. (2003). Individual therapy online via email and Internet Relay Chat. In S. Goss & K. Anthony (Eds.), Technology *in counselling and psychotherapy: A practitioner's guide* (pp. 37–58). Houndmills, England: Palgrave Macmillan.

Colon, Y., & Friedman, B. (2003). Conducting group therapy online. In S. Goss & K. Anthony (Eds.), *Technology in counselling and psychotherapy: A practitioner's guide* (pp. 59–74). Houndmills, England: Palgrave Macmillan.

Concord Consortium. (2005). *VideoPaper Builder 3*. Retrieved Jan 12, 2009, from http://vpb.concord.org/

Dudding, C.C., & Justice, L.M. (2004). An e-supervision model: Videoconferencing as a clinical training tool. *Communication Disorders Quarterly, 25*(3), 145–151.

Falvey, J.E. (2002). *Managing clinical supervision: Ethical practice and legal risk management*. Pacific Grove, CA: Brooks/Cole.

Fenichel, M. (2003). The supervisory relationship online. In S. Goss & K. Anthony (Eds.), *Technology in counselling and psychotherapy: A practitioner's guide* (pp. 75–89). Houndmills, England: Palgrave Macmillan.

Gimmestad, M.J., & Greenwood, J.D. (1974). A new twist on IPR: Concurrent recall by supervisory group. *Counselor Education and Supervision, 14*, 71–73.

Glaser, B. (1992). *Basics of grounded theory analysis*. Mill Valley, CA: Sociology Press.

Glaser, B.G., & Strauss, A.L. (1967). *The discovery of grounded theory. Strategies for qualitative research*. Chicago: Aldine.

Goss, S., Anthony, K., Jamieson, A., & Palmer, S. (2001). *Guidelines for online counselling and psychotherapy*. Rugby, England: BACP Publishing.

Goss, S., & Anthony, K. (2003). *Technology in counselling and psychotherapy A practitioner's guide*. Houndmills, England: Palgrave Macmillan.

Grafanaki, S. (2003). 'On becoming congruent': How Congruence works in person-centred counselling and practical applications for training & practice. In J. Watson, R. Goldman & M. Warner (Eds.), *Client centered and experiential psychotherapy in the 21st century: Advances in theory, research and practice* (pp. 278–290). Ross-on-Wye, UK: PCCS Publication.

Grafanaki, S., & McLeod, J. (2002). Refinement and expansion of the concept of experiential congruence: A qualitative analysis of client and counsellor narrative accounts of significant events in time-limited person-centred therapy. *Counselling and Psychotherapy Research, 2*(1), 20–33.

Gee, J.P. (1986). Units in the production of narrative discourse. *Discourse Processes, 9*, 391–422.

Gee, J.P. (1991). A linguistic approach to narrative. *Journal of Narrative and Life History, 1*, 15–39.

Gee, J.P. (2005). *An introduction to discourse analysis* (2nd ed.). Abingdon, England: Routledge.

Jencius, M., Poynton, T., & Patrick, P. (2007). *Technical competencies for counselor education: Recommended guidelines for program development*. Alexandria, VA: Association for Counselor Education and Supervision Executive Council.

Kagan, N. (1980). Influencing human interaction: Eighteen years with IPR. In A.K. Hess (Ed.), *Psychotherapy supervision: Theory, research, and practice* (pp. 262–283). New York: Wiley.

McLeod, J. (1997). *Narrative and psychotherapy*. London: Sage.

McLeod, J. (2001). *Qualitative research in counselling and psychotherapy*. London: Sage.

Mey, G., & Mruck, K. (Eds.). (2007). Grounded theory reader. *HSR-Supplement 19*. Cologne: ZHSF.

Miller, K.L., Miller, S.M., & Evans, W.J. (2002). Computer-assisted live supervision in college counseling centers. *Journal of College Counseling, 5*(2), 187–192.

Monk, A., Carroll, J., Parker, S., & Blythe, M. (2004). Why are mobile phones annoying? *Behaviour and Information Technology, 23*(1), 33–41.

Munro, K. (2002). Conflict in cyberspace: How to resolve conflict online. Retrieved May 4, 2008, from http://www.kalimunro.com/article_conflict_online.html

Nagel, D.M. (2007). Who can perform distance counseling? In J.F. Malone, R.M. Miller & G.R. Walz (Eds.), *Distance counseling: Expanding the counselor's reach and impact* (pp. 44–52). Ann Arbor, MI: Counseling Outfitters.

National Association of Social Workers/Association of Social Work Boards. (2005). *NASW & ASWB standards for technology and social work practice*. Washington, DC: NASW.

Pelling, N., & Renard, D. (1999). The use of videotaping within developmentally-based supervision. *Journal of Technology in Counseling, 1*(1). Retrieved May 19, 2008, from http://jtc.colstate.edu/v011_1/supervision.htm

Psychotherapy and Counselling Federation of Australian (PACFA). (2009). *Renewal requirements for the PACFA Register*. Available at http://www.pacfa.org.au/national register/cid/5/parent/0/t/nationalregister/l/layout

Richards, L. (1999). *Using NVIVO in qualitative research*. London: Sage.

Rogers, C.R. (1942). The use of electronically recorded interviews in improving psychotherapeutic techniques. *American Journal of Orthopsychiatry, 12*, 429–34.

Strauss, A., & Corbin, J. (1990). *Basics of qualitative research: Grounded theory procedures and techniques*. Thousand Oaks, CA: Sage Publications.

Suler, J. (2003). *Email communication and relationships*. Retrieved May 1, 2008, from http://www-usr.rider.edu/~suler/psycyber/emailrel.html

Suler, J.R. (2004). The online disinhibition effect. *CyberPsychology and Behavior, 7*, 321–326.

Trahar, S. (2008). VideoPaper and assessment. *Therapy Today, 19*(2), 41.

Walsh, M. (2003). Teaching qualitative analysis using QSR NVIVO. *The Qualitative Report 8*(2), 251–256. Retrieved July 5, 2008, from http://www.nova.edu/ssss/QR/QR8–2/walsh.pdf

Walsh, S.P., & White, K.M. (2006). Ring, ring, why did I make that call? Mobile phone beliefs and behaviour amongst Australian university students. *Youth Studies Australia, 25*(3), 49–57.

—|—|—|—|—|—

chapter twenty

Supervising Clinical Placement

John Barletta and Jason Dixon

Introduction to Internship and Practicum

Internship and practicum are the pinnacle of the therapist training experience. During these fieldwork experiences trainees are challenged to apply what they have learned in coursework and research to a real-life workplace situation. Internship is where the rigorous science of the profession and the imperfect art of the practice intersect and trainees begin to develop clinical wisdom. The trainee therapist being prepared for their responsibilities who has a successful relationship with their supervisor can optimise the gains from this integrated experience. In this chapter, an introduction to supervised internship or practicum encounters is provided with the trainee therapist and future supervisor squarely in mind.

Definition and Purpose

Supervision is a service to clients and to the trainee. In the simplest of terms, supervision is a service provided directly to trainees with an impact on the clinical outcomes for clients. Understanding the nature of supervision and internship or practicum will prepare trainees to effectively engage and profit from these experiences.

There are several definitions of supervision used in the helping professions. Some of these definitions solely emphasise the relationship between the supervisor and the supervisee (e.g., Gilbert & Evans, 2000), while others focus only on the client's experience. The tasks of supervision maybe as narrow as just administrative responsibilities or as broad as encompassing all aspects relating work as a therapist (Loganbill, Hardy, & Delworth, 1982). Bernard and Goodyear's (2004) definition of supervision is the most comprehensive as it relates to provision of therapy in that supervision is defined as a relationship between the supervisor and supervisee that is evaluative, extends over time, enhances supervisee functioning, monitors the quality of professional services and serves as gatekeeping to the profession.

In the United Kingdom (UK), the literature of Proctor and Kadushin are very influential in the field of supervision. They outline three functions of supervision being normative (administrative), formative (educational) and restorative (supportive) and these are common across the professions of social work, nursing, medicine, educational psychology and teaching (Kilminster & Jolly, 2000). In the United States (US), Bernard and Goodyear (2004) are arguably the most influential authors in the field of supervision and state that the fundamental purpose of supervision is to foster supervisee professional development and ensure client welfare. In Japan, Nojima (1997) mentions that individual clinical supervision not only functions to improve the development of a clinician and reduce any risks to clients, but that attending professional conferences is also an aspect of supervision in the broad sense. As trainees experience supervision they discover areas of proficiency and shortcomings that they will want to explore through professional development.

What to Expect From the Supervision Experience

The fieldwork experience should be organised so that it is not so effortless that it becomes tedious and not so challenging that it is overwhelming. Thankfully, in the experience of internship and practicum, trainees are very likely to have more than one supervisor who can monitor progress. This will probably be someone from the academic institution where trainees are studying and a field supervisor who will oversee work in the clinical setting. This section focuses on the collaboration trainees undertake with the field supervisor.

Approaches a Supervisor May Employ

In general, the field supervisor may employ at least three broad approaches to working with trainees. Supervisors may assist through teaching, counselling and/or consultation (Barletta, 2007). In the case of teaching trainees will have the already familiar learning role. However, unlike the classroom experience where a general syllabus is provided to outline the learning objectives, teaching in the supervisory setting will be designed to the trainee's specific needs, strengths and weaknesses (Bernard & Goodyear, 2004). Without the structure of a syllabus, the learning trainees will do in supervision is andragogic (i.e., adult learning), which means that trainees develop the way they learn and, to some extent, what they learn in, from and beyond supervision (Granello & Hazler, 1998; Marshak, 1983). This allows for greater control over learning experiences and helps develop an insight into managing professional development above and beyond supervision and internship.

The clients trainees help will personally affect them in different ways. Depending on trainees' experience, a supervisor may use a counselling approach with them. Most of trainees' encounters in helping clients will lead to a deep sense of occupational satisfaction and encouragement. However, sometimes clients will have a negative personal impact on trainees — this goes with the territory of the helping professions. Well documented is the clinician's experience of vicarious or secondary trauma of those working with people with posttraumatic stress disorder (Zimering, Munroe, & Gulliver, 2003). Sometimes less dramatic experiences can also affect therapists negatively. One of the authors of this chapter had a supervisee who was shocked at a teenage client who was questioning his sexuality and presented her with pornographic drawings. In this case, the author used counselling interventions to assist the supervisee to work through their shock and integrate this situation into her understanding of the client's case, and thus improve her effectiveness in helping him. However, it is important to remember that a supervisor is not the trainee's therapist per se and has an ethical responsibility to refer trainees to a mental health professional should they present with issues whose aetiology is independent from client work (Ladany, Lehrman-Waterman, Molinaro, & Wolgast, 1999)

Especially in the Australian context, the supervisor trainees work with may or may not be from the same profession. This will depend on which profession the trainee is pursuing. When a supervisor is from a different profession, for example the supervisor is a psychologist and the trainee is a counsellor, the supervisor may employ more of a consultation approach. Consultation is often used when the supervisee is an experienced clinician and has the purpose of handling difficult and complicated cases or for the need to retrieve objectivity (Bernard & Goodyear, 2004). It is also suggested that consultation is useful for experienced clinicians moving into a new area of clinical practice. It should be remembered that if trainees are experiencing hurdles during internship, and the field supervisory relationship only allows for consultation, trainees should consider seeking advice from the supervisor at the academic institution.

Live Supervision and Supervision With Prerecorded Work

The practice of live supervision has decades of history in the helping professions. Live supervision is a training component used across a wide range of helping professions including counselling, social work and psychology (Champe & Kleist, 2003). Live supervision, along with video and audiotape recordings reviewed by a supervisor, are ways of addressing possible conscious and unconscious distortion in the reporting of clinical work by the supervisee (Noelle, 2002)

Live supervision is delivered in different ways. Supervisors can view trainees' work from behind a two-way mirror in a clinical or training facility (Hunt & Sharpe, 2008) and give instructions via a 'bug in the ear'. The supervisor may not be on site and trainees receive guidance via teleconferencing or the supervisor can co-counsel with the trainees giving a source of clinical practice to emulate. A review of the literature on live supervision suggests that it is best when it is collaborative and supportive in nature (Champe & Kleist, 2003).

Interpersonal Process Recall (IPR; Kagan, 1975) is a counselling approach that has been applied to supervision and training. In this technique the trainee and the supervisor review a prerecorded therapy session. Either the trainees or supervisor stop the recording at any time to explore matters relating to the therapeutic process. The supervisor will establish the space to recall and examine trainees' experiences as it related to the therapeutic process. Results from an empirical study of counsellor trainees was used to draw conclusions that the IPR method of training was best suited for trainee counsellors who had masted advanced counselling skills and are ready to personalise diverse theoretical concepts to client helping practices (Crews et al., 2005). Thus this approach is suited to those who are entering the practicum and internship phases of their therapist training.

Characteristics of Effective Supervisors

When considering the role of the trainee as a supervisee one might wonder how they know if the supervision being received is effective. One of the most important core conditions for the therapeutic environment is interpersonal trust (Hazler & Barwick, 2001). One way to gauge the effectiveness of supervision experience is to consider if the supervisor is able to develop and maintain trust and a successful working alliance. This should not be dissimilar to the counselling and other intimate relationships. The supervisor should also be providing trainees with clear and useful feedback. Supervisees should feel that, in a professional capacity, they are receiving appropriate support and care. In a study of 91 educational psychologists in the UK, the most important requirements for effective supervision were problem-solving, appropriate guidance and support accommodating supervisees' needs and effective communication (Atkinson & Woods, 2007). Maintaining trust and an effective working alliance is, as in any effective relationship, a task that requires commitment and dedication from both parties involved.

Case Conceptualisation, Critical Thinking and Note-Taking

The way trainees think about a case and the notes they take are related to the way they conceptualise the client's experience and the paradigm and world-view from which they operate. By collaborating with the supervisor the trainee will develop the skills to accurately articulate, in clinical language, the client's status. The dialogue with the supervisor will assist the trainee in discovering unexplored areas of the client's experience and further the depth and spectrum of the way they conceptualise the case.

In a study of trainee counsellors, Ladany, Marotta and Muse-Burke (2001) found that the more client and supervision sessions a counsellor experiences, the more integrated and complex aetiologic and treatment conceptualisations are made. This means that the way a trainee sees the client's issues will develop in depth and sophistication through the process of supervision.

Note taking is an integral requirement of clinical practice and is an art that will improve as the internship progresses. Note taking is a central part of the clinical interview and an ongoing task of any professional work.

In the practical sense, note taking serves the functions of:

- A description of the presenting problem closely reflecting the language used by the client.
- A description of how the presenting problem impairs the client's life (e.g., social, occupational, affective, cognitive, physical).
- A history of the presenting problem (i.e., precipitating events, predisposing factors).
- A record of the primary support network, which includes family and close social relationships and the strengths and stressors of these relationships.
- A record of cultural, religious and ethnic background.
- A description of any medical condition and medication, especially those that may have an impact on the prognosis and progress of therapy.
- An accurate record of the necessary information pertaining to the client's presenting problems in relation to the approaches of the profession. (e.g., psychologists may incorporate more information on symptomology, and social workers may include more details about psychosocial aspects).
- An outline of treatment recommendations.
- A record of client and therapist goals (clinical outcomes), process (specific interventions), prognosis (prediction) and progress (actual client change toward the goals)

Once a trainee understands the basic functions of note taking, there may appear to be a tremendous amount of work involved in this task. Much of this work can be part of, but not limited to, the first clinical interview and is an opportunity to 'start establishing the therapeutic relationship between (therapist) and client, which conveys a sense of client worth and worthiness for treatment' (Faiver, Eisengart, & Colona, 2000, p. 46). Building trust and rapport with the client should take precedence over taking notes, yet both tasks need to be accomplished. As trainees spend more time with clients notes will be added to create a comprehensive clinical picture. Depending on the trainee's unique way of interacting with people they may wish to take notes during each session and/or at the end of each session. Creating clinical notes (writing) and the presentation of client material in supervision (verbal) are both ways to practise and improve how to conceptualise and articulate the client's world. Please refer to Figure 20.1 for an example of a client intake form.

Therapist Development

Supervision seen as a developmental process has a long history in the counselling literature and is useful as developmental models are not tied to any particular system of therapy (Bernard, 1979; Bernard & Goodyear, 2004). Developmental models give an insight into the development as a therapist for internship and practical training and into a career as a successful and competent professional. Stoltenberg and Delworth's (1987) Integrated Developmental Model of supervision is arguably the most popular approach to understanding the supervision experience (Leach & Stoltenberg, 1997; Bernard & Goodyear, 2004).

According to this model, in the journey as a helping professional trainees experience issues around anxiety–dependence. Simply put, they might be motivated, but experience the need to check and monitor their work as a therapist. At this stage the supervisor can provide the structure and feedback needed. As the trainee continues to develop as a therapist they will experience a dependency–autonomy conflict where they need less supervisory structure and more emotional encouragement from the supervisor. Following this the trainee will start to experience collegial supervision where they have confidence, insight and competence and the supervisor will start interact with them more in the way of a professional peer. Finally the trainee will find themselves at the integrated level where they experience autonomy, self- and other awareness, security and the ability to self-confront. This self-confrontation or self-challenging is the beginning of the ability to engage in a form of 'self-supervision' (Lowe, 2002), developing a reliable 'internal supervisor' (Gilbert & Evans, 2000) or autonomous professional development. Figure 20.2 outlines a develop-

Client: _____   D.O.B.: _____

Agency: _____   Phone: _____

Identifying Information:

Referral Source:

Presenting Concern/Goals:

Previous Treatment:

Mental Status:

Family History:

Siblings:

Education:

Employment History:

Social Development and Connections:

Marital and Dating History:

Medical Information and Current Illness:

Habits and Criminal Behaviour:

Personality:

Religious Affiliation:

Strengths and Supports:

Diagnostic Impressions:

Summary:

Treatment Plans and Recommendations:

_____   _____

Therapist   Date

FIGURE 20.1
Client history: Intake form.

	The Person (The Role)	Awareness and Skill (Affect)	Phases of Professional Development (Ronnestad & Skovholt)	Focus of Approach	Consideration and Attention (Virtues)
1	HUMAN (Accidental Helper) Observe	Unconscious Incompetence (Ignorance)	Conventional	Instinct & Experience	SELF (Hope & Will)
2	THERAPY STUDENT (Apprentice) Discover	Conscious Incompetence (Confusion)	Transition	Theory	OTHERS (Self-discipline & Responsibility)
3	EMERGING PROFESSIONAL (Novice) Hypothesise	Conscious Competence (Confidence)	Imitation of Experts	Skills	RELATIONSHIP (Competence & Fidelity)
4	THERAPIST (Practitioner) Verify	Conscious Competence (Certainty)	Conditional Autonomy Exploration	Values	THERAPEUTIC FRAME (Love & Care)
5	SENIOR PROFESSIONAL THERAPIST (Expert) Communicate	Unconscious Competence (Satisfaction)	Integration Individuation Integrity	Being with	CONTEXT & CULTURE (Wisdom & Humility)

FIGURE 20.2
The journey of professional therapists (Barletta, 2009).

mental model that integrates a range of concepts that can be further explored to describe the growth of a helping professional. It highlights the changing role, levels of awareness and skill, focus of clinical attention and associated virtues.

Critical Incidents and Case Studies
The study of critical incidents grew out of the practice of industrial and organisational psychology in the US military during World War II (Butterfield, Borgen, Amundson, & Maglio 2005). Critical incidents in clinical supervision in counselling have been defined as an incident, milestone or turning point that results in a change in the supervisee's perception of their effectiveness as a counsellor (Heppner & Roehlke, 1984). Critical incidents can be perceived as both positive and/or negative. For

example, a trainee might help a client who gives them positive feedback on the work they did with them, or the trainee might experience a difficult client who seems like nothing they do is helping. Both types of these incidents are useful for the development as a counsellor. Positive incidents reinforce confidence in competence as a therapist, while negative incidents can be an indication of what areas need further development. Heppner and Roehlke (1984) found that critical incidents can be classified in terms of counsellor development. They can be incidents related to self-awareness, professional development, competency and personal issues affecting therapy. Whether the incidents are positive or negative in essence, the field supervisor can help the trainee work with these experiences to gain the most benefit from them.

As trainees review the literature of their particular helping profession, they will routinely come across examples of case studies. Case studies are an excellent way to present, in detail, a client and the complexities that surround them (Page, Stritzke, & McLean, 2008). Client cases used in supervision can function in a similar way to Interpersonal Process Recall (IPR), which is used to recall in an experiential manner the therapeutic process by viewing a taped therapy session. Producing case studies functions in a similar way to IPR, in that the therapist recalls and articulates in writing their knowledge about a case and the therapeutic process. Critical incidents can be incorporated into the writing up of case studies and can be presented during supervision sessions. Trainees should take the initiative to write up a case study for experience, and below is a simple guide to facilitating the process.

• Describe the background to the case including the presenting problem and historical information,
• What was happening for you when working with this client?
• What do you feel was happening for the client?
• Describe what approaches were or were not effective?
• Was there anything of a personal nature, on your part, hindering or promoting therapeutic change?

As in the IPR approach, trainees need to recall how they felt, what they might have liked to have done, their thoughts about what happened and any mental imagery they had or have about the experience.

Case Presentations

Case presentations are useful if trainees are participating in group supervision, particularly if it is multidisciplinary, or peer consultation. The content presented will be similar to what one would include in writing up a case study except it is presented for feedback and discussion among pro-

fessional peers. The supervisor and/or group will have a format and procedure in place for trainees to follow. They may use specific technologies
such as presentation software or audio/visual records of client sessions to
assist in communicating to peers. Case presentations in a group setting are
an excellent supervision environment, as trainees will benefit from several
people thinking about and working with them on a particular issue. In
spite of the initial anxiety associated with presenting in front of others,
greater understandings and new ideas will invariably be the outcome.

Circumstances Requiring Immediate Action to Prevent Imminent Harm

Included in the incidents described above, trainees need to be prepared
for circumstances where their immediate action is necessary to prevent
imminent harm to the client or someone the client intends to harm.

The most obvious circumstance of imminent harm is potential suicide.
Suicide can be understood as a continuum of behaviour that includes
fleeting thoughts of suicide, suicidal ideation (a reaction to overwhelming
events), suicide planning and means (concrete preparation and access to
resources), suicidal attempts and completed suicide (Gliatto & Rai, 1999;
Kanel, 2003). The way to gain an indication of where the client stands on
suicide is to ask within the context of the therapeutic relationship. More
detailed methods to explore this clinical issue exist in a plethora of literature on the topic of suicide.

While there is still no universally accepted assessment instrument for
suicidal risk or prediction, the Suicide Assessment Scale (SUAS) has some
established reliability and validity (Nimeus, Alsen, & Traskman-Bendz,
2000). The SUAS has also been modified to an interview version and has
high reliability and established predictive validity (for manual and scale
see Nimeus, Stahlfors, Sunnqvist, Stanle, & Traskman-Bendz 2006).
Trainees can discuss the use of the SUAS, SUAS-interview version and
similar assessment instruments with their field supervisor.

In any event, at the first indication of potential suicidal behaviour the
trainee can put a suicide contract into place. While the internship site
may already have a preferred document for contracting, Figure 20.3 is an
example of a contract that can be modified as desired. Please keep in
mind that there is some degree of controversy regarding the use of suicide
contracts. For a brief review of the topic of suicide the reader is referred to
Macdonald, Pelling, and Granello (in press).

Although less prevalent than suicide, some clients will disclose their
intention to harm others or property. As with the suicidal client, a client
who threatens the safety of others presents a dilemma in the duty of care
to protect the client's rights to privacy and the trainee's responsibility to
protect society from harm (Van Exan, 2004) It is here that informed

Date: _____

I, _____, (client), hereby agree that I will take the following actions if I feel suicidal.

1. I will not attempt suicide.

2. I will phone _____ at _____.

3. If the above person can not be reached I will contact the following services in the order below:

Name/Agency	Phone
_____	_____
_____	_____
_____	_____

4. I will also seek social support from any or all of the following people:

Name	Phone
_____	_____
_____	_____
_____	_____

5. If none of these actions are helpful or available, I will present at the Emergency department at one of the following:

Hospital	Address	Phone
_____	_____	_____
_____	_____	_____
_____	_____	_____

6. If I am not able in anyway to undertake the above-mentioned actions I will phone Emergency Services on _____ if I feel I am in immediate danger of harming myself.

7. I agree to discuss any crisis leading to suicidal thoughts or planning to my therapist_____(therapist's name) during our next session together.

Client's signature: _____ Date: ___/___/___

Therapist's signature: _____ Date: ___/___/___

FIGURE 20.3
Example of suicide contract.

consent is the greatest ally as it protects the trainee's position and informs the client of professional responsibilities. For these and other legal and ethical responsibilities, it is important that trainees review the *code of ethics* relevant to the profession. Below is a brief procedure of an ethical decision-making model that can be applied to ethical dilemmas. It is good practice to keep a record of the details of this process as it relates to a specific client in the clinical notes. Please note that the field and institution supervisor must be informed of any ethical dilemmas a trainee might have during their internship and will be ready to assist them in the decision making process.

1. Identify the problem.
2. Apply the relevant code of ethics.
3. Determine the nature and dimensions of the dilemma.
4. Generate potential courses of action.
5. Consider the potential consequences of all options, choose a course of action.
6. Evaluate the selected course of action.
7. Implement the course of action.

(Adapted from Miller & Davis, 2006)

Concluding Statement

Clinical fieldwork in the training context is a critical component of the formation of the therapist. It gives the trainee, institution and professional community a sense of the potential for the novice. As trainees are challenged and supported to apply what they have learned in the classroom and from research to the workplace, they are exploring how the science of the profession becomes the art of clinical practice. This chapter provided an overview of the key elements to the supervision of placement experiences to facilitate the development of clinical wisdom in the trainee, via a quality relationship and thoughtful structured supervisory experiences.

Educational Questions and Activities

1. Activity: General Discussion. 'The Purpose of Supervision'. Prepare a specific job description including general responsibilities and the type of clients who would be served. Have students imagine what possible incidents and challenges may occur. Students should discuss this with the class group. In response to student concerns, expose them to certain supervision techniques pointing these out to students following your engagement with each student.

2. Activity: Note-taking, simulation, self-appraisal, specific and general discussion. Provide each student with a copy of the intake form in this chapter or one that you (the educator/supervisor) has designed or use. Prepare a comprehensive description of a complex clinical case.

- Step 1. Read the case to the class while students fill in the information on the intake form.
- Step 2. Allow students to ask you questions to repeat information they may have missed. (This allows students to be active and intentional in thinking about information they need from a client.)
- Step 3. In pairs, have students compare and contrast their notes, while adding information to make this record more comprehensive.
- Step 4. Engage in an open-ended class discussion including the content of their record, what information should be gathered first, what could be gathered in later client sessions, and student reactions to the note-taking process.

3. Use Barletta's developmental model shown as Figure 20.2, 'The Journey of Professional Therapists', to discuss the concept of the growth of a helping professional, with particular attention to participants' current phase, individual plans to facilitate such progress, and expectations of what the future phases might be like.

Selected Internet Resources

- CESNET-L Listserv
- http://listserv.kent.edu/archives/cesnet-1.html
- Discussion list established at Kent State University covers a variety of topics concerning counsellor education and supervision.

References and Selected Further Reading

Atkinson, C., & Woods, K. (2007). A model of effective fieldwork supervision for trainee Educational Psychologists. *Educational Psychology in Practice, 23*, 299–316.

Barletta, J. (2007). Clinical supervision. In N. Pelling, R. Bowers, & P. Armstrong (Eds.), *The practice of counselling* (pp.118–135). Melbourne, Australia: Thomson.

Bernard, J.M. (1979). Supervision training: A discrimination model. *Counselor Education and Supervision, 19*, 60–68.

Bernard, J.M., & Goodyear, R.K. (2004). *Fundamentals of clinical supervision* (3rd ed.). Boston: Pearson.

Butterfield, L.D., Borgen, W.A., Amundson, N.E., & Maglio, A.T. (2005). Fifty years of the critical incident technique: 1954-2004 and beyond. *Qualitative Research, 5*, 475–497.

Carrington, G. (2004). Supervision as a reciprocal learning process. *Educational Psychology Practice, 20*(1), 31–42.

Carroll, M., & Gilbert, M.C. (2006). *On being a supervisee: Creating learning partnerships.* Kew, Australia: PsychOz.

Champe, J., & Kleist, D.M. (2003). Live supervision: A review of the research. *The Family Journal, 11,* 268–275.

Crews, J., Smith, M.R., Smaby, M.H., Maddux, C.D., Torres-Rivera, E., Casey, J.A., & Urbani, S. (2005). Self-monitoring and counselling skills: Skills-based versus interpersonal process recall training. *Journal of Counseling and Development, 83*(1), 78–85.

Faiver, C., Eisengart, S., & Colona, R. (2000). *The counselor intern's handbook* (2nd ed.). Belmont, CA: Wadsworth/Thomson.

Gilbert, M.C., & Evans, K. (2000). *Psychotherapy supervision: An integrative relational approach to psychotherapy supervision.* Philadelphia, PA: Open University.

Gliatto, M.F., & Rai, A.K. (1999, March 15). *Evaluation and treatment of patients with suicide ideation.* Retrieved July 1, 2008, from American Academy of Family Physicians Web Site: http://www.aafp.org/afp/990315ap/1500.html

Granello, D., & Hazler, R. (1998). A developmental rationale for curriculum order and teaching styles in counselor education programs. *Counselor Education and Supervision, 38*(2), 89.

Hazler, R.J., & Barwick, N. (2001). *The therapeutic environment.* Philadelphia, PA: Open University.

Heppner, P.P., & Roehlke, H.J. (1984). Differences among supervisees at different levels of training: Implications for a developmental model of supervsion. *Journal of Counseling Psychology, 31*(1), 76–90.

Hunt, C., & Sharpe, L. (2008). Within-session supervision communication in the training of clinical psychologists. *Australian Psychologist, 43*(2), 121–126.

Kagan, N. (1975). Influencing human interaction: Eleven years with IPR. *Canadian Counsellor, 9*(2), 74–97.

Kanel, K. (2003). When crisis is a danger. In (Ed.), *A guide to crisis intervention* (2nd ed., pp. 74–90). Pacific Grove, CA: Brooks-Cole.

Kilminster, S.M., & Jolly, B.C. (2000). Effective supervision in clinical practice settings: A literature review. *Medical Education, 34,* 827–840.

Ladany, N., Lehrman-Waterman, D., Molinaro, M., & Wolgast, B. (1999). Psychotherapy supervisor ethical practices: Adherence to guidelines, the supervisory working alliance, and supervisee satisfaction. *The Counseling Psychologist, 27*(3), 443–475.

Ladany, N., Marotta, S., & Muse-Burke, J. L. (2001). Counselor experience related to complexity of case conceptualizatoin and supervision preference. *Counselor Education and Supervision, 40,* 203–219.

Leach, M.M., & Stoltenberg, C.D. (1997). Self-efficacy and counselor development. *Counselor Education and Supervision, 37*(2), 115–124.

Loganbill, C., Hardy, E., & Delworth, U. (1982). Supervision: A conceptual model. *The Counseling Psychologist, 10*(1), 3–42.

Lowe, R. (2002). Self-supervision: From developmental goal to systemic practice. In M. McMahon & W. Patton (Eds.), *Supervision in the helping professions: A practical approach* (pp. 67–78). Sydney, Australia: Pearson.

Macdonald, L., Pelling, N., & Haag Granello, D. (in press). Suicide: A biopsychoso-cial perspective. *Psychotherapy in Australia.*

Marshak, R.J. (1983). What's between pedagogy and andragogy. *Training and Development Journal, 30*(10), 80–81.

Miller, H.F., & Davis, T. (2006). *A practitioner's guide to ethical decision making.* Alexandria, VA: American Counseling Association. Retrieved July 1, 2007, from http://www.counseling.org/Files/FD.ashx?guid=c4dcf247-66e8-45a3-abcc 024f5d7e836f

Nimeus, A., Alsen, M., & Traskman-Bendz, L. (2000). The Suicide Assessment Scale: An instrument assessing suicide risk of suicide attempters. *European Psychiatry, 15,* 416–423.

Nimeus, A., Stahlfors, F.H., Sunnqvist, C., Stanley, B., & Traskman-Bendz, L. (2006). Evaluation of a modified interview version of a self-rating version of the Suicide Assessment Scale. *European Psychiatry, 21,* 471–477.

Noelle, M. (2002). Self-report in supervision: Positive and negative slants. *Clinical Supervisor, 21* 125–134.

Nojima, K. (1997). Nojima Sensei no Kangae. In *Shinri rinshoka wo mezasu hito ni nozomu koto.* Retrieved May 22, 2008, from Kyushu University Web Site: http://nojima2.hes.kyushu-u.ac.jp/nozomi.htm

Page, A., Stritzke, G., & McLean,N., (2008). Toward science-informed supervision of clinical case formulation: A training model and supervision method. *Australian Psychologist, 43*(2), 88–95.

Ronnestad, M.H., & Skovholt, T.M. (2003). The journey of the counselor and ther-apist: Research findings and perspectives on development. *Journal of Career Development, 30,* 5–44.

Skovholt, T.M., & Ronnestad, M.H. (1995). *The evolving professional self: Stages and themes in therapist and counselor development.* New York: John Wiley.

Stoltenberg, C.D., & Delworth, U. (1987). *Supervising counselors and therapists: A developmental approach.* San Francisco, CA: Jossey-Bass.

Van Exan, J. (2004). The legal and ethical issues surrounding the duty to warn in the practice of psychology. *Windsor Review of Legal and Social Issues, 18,* 123–126.

Zimering, R., Munroe, J., & Gulliver, S. B. (2003). Secondary traumatization in mental health providers. *Psychiatric Times, 20*(4), 43.

—⊢⊢⊢⊢⊢—

Appendices

Appendix A

A Framework for Developing a Supervision Contract, Incorporating Assessment Procedures

Deciding the purpose

1. Clarify the purpose of the supervision program. For example:
   (a) meeting requirements of a government licensing authority
   (b) meeting requirements of a credentialing professional association or college
   (c) meeting requirements of a tertiary course
   (d) meeting other requirements/purposes (e.g., ongoing monitoring and provision of feedback re professional practice).

2. Clarify details of requirements of relevant licensing or credentialing agencies or courses, such as:
   (a) specified content, such as a list of specifically state required competencies, or content that is implied in application forms that will be submitted at the end of the program
   (b) specified time requirements and limits, such as the number of hours required for the supervision program, and whether this must be completed within a set period
   (c) specified client contact requirements, such as the number of direct contact hours
   (d) specified breadth of experiences, such as that child and adult clients are seen, that clients include those with mental health issues and those without mental health issues, for example
   (e) specified frequency and length of supervision sections, such as requirements that supervision occurs on a weekly basis or that a certain number of direct contact hours is required
   (f) specified reporting and documentation requirements, such as practice or supervision logs, or activity logs, or lists of times spent carrying out assessments (for example) with what client age group etc.
   (g) specified supervisee entry requirements
   (h) specified supervisor credential/qualification/experience requirements.

Deciding the personnel and the setting

3. Does the supervisee meet the entry requirements for the supervision program?

4. Does the supervisor meet any specified requirements for the supervision program?

5. Does any secondary supervisor (i.e., a person involved in providing supervision for part of the overall program, perhaps because of specific expertise, or access to additional areas of practice) meet specified requirements?

6. Does the organisational or other setting meet any specified requirements for the supervision program?

Negotiating the contract

The contract may have sections such as:

(a) identifying information of parties involved

(b) description of the setting/s in which supervision will occur

(c) agreements on the length and timetabling of the supervision program

(d) agreements on the nature, frequency and purposes of supervision program activities that will be involved

(e) agreement on direct supervision activities between supervisee and supervisor

(f) agreements on record-keeping and documentation processes developed to meet relevant requirements

(g) sections on each core competency required in order to meet licensing, membership, or course requirements, or that are otherwise agreed, for example:
   (i) ethical awareness
   (ii) assessment skills
   (iii) knowledge and implementation of interventions
   (iv) cultural competence.

(h) sections that may be generic, specific to the particular setting, or specific to the supervision program, such as:
   (i) basic work requirements
   (ii) response to, and participation in, supervision
   (iii) understanding of the client population
   (iv) interactions with clients.

For each section there should be clear understanding of what skills and knowledge are expected, how these will be assessed, how feedback will be give, and how further development will then be facilitated.

Negotiating reporting or recording processes that will be used in ongoing reviews and at the end of the supervision program

As an example, a certificate of competency in ethical awareness might be formatted as follows:

Competence: Ethical, Legal and Professional Matters

Subcompetency	Possible assessment processes	Supervisor's assessment of whether competence is met	Supervisor's signature and date on which competency satisfied
Knowledge of legislation relevant to practice: List	Presentations, questionnaires, discussion, application as required in casework		
Knowledge of codes of ethics relevant to practice: List	Presentations, questionnaires, discussion, application as required in casework		
Knowledge of legal requirements of practitioners, such as: • mandatory reporting of child or elder abuse, • response to risk of suicide, • response to risk of injury to others	Presentations, discussion, application as required during casework		

(Adapted from the PRBV supervision program guidelines, with the addition of the second column about possible assessment processes).

Evaluating a contract

1. Are all relevant licensing, credentialing, professional association or course requirements addressed?

2. Are the aims and content of the supervision program clearly described and agreed?

3. Is there provision for identifying competencies and skills the supervisee brings to the supervision program?

4. Is there agreement on the kinds of activities that will be involved in the supervision program to facilitate the supervisee acquiring, practicing and demonstrating competence?

5. Is there agreement on how each competency and knowledge area will be assessed, both during the program and in terms of whether performance is satisfactory in terms of the eventual requirements of the contract?

6. Are all competence assessments planned to be based on a variety of appropriate assessment measures, using a number of observations?

7. Is there agreement on how each competency and knowledge area will be reported to licensing, credentialing or course authorities as relevant?

8. Is there provision for ongoing assessment and feedback with a view to identifying strengths and areas for further development?

9. Is there a timetable for periodic formal progress reviews against the eventual standards required by the eventual requirements of the contract?

10. Is there agreement about the grading system/s that will be used?

11. Is there agreement on what the criteria for the grading system will be?

12. Is there an appeal provision available?

13. Is there provision for ongoing evaluation of the supervision process with a view to identifying facilitative and inhibiting aspects?

Appendix B

Conducting a Cultural Audit of Supervision Practices

Relationship between Supervisor and Counsellor

1. Reflect on the potential influences of culture on establishing initial rapport in the supervision relationship.

   This involves openly acknowledging the similarities and differences in cultural identity(ies) of both the supervisor and the supervisee and exploring the potential impact their world-views may have on the supervision process. It also involves understanding the processes and goals of supervision from a cultural perspective.

2. Reflect on the potential influences of culture on the development of a supervisory relationship of trust and respect.

   The style of supervision, supervisor credibility, openness in exploring cultural issues and issues of power and expertise are all culturally-embedded. Developing trust and respect is dependent upon recognition and appreciation of the impacts of culture on the relationship.

Relationship between Counsellor and Client

3. Reflect on the potential influences of culture on establishing initial rapport in the counselling relationship.

   First impression, both on the part of the client and the counsellor, are often formed around obvious cultural factors and, without careful reflection, can lead to misinterpretation and misperception. Building rapport depends upon learning about each other's perspectives, world-view and visible and less visible cultural influences. Premature foreclosure on such exploration may lead to significant barriers in working together.

4. Reflect on the potential influences of culture on the development of a relationship of trust and respect.

   Establishing a solid working relationship is predicated on the development of a sense of trust and mutual respect. Client trust is closely linked to counsellor credibility, and credibility is built through cultural awareness and sensitivity. Flexibility and responsiveness to particular client needs and expectations of the counselling process are also central factors. Without trust and respect, the working alliance is compromised.

Counselling and Supervision Conventions

5. Reflect on the potential influences of culture on the structure and contexts of counselling and supervision.

In some cases, clients from nondominant populations may not even make it into the counsellor's office because the normative way of doing business presents barriers to accessible, effective and sensitive service. Hours of operation, location and scheduling may need to be reviewed, along with the physical characteristics of the professional environment. Similar issues in the context of supervision should also be considered.

Multicultural Case Conceptualisation

6. Reflect on the potential influences of differences in personal culture on how you view the client.

Too often counsellors are focused on understanding their client and miss the critical step of self-reflection on personal cultural, values, world-views and assumptions. How I view others is intimately related to how I view myself and how I view the world around me, which in turn is a reflection of my own cultural and social history. This type of reflection is important for both the supervisor and the counsellor since each will come with their own cultural lens.

7. Reflect on the potential influences of your personal cultures on how you each view the client's presenting issues.

One area where the counsellor's personal cultural is likely to be influential is in the assessment of client presenting concerns. How we define health, healthy and unhealthy development, and the nature of problems are all culturally embedded. The challenge for both the supervisor and the counsellor is to identify their own cultural assumptions and to develop hypotheses about client issues that are inclusive of what they know of the client's cultural perspective.

8. Reflect on the potential influences of broader social, economic and political systems on the client's presenting concerns.

Our perspectives are also strongly influenced by dominant theoretical models, which tend to locate the problem within the individual. The cultural auditing process encourages a broader reflection on the interpersonal, familial, societal and other influences on the client that may, in fact, be the primary sources of distress or barriers to career development. Thinking systemically then leads to the need to act systemically.

Goal-Setting and Intervention

9. Reflect on the potential influences of culture on the definition and negotiation of client goals.

Understanding the impact of world-view on the client's presenting concerns provides a foundation for building agreement about goals. These goals may be influenced by the client's level of acculturation or cultural identity development, and the counsellor's commitment to these goals will also be influenced by personal identity development, multicultural competency and skills for multicultural case conceptualisation.

10. Reflect on the potential influences of culture on the negotiation of counselling interventions.

    Recognition that culture impacts how a problem is defined opens the door to a broader range of options for how the problem is then addressed and requires supervisors and counsellors to expand their repertoire of both intervention strategies and targets of intervention. Supervisors must be prepared to explore alternative roles for advocacy, consultation, social justice, organisational change or community capacity building.

11. Reflect on the best ways to evaluate her progress in counselling.

    Success is a highly culture-bound concept and must be defined in collaboration with the particular client and in response to her/his cultural norms and world-view. Goal attainment and processes for evaluating progress must also be developed and implemented together. Building culturally sensitive measures into evaluation will also impact the profession as a whole as counsellors share challenges and successes with one another.

12. Reflect on the influence of culture on termination and follow-up.

    The cultural meanings attached to ending a relationship may be very different across clients and will also depend on the degree to which each client is influenced by various personal cultural factors. Active negotiation of termination and follow-up, beginning early on in the counselling process, will ensure that client needs are met and counsellor professional boundaries are sufficiently maintained.

Multicultural Competency Development

13. Reflect on the cultural learning obtained through various client encounters.

    Supervisors and counsellors are in an ideal position to observe how culture impacts the wellbeing of their clients and to search for common themes. These themes may result in identification of targets of advocacy interventions, in changes to counselling conventions or in modifications to personal theories of counselling. Clients remain our richest source of information.

14. Reflect on the counsellor's experience in counselling and her continued competency development.

    These emergent themes may also provide a mirror for further self-reflection and identification of areas for continued competency development. The cultural auditing process provides a tool for assisting in both building an effective working alliance with clients to ensure culturally sensitive and responsive practice and also in highlighting areas for further professional development.

15. Reflect on the counsellor's experience in supervision and her continued competency development.

If culture is effectively infused into the supervisory relationship then a further opportunity is provided for the counsellor to explore issues for further multicultural competency development both through the feedback of the supervisor about client interactions and counselling processes and through reflection on the working alliance developed between supervisor and supervisee.

16. Reflect on the counsellor's experience in supervision and the supervisor's continued competency development.

When approached with openness and a willingness to learn from the experience of supervision, the supervisor relationship also offers an opportunity for reflective practice on the part of the supervisor. The opportunity exists to learn in more depth about both supervisee and client cultural identities and to continue to develop awareness of one's of identity and identity development processes.